GENERAL PSYCHOPATHOLOGY

GENERAL PSYCHOPATHOLOGY

An introduction

Christian Scharfetter
Psychiatrische Universitätsklinik, Zurich

Translated by
Helen Marshall
Formerly Librarian, Institute
of Psychiatry, University of London

CAMBRIDGE UNIVERSITY PRESS

CAMBRIDGE

LONDON NEW YORK NEW ROCHELLE

MELBOURNE SYDNEY

Published by the Press Syndicate of the University of Cambridge
The Pitt Building, Trumpington Street, Cambridge CB2 1RP
32 East 57th Street, New York, NY 10022, USA
296 Beaconsfield Parade, Middle Park, Melbourne 3206, Australia

German edition © Georg Thieme Verlag, Stuttgart 1976
English translation © Cambridge University Press 1980

First published in German as *Allgemeine Psychopathologie* 1976
English translation first published 1980

Printed in Great Britain at the University Press, Cambridge

Library of Congress Cataloguing in Publication Data
Scharfetter, Christian.
General psychopathology.
Translation of Allgemeine Psychopathologie.
Bibliography: p.
Includes index.
1. Psychology, Pathological. 2. Consciousness.
3. Ego (Psychology) I. Title. [DNLM: 1. Psycho-
pathology. WM100.3 S311a]
RC454.S313   616.8'9'07   79-52853
ISBN 0 521 22812 3 hard covers
ISBN 0 521 29655 2 paperback

*To all patients
from whom I learn
and to all those
who are concerned
with their care*

CONTENTS

Contents

Contents

Contents

PREFACE

Everything we see could equally well be something else.
(Wittgenstein, *Tract 5*, 434)

This introduction to general psychopathology arose from my contact with patients and with students, both undergraduate and graduate – with the former in a setting of treatment and research, with the latter in the course of teaching and conversation

The time seemed ripe to take another look at general psychopathology and sift out what in it appeared to be of use to our specialty. Now that the World Health Organization has completed its *International Classification of Diseases* with its accompanying *Glossary* (for the literature see under WHO), the time is more than ripe to develop internationally acceptable definitions of psychopathological concepts, a task that becomes all the more pressing as psychiatry throughout the world draws closer together. And the time is always ripe to look beneath the multiplicity of theories for the simple common factor of the patient himself.

I have included everything that seemed to me worthwhile – drawing on the work of many psychiatrists as well as on my own views. Jaspers' *General Psychopathology* (1st edition, 1913, later editions to 1942, thereafter only re-issues) is still of methodological importance. Freud's work still influences us in its passionate search for meaning, its desire to understand, and its capacity to raise questions. Phenomenologists before and after Heidegger have made us aware of the importance of 'the matter' and have opened up for us hermeneutic ways of thought. Clinicians have given us the benefit of their personal expertise. Research workers with an empirical, experimental and statistical orientation have made us see the value and limitations of a numerate approach to the study of man. Such, then, is my understanding of the situation. And since understanding is first and foremost a question of *oneself* understanding something (Gadamer, 1972, p. 246), it becomes necessarily a personal affair, which means that there can be no absolute agreement with other

xiii

people. There is much in the present book that has still not been subjected to sufficient questioning, in the sense of 'laying the matter open' (Gadamer, 1972, p. 283), while remaining open to the demands of 'the matter'; this entails a true understanding of the existence of our patients, if appropriate answers are to be obtained. We must concern ourselves very closely with the cautious 'attack' (*Angriff*) 'which in nature is given verbal expression' (Heidegger, 1959, p. 71). Our task is to understand this verbal expression and to make sense of it.

The style has deliberately been kept terse and the text is intended to be used as a basis for seminar discussions. Statements (Protocols)[1] from patients' records, which include their own depositions and deal with the reality of their lives, are more important than a repetition of the opinions of other authors, no matter how wide their range of neologistic terms and constructs. It is not my intention to examine in great detail other similar works. The bibliography, which is arranged by chapter, covers earlier studies and other points of view.

The plan of the book can be seen from the table of contents. The chapters are in a lexical form. The work does not present any clear unity (such as H. Ey tried to achieve, for example, in his significant work on *Consciousness*, 1963). The sections covering different aspects and functions are therefore disconnected: they do not add up to a whole. The question put to me by a patient (*Protocol 7*): 'Does the psychiatrist understand anything about people? What are his guidelines?' must always be borne in mind as a serious question, a warning (see Keller, Kunz, Bräutigam, Tellenbach, all quoted in Gadamer and Vogler, vol. VI, 1974). The most important chapters in the book are those on Consciousness especially Ego-consciousness or self-awareness, Delusions and Perception. Some therapeutic indications have been included, when they arose from the views under consideration.

The findings and normal psychology[2] and neurophysiology[3] which underly the concepts discussed are only briefly indicated, as are technical methods of examination.[4] Test psychology[5] and experimental psychopathology[6] have become independent disciplines which still, however, must base their formulations and methodologies on careful observation and description.

xiv

FOREWORD

No book called *General Psychopathology* can escape comparison with Karl Jaspers' major contribution to modern psychiatry, first published under that title in 1913. The most immediately accessible section of Jaspers' volume is devoted to a detailed, descriptive account of the clinical phenomena of mental disorders, a task which he regarded as constituting one of the scientific foundations of the discipline. Professor Scharfetter's introductory text is very much in the spirit of this tradition. In it he concentrates on the phenomenological basis of psychiatry, drawing also on contributions from psychology, psychoanalysis and philosophy where relevant. How successful he has been in compressing a great deal of information and experience into a relatively small compass may be gleaned from the range of his extensive bibliography.

Half a century was to elapse before Jaspers' book appeared in English. If Professor Scharfetter has had to wait only three years this is attributable not only to the quality of his detailed and concentrated text but also to its relevance to the recent and growing interest in psychiatric diagnosis and classification among anglophonic psychiatrists. An accurate and readable translation should help ensure its place in the reading-list of clinical and non-clinical students of psychological medicine.

Institute of Psychiatry,   Michael Shepherd
London   Professor of Epidemiological Psychiatry
June 1979

INTRODUCTION

1.1 Task, goal and attitude of the psychopathologist

It is only with the heart that one sees well

(Saint-Exupery)

The task of general psychopathology

Psychiatry – no matter what the underlying assumptions of its practitioner – seeks always to help the patient. That it can translate this worthy aim into successful action is, unfortunately, not always the case, even though much good may be achieved. We still know too little of the origin of the many afflictions which confront the psychiatrist and the clinical psychologist, of how we can modify these conditions, how we may best alleviate, cure or even prevent them. The more we learn to explain and understand, the easier will it be to succeed. Our first requirement, therefore, is to achieve as accurate a grasp as possible of those forms of human experience and behaviour which we designate as morbid in the context of an individual's life history and social and cultural background.

There are no generally accepted criteria for professional aptitude in psychiatry and the selection criteria for professional training are in general irrelevant. The Menninger Clinic (which is psycho-analytically oriented) developed selection procedures for its candidates in training, who were assessed by a selection committee on the basis of one interview (or more) and the results of psychological tests (Rorschach, TAT, Association Tests). The relationship between success and personality traits was later evaluated. It proved very difficult to carry out a good initial assessment, and an unstructured interview with an experienced psychiatrist, supplemented by test data, appeared to be the best procedure. It was less a question of seeking signs of gross psychopathology (neuroses, perversions, psychopathies, psychoses), than of detecting personality traits that lay within the broad spectrum of the non-morbid. Personal integrity, genuineness vs. facade, opportunism, seriousness, honesty, etc. were best detected in the unstructured interview. Controlled or somewhat overcontrolled behaviour was prognostically a more favourable finding than impulsiveness and frank extraversion. Emotional appropriateness was particularly significant, if hard to define. Emotional warmth proved to be a better feature when it was unobtrusive and indirect than when it was strongly manifested either verbally or in mimicry. Motivation was particularly difficult to assess: a genuine desire to help arising from compassion and an ability to identify with others (without suffering oneself or over-reacting) had to be distinguished from a pseudo-altruism arising from guilt or as a form of response to hostility, and sado-masochism arising from a desire to dominate. Obvious self-confidence expressed as arrogance is not a good sign. Curiosity in the sense of thirst for knowledge should be free from sexual overtones (voyeurism). A genuine interest in research is favourable. A high IQ on HAWIE (over 119) is desirable. Objectivity and freedom from status-mindedness in relation to authorities, paraprofessionals and subordinates are further assets. Practical work in general psychiatry yielded particularly good (global) criteria (details in Holt and Luborsky, 1958).

Psychiatry calls for both an ideographic-casuistic[1] empathy and a nomothetic[2] search for regular relationships. Its practitioners must have an effective empathic relationship, even to the point of enduring affective confusion and shock, but must at the same time learn to take intellectual and rational cognizance of the situation and to make use of it.

The subject matter of psychiatry is always a human being *in toto*, in the context of his life history. We can get to know this subject matter only if we take the patient seriously and proceed with care towards an understanding of his condition. These tasks belong to psychopathology. To learn them is part of the training required by everyone who has to do with psychiatric patients. Such training must teach us to hear, experience and describe, before we attempt to consider either diagnosis or indications for treatment, and before we undertake any research.

Psychopathological insight brings us closer to our fellow-men

Psychopathological symptoms are signs, the significance of which we must understand in the same way as we understand everything else we encounter. That is our goal, though it cannot always be attained in the individual case. The first step is to detect the signs and to describe them. Describing and labelling, correctly understood, are not just pinning down an individual's experience and mode of behaviour. Descriptive psychopathology is frequently criticized (unfortunately with justice sometimes) as a method of seeking out and pinning down only what is morbid. This is a false path to follow, for psychopathological skills should lead us closer to the whole man; they should not reveal merely his abnormal experiences and forms of behaviour, but should make it possible to observe what is still healthy, so that we may know what to work on therapeutically and in what direction to proceed.

When we approach in this way those whose lives have gone badly, a psychiatric examination is not a 'degradation ceremony' (Garfinkel, 1956). The 'choice of syntax and vocabulary' does not then become a negative 'political act' (Laing, 1967, p. 54). We have, after all, long been aware of Nietzsche's 'seductive power of language' (1955).

Psychopathology as the study of experience

The patient does not 'have' symptoms. He undergoes certain experiences and therefore behaves in a way that deviates depictably from the norm of his group. Nothing in his behaviour can be written off simply as nonsensical. This is not a scientific statement but an acknowledgement of psychopathology as the study of experience and as a signpost to treatment. It embodies the attitude that alone enables us to deal justly with our patient.

Descriptive psychopathology as the basis of psycho-dynamics

Descriptive psychopathology is not static psychiatry. Anyone who has learned carefully and self-critically to observe and describe will recognize clearly that psychopathology is not a static subject but one that moves unceasingly; that there is no contradiction between descriptive psychopathology and so-called psycho-dynamics, since clear descriptive psychopathology is the basis for any history of living which is not to lose itself in speculation.[3] Even observation for purposes of classification has to take account of the information content of the symptoms observed. Observation is thus a prerequisite of any examination of the individual in his life situation, which always includes the individual as a socially determined being.

The interactional, social and cultural aspect

To the psychopathologist it is clear that a person's experience and behaviour are subject to many active and changing relationships. An individual must always be viewed in his social context, never in isolation. Therefore all good psychiatry is social psychiatry. Personality can develop only in a community (process of socialization) and this applies as much to the healthy as to the sick. Personality development and social evolution can no more be separated than physical and mental development, because the two belong together in the living man (for the literature see Baltes and Schaie, 1973). This view excludes neither the contribution of heredity, difficult as it is to pinpoint (see in particular studies of adoption),[4] nor the comparative animal behaviour models which are equally characteristic of *Homo sapiens* (see Eibl-Eibesfeld, 1969, 1972, Lorenz, 1963).

A patient's experience and behaviour can change according to his interpersonal milieu, according to the success or otherwise of discussions with him, according to how well an interviewer is able to make contact with him and help him to acquire insight. Personal contact and understanding constitute a continuous process. If the dialogue is successful, many so-called psychopathological symptoms recede – only to return when the individual in question is left alone or has to live in an unhealthy, and particularly in an isolated, environment, or when he is faced with alternatives and sees no way out. One must therefore never look at the patient in isolation. The question is not: 'does schizophrenia exist?' but in what type of environment and under what conditions does a person behave in a way which we by consensus call schizophrenic?[5] The patient's ability to achieve insight depends not only on his state of consciousness and his intellectual capacity for self-examination, but varies according to his social origin and ties, his education and his social and cultural background. It is hardly possible for either the patient or the psychopathologist to free himself entirely from the attitudes of his own cultural group and its point of view.

Transcultural psychiatry has shed light on the part played by culture in human experience and behaviour and has demonstrated the impossibility of looking at the individual from the point of view of generally valid norms.[6] What is normal in one situation and in one culture, may be abnormal in another.[7] On the other hand transcultural, comparative psychiatry also shows that people the world over may, without any gross overt ill-treatment, suffer to a degree that is abnormal for their group and for the generality of mankind.

1.2 The problem of normality, health, abnormality, morbidity

Normality. There are two main concepts of normality: the concept of the statistical or average norm and the concept of the ideal norm. Normality in the former sense means, in general, behaviour that is appropriate to the majority of members of a given socio-cultural sphere in given situations. Normality means, in particular, what such members always have in common in regard to a given aspect of behaviour. There can hardly be one norm that is valid for all men in all cultures. This average norm is different for individuals of different cultures and different social class and religion, and in different situations (e.g. war as opposed to peace). The average norm means the behaviour (how men must, should, can, may behave) that is accepted within a culture in relation to a given situation. Custom and usage provide the norms that serve as models for the When (following What) and the How of behaviour. What determines new ways of behaviour and new patterns that then come into being is recognized within a culture: it is even prescribed, legitimized and in some circumstances institutionalized (Devereux, 1974).

It is also social legitimate, and thus to a certain extent normal, to adopt the role of being sick. The legitimate criteria for a social definition of psychiatric illness are vague and blurred. Through illness an individual achieves freedom from duties and obligations, he receives consideration, he is treated leniently, he is cared for, and in the case of a physical illness there is usually no discrimination against him. This does not usually apply to mental illness, at least when the illness has no clear physical basis such as a cerebral disease. The temptation inherent in such advantages depends also on what else society offers (e.g. social insurance payments, compensation) (see Fischer-Homberger, 1970).

The *statistical norm* is the easiest to keep free of value judgements, but it is also the most liable to misuse in a way that singles out and isolates individuals who are different. The chief danger is that anyone who deviates from the statistical norm (not only patients in the strict sense, see below) is 'mentally ill' and therefore in need of treatment if possible. (For the danger of compulsory psychiatric treatment for deviant thinkers, the danger of labelling those whose life style is different and of pushing them into a career of 'stigmatization', see Scheff, 1973.)

Abnormality in the statistical sense is anything in a given mode of behaviour at a given time that deviates from the norm of the group at that given time. Such deviations or 'abnormalities' may lie in either of two directions:

(*a*) In the positive direction such abnormalities are: talent, special gifts in a field of reasoning or of art, special intuitive gifts, and so on. The term abnormality is not commonly applied here, being reserved more for the negative sense.

(*b*) Abnormalities in the negative sense: behaviour which differs from the national or group norm in a negative sense: lagging behind, failing, grieving, disturbing,[8] bringing suffering to others. Many individuals are abnormal both in a positive and in a negative direction.[9]

This statistical concept of normality certainly leaves room for the view that experience and therefore behaviour (as a function of experience) in a technological civilization is alienated from 'the structure of being', though such a notion is difficult to define (Laing, 1967) (see also Jensen 1951, Hallowell, 1955, and other ethnological works). Hence Laing's *kerygma*: 'what we call normal is a product of repression, distortion, isolation, projection, introjection and other forms of destructive action against experience' (p. 21). And: 'the forms of alienation outside the valid norm of alienation are labelled by the "normal" majority as "anti" or "insane"' (p. 22).

The second important concept of normality is the *ideal* norm, the norm of optimal fulfilment, self-realization, capacity for enjoyment, the norm of attitude and ethics. Such a concept of normality is of course implicit in many of the goals set in psychotherapy, or for example in judging family communication and similar matters, but it is of little use clinically because its boundaries cannot be defined. An ideal norm of self-realization presupposes an adequate understanding of what this is. That is perhaps approximately possible in psycho-analysis but not with the limited possibilities of communication and understanding that are available in general clinical practice.

Too little consideration is usually given to the fact that we cannot define reasonably valid norms for all mankind, and that even within our own society and its standards the norm is not clearly established. We do not, for example, know how to define normal family interaction or normal personal development, or what degree of suffering and conflict can 'normally' be tolerated in life. This is, however, of practical importance, for example in setting our goal in a course of psychotherapy in which the aim extends beyond freeing the patient from symptoms.

Abnormality is not synonymous with sickness. There are many abnormalities which are not morbid, e.g. a slightly low level of intelligence and many personality traits. Much that is 'abnormal' has nothing whatever to do with illness, but is quite healthy and vigorous (e.g. to climb to a high mountain alone in winter and/or at night, to live in the Himalayas without shoes or clothes and with a minimum of food, to lead a life of spiritual meditation, etc.). It can even be pathological (e.g. neurotic) to wish always, in all circumstances, to behave 'normally'. In certain circumstances it can also be 'normal' to be sick (e.g. after food or drink contaminated with amoebae).

It follows that the concepts of normal and abnormal are not suitable for use in classifying individuals within the framework of medical psychology or psychotherapy. There it is a question of being sick or not sick.

The dichotomy, 'healthy or sick', provides a pragmatic reference point for a particular course of action (examination, diagnostic procedure, care, therapy, rehabilitation). From the standpoint of social role playing, the question is whether an individual is permitted by his social group to adopt a sick role (free upkeep, lenient attitude, care, treatment).

Health implies globally the total condition of an individual and, unlike the concept of normality, does not refer to a particular aspect of behaviour. The concept of health is even more difficult to grasp in psychiatry than that of normality. It is untenable to base the concept of health solely on a feeling of well-being (WHO). (This assumes a state which an individual can in any case achieve only sporadically. Many brain-damaged patients do not suffer.) One can try to come closer to a definition of health: a healthy individual is one who succeeds in living *his* life – sometimes in spite of suffering from a physical illness and/or in spite of the normal pressure of his society – one who can meet the demands of his own being and of the world, who can cope satisfactorily. This mastery of life also depends of course on the circumstances in question. Such an understanding of the concept of health may seem obvious to some, but it is of little use as an operational formulation that would enable us to measure what is healthy and what is not.

The concept of sickness in the broader sense (in which it is used in psychiatry) is based on suffering and failure. A sick person, in the judgement of the patient himself and of those around him, is one who for whatever reason *suffers* from himself and from the world (the suffering aspect) to an extent that is qualitatively and quantitatively beyond the average for his country and group,[10] and who is unable, to a degree that adversely affects his life, to cope with not very extreme circumstances, who fails to maintain himself in the world (the failure aspect) and who, because he is to a considerable extent different, cannot live in a warm relationship with his fellow men (the relationship aspect). It is in this broader sense that the deranged are ill; they are non-empathic, strange, shut out from common human reality. Examples of illness in this sense are the severe neuroses and the so-called endogenous psychoses. This concept of illness in the broader sense already contains the idea that the signs (symptoms) of illness occur with a certain degree of regularity (type, model) and in regular association with a certain basic reason (motivational context) for becoming ill. We will discuss theories about these 'basic reasons' later (cf. p. 26).

It is obvious that this further concept of illness is imprecise. It cannot be made more precise, however, and yet it is impossible to dispense with it. We must therefore never lose sight of the problematic nature of these concepts.

In the medical tradition the decision to designate health or sickness is generally made in regard to a given individual as an individual case. It is already a different use of the concept of illness when we say that a marriage, or a family, or a group, or a society is sick; what we are speaking of here is a sick form of communication. To make pathogenesis synonymous with pathology in this way is wholly false. A family whose intersubjective communication might, according to certain theories, be conducive of sickness is not necessarily in itself sick. A society in which a certain percentage of members are sick (e.g. 1 per cent schizophrenic) should not on this account be called sick.

The general notion of illness (which is the one most commonly used) is a mixture of various models and concepts, partly explicit and well-considered, partly implicit and then often poorly considered. It is, however, important to realize what the different concepts are, since in our practical dealings with a potential patient and his relatives it is a matter of some importance to which view of illness a particular therapist adheres (Siegler and Osmond, 1974).

(1) *Medical-somatic model.* This is based on pathological findings in anatomy and physiology. It seeks correlations between particular physical illnesses, especially cerebral disorders (genetic, enzymatic, biochemical, toxic, morphological in nature) and particular mental illnesses. Research and diagnostic efforts in biological psychiatry have as their goal the discovery of causes, while the goal of treatment is to correct the causes.

In psychiatry the medical model of illness can be used only in those mental disorders which are associated with physical illness (especially cerebral disease): acute exogenous reactions, amnestic psychosyndromes, the dementias, the organic psychoses (brain syndromes). The medical model is thus applicable only to a proportion of the many and varied patients who need psychiatric care. It does not take account of the standpoints of developmental psychology and social interaction, which it can accommodate at best in only a secondary and complementary fashion (a multiconditional point of view).

In so far as a physical basis is postulated for the aetiologically obscure, so-called endogenous psychoses, the medical concept of illness is applied to these illnesses too, but this a particularly controversial issue.

(2) *Sociological aspect.* This turns on the relationship between the person seeking treatment and the therapist supplying it. The patient, whose awareness of illness is socially and culturally determined and whose need of treatment is likewise socially and culturally determined, has recourse to a healer, a therapist, a person who places at the disposal of others and/or offers to others his diagnostic and therapeutic knowledge: the medicine man, the shaman, the priest-doctor, the doctor, the psychiatrist, the psychotherapist, as well as members of the paramedical professions. Since the dawn of human history the healer has possessed a diagnostic and therapeutic authority; his experience, knowledge and qualifications have given him a power which he claims and which is socially conceded to him, and he exercises this power in relation to the patient, playing his socially determined role with its obligations and privileges. Society has provided norms of behaviour for both the patient and the healer, and for their interaction.

(3) *Psychological models.* According to this view, life experiences, by virtue of their influence on development, lead to vulnerability, predisposition to illness and finally to illness in the form of neurosis or psychosis. There are various and very different psychological models.

(i) *Psycho-analytical model.* Freud gives no explicit definition of the normal, the sick and the healthy. Basically, according to psycho-analytical theory, the same dynamic processes and (in topical parlance) apparatuses may be involved in all three, depending on the stage of development and the ego-formation reached (see also p. 18). The early psycho-analytical view of the isolated individual, regarded in an exclusively intrapsychic way, has had to be supplemented (Sullivan, 1953; Erikson, 1959).

(ii) *Communication psychology applied to the family delegation model.* This concept interprets mental disorder (meaning schizophrenic, narcissistic and neurotic people) as a consequence of disturbed modes of communication, originally between the mother and the eventual patient (e.g. the 'schizophrenogenic' mother, Frieda Fromm-Reichmann, 1950; Arieti, 1955), and then generally between all members of the family. This has led to the discovery of pathogenic family relationships (Alanen, 1966; Bateson *et al.*, 1956; Lidz, 1973; Richter, 1972; Stierlin, 1975; Watzlawik *et al.*, 1967; Wynne *et al.*, 1958). The concept was thus broadened from an exclusive consideration of the single individual to an examination of his entire family, viewed as an interdependent system and at times extending over more than two generations. The pathogenic family, in order to maintain its precarious balance, needs one member who is there to act as the symptom carrier or who can be permanently or temporarily excluded from the family.

(iii) *Behaviourist model.* According to this view 'sick' behaviour is learned: unpleasant experiences with people give rise to attempts to escape (e.g. social withdrawal, autism, confused talk, bizarre behaviour). These avoidance attempts may be modelled on ethnic and culturally appropriate patterns of insanity (Devereux, 1974). The behaviourist model is important not only for its interpretation of the first manifestations of insanity but also for the long-term course of mental illnesses (secondary damage, institutionalism, hospitalism, see Goffman, 1967). Its therapeutic consequences are behaviour therapy and preventive measures (against institutionalism).

(4) *Mental illness as deviation from the norm.* Anyone who flouts socially prescribed norms that are accepted, tolerated and defended, who does not conform to the 'law', may be rejected by the community as deviant, aberrant, an outsider, an eccentric. This fate of rejection unites in one undifferentiated global judgement saints and fools, ascetics and philosophers, the mentally ill and witches, seers and prophets, the poor and the voluntarily dispossessed, vagrants, outlaws and criminals. What they have in common is that they are deviants, embarrassing individuals, who pose a threat to the apparently secure norm. Originally the measures adopted by society in regard to such people were equally undifferentiated: banishment, death, torture, incarceration could be the fate of a member of any of these groups. It was only much later that distinctions were made between different kinds of deviant individuals and between the institutions and professions dealing with them (Szasz, 1961a, b, 1970).

Which forms of deviant behaviour are finally recorded as mental illness depends on the situation and on the image that society forms of what constitutes mental illness and of how it manifests itself. How this image is formed is not yet clear but includes the part played by public helplessness, the loss of voluntary action, and the implict appeal to charitable feelings.

The equation of many heterogeneous forms of deviant behaviour with mental illness is still very common today and affects much research (e.g. sexual deviations as a topic in psychiatry).

(5) *Mental disorder as social labelling.* This concept is concerned mainly with the validity and power of social norms, pointing to the social definition, the 'normalization' of what may be regarded as sick. The question of whether the concept of mental illness can be objectively justified is, on the other hand, always in the background. The patient is declared by his society (which registers him, labels him, stimatizes him) to be mentally ill, mentally abnormal, sick, and is in this way pressurized into following a particular career (Scheff, 1973). Mental illness is a social myth, its function being to enable society to expel its unwelcome members (cf. in former days the idea of witches and the Inquisition).

When a person is stigmatized as mentally ill, his subsequent fate is to all intents and purposes sealed and this frequently means social invalidism, which includes an expectation of relapse, a need to be looked after and to have allowances made for him, disparagement, repudiation of personal and professional relationships, the uniform interpretation of even healthy forms of behaviour and reaction as signs of sickness and long-term hospitalization with institutionalism (Goffman, 1967; Wing and Brown, 1970).

(6) *Psychedelic model.* According to Laing (1967), mental illness is a 'normal' or 'healthy' reaction to an impossible society which suppresses self-realization and is alien to the true essence of humanity. The psychotic is then seen as the 'truly healthy man' on an 'inward journey'. What society calls psychosis is a special strategy which the individual uses to enable him to avoid the unpleasant influences of his fellow men.

(7) *Magical, astrological, moral concepts of illness.* Even in our supposedly enlightened civilization these continue to play a world-wide role. The magical concept of illness interprets disease as the result of magic influences – abjuration, bewitchment, curses, the influence of spirits, the violation of taboos – or it may be the constellation of the stars (astrological concept of illness), or the consequence of guilt and transgression (moral concept of illness).

(8) *Forensic concept of illness.* A distinction must be drawn here between questions of civil rights (responsibility, ability to conduct a business, to have charge of one's own income, to look after one's own affairs), questions of criminal justice (soundness of mind, criminal responsibility, capacity to endure punishment and imprisonment) and questions of social insurance (disablement entitlement, need of support, etc.).

(9) There are other possible concepts of illness, such as, for example, the cybernetic concept, according to which illness is a deviation in intricately regulated organisms: both the deviation and the organisms behave and react according to regular laws.

1.3   Symptom and syndrome

Psychopathological symptoms are not merely signs of morbidity

Psychopathological symptoms[11] are the same as or similar to recognizable forms of experience and behaviour which stand out against the ordinary, everyday background of an individual in a particular culture. No one psychopathological symptom is of itself simply abnormal or even morbid, for all such phenomena may be encountered in healthy people in special circumstances.[12] Psychopathological symptoms are not therefore necessarily signs of morbidity. Many describable experiences are indeed unusual, but can nevertheless be present as isolated parts of general human experience, as can be seen from careful observation of oneself and of others, and particularly from ethnic comparisons. This is true even of such extraordinary phenomena as hallucinations or altered bodily experience, which become signs of illness only when they occur in a certain degree of severity, density, frequency, association and duration – always taking account of the patient's life history and current situation and his social and cultural background – and when they make the patient suffer and hamper the conduct of his life within his group.

From symptoms to syndrome

The symptom is the smallest describable entity with which psychiatric examination has to deal. In clinical experience we see typical clinical pictures which keep on appearing and which form constellations of symptoms that frequently occur in association one with another. These clusters of symptoms are called syndromes. *A syndrome is therefore a phenomenologically typical but not necessarily causal combination of symptoms.* The concept of the syndrome is used in varying ways (in the broader sense it is also called a symptom complex, which is, however, linguistically of little value). Most psychiatric syndromes are *noxiously non-specific*, i.e. there is no close correlation with a particular, constant causal factor.

EXAMPLES

A catatonic syndrome may occur in a psychogenic psychosis, in schizophrenia, in LSD intoxication, or in encephalitis. A depressive syndrome may appear in cerebral disorders (e.g. progressive paralysis) or equally in phasic or neurotic affective reactions. A manic syndrome may occur in mania, in intoxication (e.g. drunkenness) or in schizophrenia.

Several such syndromes are encountered in clinical psychiatry:

Disturbances of consciousness (*Benommenheit*) include stupor, coma, delirium, and twilight state.

Disturbances of memory include the amnestic syndrome which, when accompanied by confabulation, constitutes a Korsakoff syndrome.

Psychomotor syndromes include stupor, excitement and catatonic syndromes (hypokinetic, akinetic and hyperkinetic syndromes).

Affective syndromes include the depressive syndrome, the hypochondriacal syndrome, the manic syndrome, and the anxiety syndrome.

Perceptual syndromes include derealization and depersonalization syndromes, the hallucinatory syndrome, and hallucinosis.

Delusional syndromes include the paranoid syndrome and the paranoid-hallucinatory syndrome.

Obsessions and phobias characterize the anancastic syndrome, the phobic syndrome and the phobic-anancastic syndrome.

Empirical support for some clinical syndromes (symptom clusters, factorial groups) come from statistical and factorial analysis based on formal operational concepts (see, for example, the AMP Manual, 1972), standardized schedules (e.g. Lorr *et al.*, 1963; Lorr, 1966, 1967; Mombour, 1972; Wing, 1970, 1974) and documentation. This has led to the construction of a number of psychopathological scales (for the literature see Baumann, 1974; Mombour, 1973, 1974). An immediate task is the development of *nuclear axial syndromes* (e.g. devitalization in depression, disturbance of consciousness in acute exogenous reactions) and *marginal syndromes* (e.g. the paranoid syndrome in melancholia). Finally the study of syndromes seeks to determine interrelationships between the syndromes (recorded as accurately as possible in individual descriptions of the symptoms) and certain regular and demonstrable findings that are possible causes (findings from various fields of research: neuro-anatomy, neuro-physiology, biochemistry, experimental psychology, life history, psycho-dynamics, etc.). Syndromes may to some extent be summarized as certain 'basic forms' of psychiatric disturbance, e.g. organic psychosyndromes, localized brain syndromes, psycho-endocrine syndromes (Bleuler, M., 1954, 1964; Bleuler, E. and M., 1969), reversible amnesic syndromes (Wieck, 1967).

Approach to symptoms/syndromes

We can formulate our approach to symptoms in various ways and with various aims in view, with or without any preconceived theoretical basis. It is necessary, however, always to begin with the most objective possible observations and descriptions. This is the starting point for all treatment and research.

Observation may take the form of free clinical dialogue and observation of behaviour, or of standardized (or semi-standardized) schedules to be completed by the patient or by others (see p. 22). Self-evaluation scales have so far not been of much significance in clinical psychiatry, because severely ill patients are on the whole unable to complete them (see Mombour, 1972; Pichot and Olivier-Martin, 1974).

Once symptoms have been delineated, we can assess the findings in the following ways:

(1) By examining the characteristic (pathognomonic) significance of a symptom in relation to the illness and its course.[13]

(2) By examining the pathognomonic significance of a symptom is relation to diagnosis in the pathogenetic, aetiological sense (unity of clinical picture, cause and mode of occurrence).[13]

(3) By examining the significance of a symptom in relation to the patient in question, using the life history and subjecting it to hermeneutic analysis and interpretation to establish which internal and external experiences are reflected in his symptoms, for example, over-activity as an expression of despair and one's own impending doom (see *Ego-consciousness*). This approach seeks to understand the essence and meaning of a particular form of behaviour e.g. genetic, so-called 'psycho-dynamic' phenomenological, hermeneutic and deep-hermeneutic understanding, e.g. delusion as a form of self-preservation.

Psycho-analytical explanations are dominated by a functionally reductionist approach: symptoms are seen as defence mechanisms (defence against instincts, avoidance of conflict, with fulfilment at regressive levels). A deterministic chain of causality is then constructed from the psychological meaning and context.

(4) By examining the communicative context of a symptom in terms of interactional psychology, e.g. asking what the patient tells us by his behaviour, either intentionally or unintentionally (communication and metacommunication).

It is also necessary at all times to keep in view the approach and purpose of one's personal formulation. We may think we have understood a symptom by uncovering its motivational aspect, but we still do not know how the patient has arrived at that symptom, nor do we know that it was absolutely necessary for him to adopt such modes of experience and behaviour. For example, though we may understand how depressive devitalization can be translated into delusions of disaster, this does not account for the origins of the depression itself.

Theories of the origin of symptoms/syndromes

(1) When there is clear evidence of pathogenesis, the relationship between illness and symptom is a simple one of cause and effect,[14]

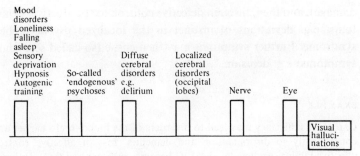

Fig. 1. Visual hallucinations.

for example, aphasia in a case of left temporal damage in a right-handed patient, dementia in a case of diffuse cerebral disease. With most psychopathological symptoms, however, there is no clear relationship between demonstrable damage and the symptom in question (especially in the case of hallucinations and delusions).

EXAMPLE

We do not know why one patient with cerebral syphilis (general paralysis) develops simple dementia, while another is euphoric, depressive, hallucinated or delusional. Nor do we understand why visual hallucinations (Fig. 1) may arise in very different circumstances even although the nature of the hallucination may be identical.

(2) Symptoms and syndromes are *reactive patterns* uniformly produced by the most varied (physical and mental) 'injuries'. Examples include *localized cerebral reaction patterns*, such as certain focal epilepsies like temporal lobe epilepsy; *humoral reaction patterns* in the sense of the psycho-endocrinological syndrome (M. Bleuler, 1954, 1964); *hereditary reaction patterns*, thymopathic, schizophrenic in nature (see, for example, C. Schneider, 1942); *psychomotor phenomena* (death-like stupor, extreme motor excitement) in very severe anxiety states of varied origin (Kretschmer, 1953, 1958).

(3) According to the Jacksonian notion of integration (1932), higher (i.e. phylo- and ontogenetically more recent) functions are destroyed by injury and older layers come to the surface (see Palaeopsychology). The psycho-analytical theory of regression also follows this model. According to this theory, the injury quickly leads to symptoms of deficit (e.g. memory disturbances, dementia in cases of brain

damage), and then, through defective control, to 'productive' symptoms, e.g. deviations of instinct in the localized psychocerebral syndrome. Further symptoms may then ensue (so-called secondary symptoms) e.g. delusion.

EXAMPLE

Cardiac insufficiency may lead to disorders of the blood–brain barrier and consequently to disorientation and dementia, loss of affective control, affective lability, excitement, etc. Life becomes insecure and this, combined with other factors such as social isolation, sensory deterioration, etc., can lead to the development of delusions of harm (e.g. being robbed) which are further elaborated according to the situation and circumstances of the patient (the pathoplastic process).

(4) Many symptoms may be viewed as an understandable *reaction* to experience.

EXAMPLE

A delusion of reference may occur in a depressed patient who believes he is rotting and that his body smells like a corpse; he then thinks that everyone wrinkles his nose at him and shuns him.

(5) According to the psycho-analytical view, the underlying causes of neuroses and psychoses are conflicts between the ego, the id and the super-ego, which together form the psychological 'apparatus' that deals with the external world ('external reality' in the Freudian sense). While neurotic symptoms reflect a conflict between the ego and the id, with the ego repulsing the demands of the id for the sake of maintaining contact with reality, the ego of the psychotic is too weak to repel the id in this way (Freud, 1924). If the id is to triumph over the ego, then for the ego (which maintains relationships with the external world) the external world must disappear: the ego in its flight into psychosis (Freud, 1894, 1896) withdraws or regresses from the objects of the external world, external reality disappears, the self is taken over by the libido (megalomania). The defence mechanisms of regression, projection, denial give rise to symptoms that are at times attempts at cure and reconstruction. The experience of world catastrophe shows, for example, the loss of object relations and is a projection of an inner catastrophe, while delusions of persecution

reflect projected hatred which itself is inverted (homosexual) love (Freud, 1911).

The turning point in the development of a psychosis occurs very early, at a stage of development when the libido is not yet fixated on external objects (phase of auto-eroticism-narcissism, Freud, 1914). (For further details see the chapters on *Ego-consciousness* and *Delusion*.)

(6) Those who favour a psychosocial genesis for many psychoses of the schizophrenic type believe that numerous symptoms are learned under the influence of the environment (intra-familial style of communication – Arieti, 1971; Bateson, 1956; Lidz *et al.*, 1957, 1973; Wynne, 1959; Alanen, 1970). It may be observed that hereditary dispositions, particularly data from studies of children in institutions or adopted children, are not always taken into account in these studies (Heston, 1966; Karlson, 1966, 1974; Rosenthal *et al.*, 1968; Rosenthal, 1970).

(7) To take these views a stage further, 'being psychotic' (used in the sense of being mentally disordered or mentally ill) is seen as a normal and even healthy reaction to an intolerable environment which suppresses self-realization (flight into one's own world), and the psychotic (who recognizes his need fully) is the only truly healthy man 'journeying inwards' in an insane world (Laing, 1967 and many others). The scapegoat is no longer merely the schizophrenogenic mother or the schizophrenogenic family, but society as a whole. This leaves unanswered the question why some (1 per cent) of the population succumb (and in so typical a fashion) to the destructive force of the accepted contemporary social norm at any time (no matter how alien that may be from the individual's real being and no matter how it may restrict the potentialities of his existence) while others do not need to adopt any such special strategy (Laing, 1967).

Mental illness is a myth, but unfortunately it is not a μῦθος πλασθί'ς (manufactured myth), it is not a fabricated or satanic invention such as Szasz (1961) depicted in his misinterpretation of the true nature of a myth. It is rather μῦθος αληθή (a real myth) in which the sad reality of many lives unfolds itself and speaks to us.

Possible ways of classifying symptoms
Classification may be in terms of diagnostic or pathognomonic
significance

(*a*) Symptoms which are diagnostic signposts: *leading symptoms, core symptoms, first-rank symptoms* (K. Schneider, 1967), *axial symptoms* (sometimes referred to as basic symptoms, though this is a bad term and leads to misunderstanding): e.g. amnestic symptoms pointing to cerebral disorders, certain kinds of auditory hallucinations, hearing voices (q.v.) indicating schizophrenia. Such diagnostic pointers have been established on the basis of clinical empiricism or statistical research (see, for example, WHO, 1973).

(*b*) Many other psychopathological symptoms have no such diagnostic implications (*second-rank symptoms*, K. Schneider, 1967; *accessory symptoms*, E. Bleuler, 1911); for example, the slowing down of thought processes, disturbed concentration, depressed or heightened affect, delusion.

Primary and secondary symptoms

Eugen Bleuler (1911) drew a distinction in the schizophrenias between primary symptoms, which were the expression of a hypothetical disease entity in the medical sense (the basic disturbance) and which could be interpreted as physiogenic (e.g. disturbances of thought and affect) and secondary (or accessory) symptoms which represented the reaction of the personality to the illness. These secondary symptoms may be interpreted psychologically (chiefly as 'Freudian mechanisms', according to Bleuler). The notion of primary symptoms is thus given a new meaning: physiogenesis is postulated only for those features which are psychologically irreducible and inexplicable.

1.4 Diagnosis

Concept and meaning

Diagnosis is the recognition of a clinically observable psychopathological picture (symptom, syndrome, presenting state, or a combination of clinical state and course) which is typical, and occurs repeatedly in the same form. Diagnosis means identifying this picture with the concept of a certain illness.

The diagnostic process – the process of recognition and association – is today often misunderstood and unjustly disparaged as labelling.[15] However, we need diagnosis whenever we have to form an opinion of the presenting state of a patient, i.e. his mode of experience or behaviour seen in relation to its background and in relation to the need to decide what, in the present stage of our knowledge, should best be done about it. *The essence and aim of diagnosis is to point the way to therapeutic and prophylactic action.* Unfortunately in the present state of our knowledge regarding pathogenesis and methods of treatment, diagnosis does not always lead to satisfactory treatment and prophylaxis.

The diagnostic process as a process of recognition (*Fig. 2*)

Diagnosis means the development of the process of recognition, a complex process of decision-making that involves the most varied data (for the literature see Gauron and Dickinson, 1966; Nathan, 1967; v. Zerssen, 1973). It ranges over different dimensions: concept formation, reliability, validity and processing of information, acquisition of knowledge – all of which must be constantly borne in mind.

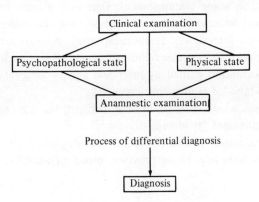

Fig. 2. The diagnostic process.

Clinical examination

This covers:

(1) *The psychopathological state:*

(*a*) First comes the recording of the experiences (the complaints) which the patient himself communicates spontaneously or which are obtained by questioning and observation of his behaviour. The examination may take the form of a free clinical dialogue (diagnostic interview)[16] or it may be conducted in a standardized or semi-standardized fashion (Mombour, 1972; Richot and Olivier-Mártin, 1974). In clinical psychiatry assessment by external observers is to be preferred to self-assessment.

An unstructured clinical dialogue has the advantage of greater flexibility and spontaneity, but in some circumstances, e.g. when the interviewer is insufficiently trained and is lacking in self-criticism, it has two disadvantages: first, it may be incomplete and, secondly, the information gathered depends not only on the patient (which is true of standardized questionnaires, whether self-administered or not) but also on several characteristics of the interviewer – his motivation, his interest, his nosological standpoint, the kind of interview situation he sets up, his intonation, the formulation of his questions and the order in which he asks them. Standardized methods have the advantage of completeness and uniformity (comparability) and the disadvantages, in some circumstances, that information may be unavoidably lost because of a lack of flexibility and spontaneity and that the patient–interviewer relationship may be hampered or paralysed so that a therapeutic relationship cannot be developed.

(*b*) The information gained by interview and by observation is described and labelled (symptom-diagnosis).

(*c*) Symptoms which coincide in time, content, etc. are regarded as forming syndromes (syndrome-diagnosis).

(2) *The physical state:* Physical (including neurological) examination and laboratory tests (e.g. blood pressure, blood sugar, EEG, c.s.f., etc.).

Anamnesis

This covers:
- (*a*) General history.
  Biographical, social, medical data.
- (*b*) Special history of illness.
  Development of the present clinical picture, course of illness.
- (*c*) Family history.
  Social and medical data, heredity.
- (*d*) Patient's own account.
  Information supplied by the patient under (*a*)–(*c*), above.
- (*e*) Other accounts.
  Information from other people (mainly relatives, friends, colleagues, guardians, welfare workers, under (*a*)–(*c*), above).

The process of differential diagnosis

How should we co-ordinate the clinical picture described with the findings obtained and the information revealed in the case history? Do these indicate the presence of physically-based psychological disturbances?

Are there leading symptoms or syndromes which enable us to classify the illness (to recognize the model)?

Which diagnoses may be eliminated (diagnosis *per exclusionem*)?

What information derived from the clinical examination and from the case history, sometimes supplemented by information obtained subsequently, makes it possible to formulate a provisional diagnosis? What additional data do I need in order to confirm this *heuristic diagnostic hypothesis*?

In practice an immediate intuitive diagnosis, often made in the first few minutes (a good clinical 'nose'), plays an inordinately important role.

EXAMPLE

(1) Psychopathological state:
   (*a*) Symptom level: loss of activity, depressed mood, thought inhibition, anxiety, etc.
   (*b*) Syndrome level: depressive-inhibited syndrome.

(2) Physical state: fixed pupils, disturbed reflexes, disturbed speech.

(3) History:

    (*a*) Course: chronically increasing severity of illness.

    (*b*) Biographical: no special features, until the start of the illness in middle age. Nothing in his life history to suggest a recognizable cause.

    (*c*) Social: lives in a well-ordered, socially secure family environment.

    (*d*) Medical: 15 years ago had a genital infection, treated by several injections.

(4) Suspected diagnosis: chronic depression in progressive paralysis.

(5) Supplementary examination of blood and c.s.f.: positive reaction for syphilis.

(6) Diagnosis: chronic depression in progressive paralysis (neurosyphilitic); diagnosis of clinical state and aetiological diagnosis.

Diagnosis and nosological classification

The purpose of making a diagnostic decision is to co-ordinate the clinical phenomenological picture with diagnosis in the sense of an aetiological and pathogenetic designation of illness. Because of the incomplete state of our knowledge of the causes of mental illness at the present time, however (especially in the area of the so-called endogenous psychoses), this goal is still remote. Our diagnostic activities must therefore be limited to the establishment of a typology compounded of clinical state and course of illness.

In psychiatry, however, clinical pictures and courses of illness that seem to be alike are often heterogeneous in respect of both aetiology and pathogenesis. Different noxae (physical and mental) can lead to similar clinical pictures (e.g. schizophrenia-like psychoses in stressful life situations, in temporal lobe epilepsy, in LSD intoxication, etc.). And the same noxae can lead to different clinical pictures (e.g. chronic alcoholism may lead to delirium, to hallucinosis, to dementia or to epilepsy).

Basic forms of mental disturbance (*nosological schema*)

(1) Psychoses accompanying physical illnesses:

    (*a*) diffuse – organic psychosyndrome (Bleuler, E. and M., 1969).

    (*b*) local – localized cerebral psychosyndrome (Bleuler, E. and M., 1969).

(c) acute – acute exogenous reaction type (Bonhœffer, 1910).

(d) chronic – chronic organic psychosyndrome, dementia.

(2) Abnormal reactions and developments. Sequelae of distressing life events and experiences:

(a) Immediate reactions (e.g. reactive depression).

(b) Neuroses: abnormal forms of development, mostly associated with childhood trauma which are often covert until exposed by psychotherapy, unresolved conflicts, passions, perversions, etc.

(c) Psychosomatic illnesses: neuroses manifesting themselves predominantly in the somatic field.

(3) Abnormal predispositions:

(a) Intelligence: oligophrenia (mental retardation).

(b) Personality: psychopathy (personality disorder). (This can be difficult to distinguish from neurotic forms of development.)

(4) So-called endogenous psychoses (functional psychoses):

(a) Affective psychoses.

(b) The schizophrenias.

The World Health Organization has produced an *International Classification of Diseases* which includes psychiatric diseases in the broad sense and, to go with it, a *Glossary of Mental Disorders*, both of which contribute to international agreement and compatibility in diagnostic practice and therapy. (For the literature see WHO, 1971, 1974.)

For the purposes of empirical statistical research there are numerous instruments available for standardized documentation and the collection of data, and also for standardized handling of data and computer diagnosis (for the literature see Cooper, J. E., 1970; Kreitman, 1961; Mombour, 1972; Pichot and Martin, 1974; Sartorius, *et al.*, 1970; Shepherd *et al.*, 1968; Spitzer and Endicott, 1969; Wing, 1970, 1974; Zubin, 1967).

For the treatment of the individual patient, however, we must still establish an 'individual diagnosis' (Curtius, 1959), that is to say, we must always take into account the personality of the patient seen in its historical development, its life history and situation. This always implies a social context – the context of the patient's economic, family and home situation.

Diagnosis as a pointer to treatment

Diagnosis is essentially a pointer to treatment and prevention. If the symptoms are not carefully and correctly assessed, then the correct diagnosis is missed and with it the appropriate treatment in terms of the current state of knowledge. If, for example, we fail to recognize a depression in progressive paralysis but mistake it for a reactive depression, then we will fail to give the life-saving penicillin therapy. If disturbed development in adolescence is not recognized as the first sign of a manic psychosis, then we may fail to prescribe prophylactic lithium. If a schoolboy's inattentiveness is not recognized to be a disorder of consciousness, then we will fail to carry out the appropriate EEG examination and to administer anticonvulsant therapy. If apathetic indifference and dullness are attributed to a lack of social stimulation, to isolation and to middle age, then in some circumstances a brain tumour may be allowed to develop unrecognized. If we fail to spot thyrotoxicosis in a state of changeable excitement, then we will fail to give the required treatment. If a patient with a periodic depressive illness is regarded as a neurotic depressive, then he may not receive the help of antidepressant medications. If a schizophrenic is not recognized as such but 'put on the couch', then his psychosis may be exacerbated.

1.5   Theoretical considerations

> The greatest achievement would be to realize that everything that is a
> fact is already a theory.   (Goethe)

In psychotherapy different schools exist side by side with no attempt at integration. For the most part they are applied unreflectingly in a confused and contradictory manner.[17]

   While every piece of empirical research in the natural sciences begins with observation and description, this does not take place without an element of theory in the general sense of a point of view. In Popper's words: 'Clinical observations, like all other observations, are interpretations in the light of theories' (1959). All the different phenomenological studies have their starting point in individual observation, even though they seek by so-called reductionism to exclude as far as possible everything that is only suppositional, or assumed, and try to find the kernel (the phenomenon) of a given matter, the invariant in the individually varying (Husserl, 1913). It is an ideal goal, this exclusion of everything theoretical, this letting the matter speak for itself, for all our understanding is itself no more than theory! Phenomenological hermeneutics, however (Heidegger, 1927; Gadamer, 1972), has introduced a new development.

Phenomenological hermeneutics should not be confused with the 'deep hermeneutics' (Habermas, 1973) of psycho-analysis, an explanatory hermeneutic method clothed in the terminology of the natural sciences. It is Freud's great achievement that he opened up paths to this understanding.[18] Unfortunately he soon abandoned what was there to be discovered. 'The phenomena that are perceived must in our opinion yield in importance to trends that are only hypothetical' (*Gesammelte Werke*, vol. XI, p. 62). Therein lies the danger: the temptation, for the sake of theoretical consistency, to abandon the matter prematurely and, interpreting from a creative fantasy, to evade the obligation to supply demonstrable evidence by the process of hypostatization.[19]

Empirical nomothetic research also seeks in various ways to establish supra-individual, general validity and constant relationships. At times this approach employs idiographic and hermeneutic-analytical interpretation, at other times it applies statistical methods to operational concepts by means of standardized data-collection and documentation. These methods should not be regarded as mutually exclusive. Hermeneutics constitute a search for an understanding of the individual and of what in his existence is of general human validity. 'Hermeneutics are effective history' (Gadamer, 1972, p. 283). Empirical statistical research, which does not concern itself with the individual patient, can, by testing the regularity of their occurrence, help to check the general validity of results obtained by other methods (Fig. 3).

Once the factual material (which already contains a theory) has been established, the formation of hypotheses begins. Plausible hypotheses are valid until they have been proved wrong or are replaced by better ones. Science constructs explanatory theories out of relationships and in so doing develops its own idioms. This is where the different approaches part company: psycho-analysis, behaviourism, learning theory, Gestalt psychology, communication psychology and much else besides, all follow their own separate

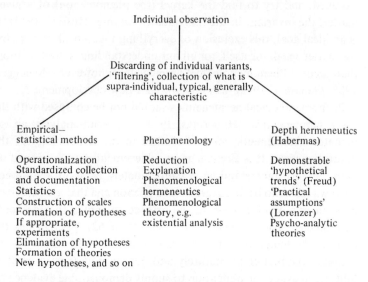

Individual observation

Discarding of individual variants, 'filtering', collection of what is supra-individual, typical, generally characteristic

Empirical–statistical methods	Phenomenology	Depth hermeneutics (Habermas)
Operationalization Standardized collection and documentation Statistics Construction of scales Formation of hypotheses If appropriate, experiments Elimination of hypotheses Formation of theories New hypotheses, and so on	Reduction Explanation Phenomenological hermeneutics Phenomenological theory, e.g. existential analysis	Demonstrable 'hypothetical trends' (Freud) 'Practical assumptions' (Lorenzer) Psycho-analytic theories

Fig. 3. Approaches to empirical research in psychiatry.

paths. Theoretical pluralism is inevitable and is fruitful if its methodology is kept pure, i.e. so long as we do not use the idiom of one theory to argue against another.

See Bochenski (1954, p. 139): 'In view of the findings of contemporary methodology, different modes of thought are not mutually exclusive but are complementary aspects of thought.' The choice of ways of thinking, or even of the goal of thinking, is a decision that precedes knowledge; even his philosophical mode of thought is an expression of a man's essential being. The 'psychology of philosophy' has not yet been unravelled (see Jaspers, 1925).

Theories are attempts to bring together in a meaningful way subject-matter which is designated as inter-linked, so as to form the one systematic, consistent set of propositions that best suits the matter in question (formulation in line with Bochenski, 1954).

The value of a theory is assessed by the following criteria:

(1) How much does it enable us to explain and understand in as simple (economic) a way as possible? All complex theoretical systems should be evaluated in terms of which parts of them are necessary and should be retained (reduction of theories).

(2) What predictions are made possible by a particular theory, i.e.

what is the value of the therapeutic implications of the theory for our therapeutic activity?

The starting point and proving point of all theoretical systems must be a careful description of the subject-matter itself.

All research must be based on individual observations. The point of view of the individual observer is, however, not easy to eliminate. We always hope, but we can never be sure, that what is observed is seen unambiguously in its own right, so that our testimony is absolutely unbiased and is concerned with the subject-matter alone. What is individual can be understood only with the help of a general concept which is itself in the nature of a theory (whether this is consciously realized and formulated or not).

It is a danger inherent in general concepts that we assume knowledge when we have nothing more than ideas or imaginary notions and perhaps not even these. This is the case, for example, in the concepts of structure and dynamics which are used so abundantly in the most diverse theories. Again and again complicated concepts and constructs, which should be used to help us interpret a matter theoretically, are used for purposes of description. And description is often falsely equated with phenomenology.

Our grasp of the world is effected by means of constructs and images. We can only hope that with honest endeavour we will to some extent come to achieve a generally acceptable grasp of our material.

Lorenz (1973) is convinced that man's 'apparatus for perceiving the world', i.e. his mode of thought and point of view, make it possible to form 'a true picture of reality' or at least one which 'is simplified in a grossly utilitarian way' (p. 17). 'The physiological apparatus, whose task it is to recognize the real world, is no less real than the world' (p. 32).

The world is already complicated enough for our understanding. We have every reason to burden ourselves only with those constructs which we regard as necessary to enable us to survive in the present state of our knowledge.

We have every reason to strive after unambiguous and clear concepts and not to use a confusion of descriptive and interpretative terms, or words, that have different levels of meaning.

As a patient put it, 'Even God himself cannot use words with two special contradictory meanings, just to teach us in an understandable manner' (*Protocol 149*).

2

CONSCIOUSNESS

(*Bewußtsein*)

2.1 Definition

The use of the abstract term consciousness should not mislead us into thinking that consciousness cannot be substantialized in the sense, for example, of Descartes' substantialization as *res cogitans*. Consciousness is to be conscious (Ey, 1963: *être conscient*), to know about oneself and the world. In other words, the conscious man does not possess consciousness, but is a conscious being, he is himself conscious in an unmistakable way – aware, sentient, experiencing, feeling, affectively disposed, rationally knowing and taking action.

Consciousness as *conscientia* always implies in the broad sense understanding and knowing something; it is always related to something.[1] This is what is meant by the social dimension of consciousness, in the sense of being in tune with people and things, of being in touch. The conscious man and the object of his consciousness belong together. It is not necessary to construct a distinction between the act and the content of consciousness.

2.2 Areas of functioning

'Consciousness is awareness of self and environment.' This formulation of Cobb (1957) encompasses in its brevity three large areas which may be defined as follows:

(1) *Wakefulness (vigilance)*. To be vigilant is a necessary condition of clear consciousness.

(2) *Clarity of consciousness, lucidity*. This enables man to experience as such those objects which are within his horizon: perceptive and cognitive functions.

(3) *Consciousness of self (ego-consciousness)*. The healthy man knows himself as an experiencing, action-taking person. He is aware of himself as a biographically continuous ('enduring' – Boss, 1971), integral self (see also p. 41). This embraces the consciousness of experience and of reality and also the experience of time.

30

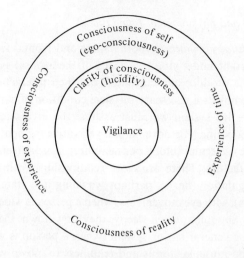

Fig. 4. Areas of consciousness.

The diagram (Fig. 4) gives an overall view of the areas of consciousness. The inner areas (looked at concentrically) must be functioning before the more outlying areas can come into play. Without vigilance there can be no clarity of consciousness, and without clarity of consciousness there can be no clear consciousness of self, no consciousness of experience, no consciousness of reality and no experience of time.

2.3   Wakefulness (vigilance)

Vigilance is not a constant but a fluctuating state. It is subject to changes (degrees of vigilance) which (*a*) are regulated by the organism itself (self-regulation of the rhythm of sleep and waking and of drive or basic activity); (*b*) depend on the state as a whole (e.g. health, mood, etc.). For example, anxiety, terror and joy arouse the organism and keep it awake; pain, cold water and noise stimulate wakefulness; by contrast, monotony, lack of stimulus and boredom induce sleep.

Anatomical and physiological foundations[2]

The *substantia reticularis*, hypothalamus and frontal lobes are the most important underlying structures of the arousal system. They cannot alone produce consciousness, but their interaction with the brain as a whole is a necessary physical condition of consciousness. To activate this system we must assume the involvement also of humoral-endocrine (e.g. adrenaline), vegetative (sympathetic, parasympathetic), vascular (blood permeability), sensory (sensory influx) and other factors. There are close relationships with central respiratory regulation (hence, perhaps, yawning in a state of reduced wakefulness), with eye movements (when a person is wide awake, eye movements are quick; when sleepy, they slow down, the lids close), and with the general motor system (when a person is wide awake, there is good muscular tonus and readiness to move; when sleepy, tonus is slack and movements sluggish). The degree of viligance is mirrored in cerebral electrical activity and can therefore be measured objectively by means of the electroencephalogram (EEG).

Examination

The degree of wakefulness can be assessed (*a*) by self-observation; (*b*) clinically by questioning and by observation of behaviour. A person who is fully awake gives active attention to another person or to an object (by seeing, hearing, feeling, thinking, speaking, etc.) and is always ready for action.

From full wakefulness there are various stages of drowsiness on the way to sleep: turning away from the environment, closed eyes, lack of attention, reduced muscular tonus, reduced motor activity, reduced reactivity, altered rhythm of breathing, etc. A sleeping person can be wakened by sensory stimuli, an important observation when differentiating between sleep and disturbances of consciousness.

2.4 Lucidity (clarity of consciousness)

Lucidity is closely associated with degree of vigilance. Only a person who is fully awake has his perceptive, cognitive, intellectual and sensory functions clearly at his disposal.

Degrees of lucidity range broadly from pre-reflexive (pre-predicative and therefore verbally incommunicable) perception (diffuse expectation, protopathic), through increasingly clear, conscious perception, with attention and concentration, and finally to reflection, understanding and knowledge (epicritic).[3]

Most intellectual activities are thus already covered: comprehension and recognition, orientation, understanding, connecting, logical judgement, communication by speech, purposeful and sensible action. Previous experience (everything we learn) also contributes to these processes, helped by memory.

When a situation is fully considered in the context of one's total life history, this is called rational reflection (*Besonnenheit* – Stoerring's *Besinnung*, 1953).

When we consciously recognize something clearly, our 'object-awareness' (Jaspers, 1959) tells us whether what we recognize is objective or non-objective (see chapter on *Perception*) and our consciousness of experience and of reality (q.v.) tell us whether what we are experiencing is thought, assumed or visualized by us, or is actually presented to us.

Anatomical and physiological foundations

Apart from the structures already mentioned in connection with vigilance, lucidity, especially at the higher stages of rational reflection, requires the integrative functioning of the total brain.

Examination

The clinical examination of lucidity can be made by questioning the patient about and by observing his sensory functioning (the sensorium), his orientation (q.v.), his attention and his ability to give an orderly verbal account of sensible, appropriate and goal-directed action.

2.5　Pathology of consciousness – disturbances of consciousness – disturbances of vigilance and lucidity

Disturbances of total experience and behaviour occur in varying degree. They include disturbances of sensory apperception, of alert and purposeful reaction to environmental stimuli, of attention, of orientation in place, time and one's own person and situation, of orderly thinking, will and action, of clarity of intention and of purposefulness in attending to and coming to terms with the environment. Often there are changes in degree of arousal or shifts in vigilance. Qualitative disturbances (changes, shifts) of consciousness are usually associated with quantitative changes in intensity (stages of vigilance).

The categories are:

Predominantly quantitative reduction in consciousness – clouding of consciousness, loss of consciousness (Bewußtseinsstörungen, Bewußtlosigkeit)

Stages:
　　Clouding, obnubilation (*Benommenheit*)
　　Drowsiness, somnolence
　　Sopor
　　Coma
　　(See below)

Qualitative disturbances of consciousness

　　Delirium tremens
　　Twilight state
　　Dreamlike state (*Oneiroid*)
　　Confusion (*Verwirrtheit*)
　　Parasomnia, coma-vigil (*Parasomnische Bewußtseinlage*)
　　(See below)

Heightened (broadened) consciousness

(See below.)

Clouding, obnubilation

Lucidity (clarity) and vigilance are slightly affected. Generally there is sleepiness, lack of spontaneity, sluggishness. Though in the absence of stimulation (if left alone), the patient often seems to be asleep, he can still move about and to some extent act appropriately. The patient can be aroused when spoken to or by physical contact. He understands simple requests (give me your hand, show me your tongue) and can obey such instructions, although very slowly. In general he is in poor touch with the environment and is often partly disoriented. There is little spontaneous speech; silence or whispers are the rule.

Somnolence

The patient is very apathetic, slow and sleepy. If left alone he continuously falls asleep, though he can easily be aroused when spoken to loudly or by physical contact. He is then at first bewildered, though still to some extent orientated. If the patient can still speak, his articulation is generally bad and he tends to mumble. He no longer speaks spontaneously and makes few spontaneous move-ments: if painful stimuli are applied, he makes defensive or avoiding movements and corrects his posture. His reflexes are maintained, though muscular tonus is somewhat reduced. Swallowing and often also coughing reflex movements are reduced.

Sopor

The patient can be roused only by strong stimuli (such as shaking, pinching, tweaking). Verbal responses can no longer be elicited, nor can expressions of pain. Posture is generally not corrected. Reflexes are still present, muscular tonus is reduced. Breathing is slow, deep and generally rhythmic, as in sleep.

Pre-coma (sub-coma) and coma (I–IV)

The patient can no longer be aroused. Even the strongest stimulus produces no defensive or avoiding movement. Muscular tonus is severely diminished and the muscles are flabby. Sub-coma and the four stages of coma are distinguished on the basis of neurological and EEG findings. In sub-coma the pupillary reflex to light and the corneal reflex (blinking when the cornea is touched) are still present, but the plantar reflex and the peripheral tendon reflex are lost. In coma the corneal reflex and, lastly, the light reflex also disappear, the pupils usually being wide open. Breathing is also usually altered, with slow, apnoeic pauses and irregular respiration.

Causal associations. Clouding of consciousness, from obnubilation to coma, is always caused by disturbed cerebral functioning in which the brain is directly or indirectly involved. The diagnostic possibilities are:

Cranial trauma
  Commotio cerebri (cerebral shock)
  Contusio cerebri (cerebral contusion)
  Compressio cerebri (cerebral compression, e.g. caused by haemorrhage)
  Increased cerebral pressure due to various causes, e.g. tumour, intracranial haemorrhage, etc. Increased cerebral pressure leads to disorders in blood supply and to lack of nutrition in the nerve cells.

Ischaemia
  In arteriosclerosis, in embolic or thrombotic occlusion (apoplexy), in cerebral haemorrhage involving the blood vessels of the brain or the brain surface or meninges (subarachnoid haemorrhage). Other vascular disorders (Bürger's disease, aneurysm, migraine).

Lack of respiratory oxygen, following strangulation (choking, hanging), collapse, severe loss of blood, carbon monoxide poisoning.

In epileptic attacks there is a sudden and complete loss of consciousness followed by a post-convulsive disturbance of consciousness of varying duration.

Severe inflammation of the brain and meninges (encephalitis, encephalomeningitis).

Toxic cerebral damage
  Exogenous poisoning, e.g. severe infectious illnesses such as typhus, soporific drugs, alcohol, narcotics, carbon monoxide.
  Endogenous poisoning, e.g. metabolic failure in hepatic coma, uraemia, hypoglycaemia, eclampsia, endocrine disorders, such as thyrotoxic coma.

Delirium tremens

Here we find severe disturbances of consciousness, both qualitative and quantitative, with increased psychomotor activity. Partial or total disorientation (confusion), incoherence of thought (confused thinking, bewilderment), misidentification of surroundings, hallucinations (especially visual, but also vestibular, auditory and sometimes tactile). The visual hallucinations are often suggestible. The patient is still usually accessible when one talks to him or addresses him by name, but his mind soon wanders again. The rhythm of sleep and waking is disturbed; the delirium often begins in the evening and at night there is unrest and increased confusion. Vegetative symptoms which often accompany the disorder include sweating, tachycardia, sebaceous secretion, flushing, coarse tremor, raised temperature and dehydration. In the classical form of alcoholic delirium the basic mood is often one of gaiety and excitement, but occasionally the patient is filled with anxiety. This happens particularly when he suffers from a mixture of delirium and hallucinosis. Less severe stages of delirium are known also as *sub-delirium, pre-delirium* or *abortive delirium*.

EXAMPLES

A 55-year-old building worker who had been in hospital for one day with inflammation of the lungs, got out of bed towards evening, became restless, roamed around the room, went to the window and conducted a loud, blustering conversation with imaginary figures whom he saw in the park at night, making signs to him and speaking to him. When addressed, he was surly and unco-operative and was disoriented regarding his situation.

Another man saw in his room nothing but threads of glass hanging from the ceiling and moving as if in the wind. He felt as though he was being rocked in his bed (vestibular hallucinations).

Another patient saw a whole crowd of elephants (as small as hares) moving across the wall of the room. Another read a few words from an empty piece of paper. Another collected beetles in the drawer of a bedside cupboard. Another saw little coloured birds on his bedspread, touching each other with the tips of their wings; he found this sight entrancing and smiled and beamed; his temperature was raised, he was sweating, his skin was flushed, and on questioning he was found to be disoriented in time, place and situation.

Causal associations. Delirium not only occurs as a complication of chronic alcoholism but is found also in non-alcoholic intoxication, e.g. with various drugs such as atropine, drugs used in Parkinsonism, antidepressants, cocaine, poisonous mushrooms, etc. Endogenous noxae (such as metabolic errors) may give rise to delirium-like states.

Clinical pictures that resemble delirium can also be found in acute, confused endogenous pyschoses (so-called schizophrenic delirium, a term which is only rarely used).

Twilight state

This state is characterized by a narrowing of the field of consciousness, with exclusive concentration on certain inner experiences and suspension (or decrease) of interest in the environment. There is a decrease in accessibility to external stimuli. Attention to the environment diminishes or may even cease. Thinking is unclear to a varying degree, even to the point of confusion.

Misidentification of the environment is frequent and hallucinations occur in all sensory fields. Mood is coloured by anxiety, but may also be blissful to the point of ecstasy. Psychomotor activity may be normal, heightened or reduced. Twilight states do not usually last long, often ending in sleep and being followed by total amnesia.

In the so-called *orientated twilight state*, attention, thinking and judgement are narrowed. Thoughts may still be orderly, and outward activity may seem also to be normal.[4]

Causal associations. Twilight states may be divided according to their cause into organic and psychogenic.

Organic causes are epilepsy (psychomotor epilepsy, post-paroxysmal twilight state), cerebral trauma (post-commotional twilight state), disorders of circulation (arteriosclerosis), hypoxic (lack of oxygen) and toxic (endogenous and exogenous) states.

Psychogenic twilight states (synonym: psychogenic stress reactions) occur in terror, shock, panic, when immature and ill-balanced persons are thrust into a completely strange environment and cannot come to terms with it. Hysterical twilight states also belong to this group.

Dream-like or oneroid state

This term covers a dream-like, disoriented, confused state, in which the patient has a hallucinatory experience of dramatic and fantastically elaborate scenes in which he participates with deep and appropriate emotional involvement, as if under a spell, at times misidentifying elements in his environment. Patients no longer pay attention to their surroundings, though they can still at times be recalled to them for short periods, if energetically addressed; they are then, however, bewildered, surprised and disoriented, though there is no amnesia for what they experience. To outward appearance they are either sunk in stupor or in a state of great excitement. An oneiroid patient usually comes to the clinic after a period of disturbed sleep and in a state of excessive fatigue, often associated with excitability.[5]

EXAMPLES

Such patients experience catastrophes, battles, floods, festivals, a Heaven and Hell in which they are physically torn asunder between good and evil powers. They also experience the end of the world and in a state of religious ecstasy they may see and speak with God.

Causal associations. Dream-like states occur in many acute and dramatic forms of schizophrenia, in epilepsy (psychotic twilight state) and also in cases of drug intoxication.

Confusion (amentia)

This term is no longer commonly used today. It describes a syndrome of severe confusion of thought (incoherence) accompanied by general disorientation, hallucinations, delusions, and a mood of anxious bewilderment.[6]

It is not possible to draw a clear distinction between this syndrome and acute severe delirium or a dream-like state.

Causal associations. States of amentia are found not only in acute exogenous reactive states (e.g. cerebral arteriosclerosis) but also in schizophrenic psychoses of acute onset and dramatic course (so-called schizophrenic delirium), in puerperal psychoses and in so-called affective psychoses.

Parasomnia

(Synonyms: apallic syndrome (Kretschmer, 1940; Scharfetter, C. and F., 1968), akinetic mutism, coma *vigile*.) The patient, although mute and motionless, seems to be awake. He stares straight ahead or his gaze wanders, but he takes nothing in. He does not react to verbal or other stimuli, e.g. being touched or having objects held up before him. Normal reflex movements of avoidance or defence may also be absent. He may become rigid in any posture and make no corrective movement. The elementary vegetative functions of cardiac rhythm, breathing, sleeping, waking, are maintained.

The syndrome should not be confused with coma or with catatonic stupor. In addition to psychopathological and neurological findings, the EEG findings are important.

Causal associations. The syndrome is associated with very severe damage to, and functional impairment of, the pallidum, for example in cerebral trauma, cerebral haemorrhage, cerebral inflammation, and after cerebral venal thrombosis.

State of heightened consciousness

This is a vague concept which is supposed to describe an experience in which an individual feels himself stretched, his existence is broadened, his impressions of the external world are more vivid and more alert, his understanding is richer and his faculties of association and memory are more active. The state is sometimes accompanied by changes in the experience of time. The perception of objects seems to be more brilliant and is accompanied by stronger emotional response and perhaps by synaesthesias. Experiences are focused afresh on things other than the usual everyday objects.

Causal associations. Such feelings of heightened awareness ('being high') can occur under the influence of hallucinogenic drugs (LSD, mescaline, hashish, etc.) or of stimulants (amphetamine). Occasionally in mania, at the beginning of schizophrenia, a patient may have the feeling that he is inspired or ecstatic, that he is experiencing the world in a more vivid, penetrating, clear and intelligent way. The mood is accompanied by a feeling of being stimulated.

EGO-CONSCIOUSNESS

3.1 Definition

Ego-consciousness is the certainty with which the conscious, lucid individual is able to say 'I am myself'. The ego is therefore the conscious, lucid man who is fully aware of himself, who experiences himself in harmony and with a purpose, a person with wishes, needs, instincts, longings, perceptions, sensations and thoughts, acting throughout his life history in an unbroken continuum. We use the substantive abstract 'ego' to designate this being one's own self, and in so doing we do not forget the intimate relationship between the ego and the external world.

3.2 Dimensions

When we speak in what follows of dimensions of ego-consciousness, we do not mean independent mechanisms of an apparatus. We refer rather to what should be thought of as aspects of our own inner experiences, of which pathology makes us aware, and aspects of morbid modes of self-experience which can be recognized in the experience of patients. Frequently the two overlap.

The table of dimensions (Fig. 5) which we have drawn up (for didactic purposes only) is derived more from the experience of patients (see *Pathology*) than from the self-analysis of 'normal people' who are of course inclined to take the basic dimensions (see dimensions 1–5 below) for granted and entertain no doubts about them provided that their relationships to the people and things around them are natural, i.e. in physiological terms, provided that they experience the ordinary pattern of stimulus-response. It is of decisive importance in psychopathology that the dimensions in question are qualities in the self-experience of patients, whose presentation of them helps us to see their nature and strength and to find a therapeutic approach to them. The dimensions discussed below may be viewed as a series of concentric circles whose 'inner',

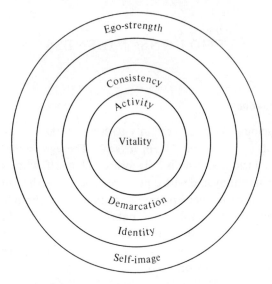

Fig. 5. Dimensions of ego-consciousness.

'lower', 'leading' members must exist before the 'outer' and 'upper' members can come into being: the terms 'inner-outer', 'upper-lower' refer, of course, only to the graphic representation. The dimensions should not be regarded as uni-dimensional, e.g. as strata or onion layers, since the 'inner' dimensions, such as vitality, permeate all the others, of which they are prerequisites.

1. Ego-vitality

We experience ourselves – in full consciousness – as sentient, somatically alive, real. This 'I am' experience is already a form of mood or affect (feeling of vitality).[1]

2. Ego-activity

The healthy man takes it for granted that it is he himself who lives, experiences, perceives, feels, has moods, thinks, speaks, moves and acts. We experience ourselves as doers, as functioning independently (self-driven) in our conduct and actions.[2]

3. Ego-consistency

We experience ourselves always as being one unit, as being consistent within our own being. This is true even if inner divisions and conflicts make us creative (Goethe's 'two souls').

4. Ego-demarcation

We are aware of ourselves as ourselves and at the same time we know what is external to ourselves: we distinguish between the ego and the non-ego, drawing a demarcation line between the two. We can thus determine what belongs to the ego and what comes to us from the non-ego, e.g. we distinguish in the sensory field between a seemingly living image or visualization and a perception. Ego-demarcation is closely associated with the ability to achieve so-called *reality control* (q.v.).

Demarcation line is a figurative expression which should not be viewed as mechanical. It implies a two-way border traffic, i.e. in association with other people and with objects. Such a free border passage makes possible an interplay, a to-and-fro movement between the ego and the non-ego. In pathological cases the boundary can become a wall, a barrier which imprisons the individual in a state of loneliness (restriction of existence, alienation, autism), or the boundary can break down and the defenceless individual is overrun by the non-ego, from outside.

5. Ego-identity

Consciousness of one's own identity[3] and continuity (individuality) in the face of changes in oneself and in the external world in the course of life: a man knows that from birth to the present day he is the same man, who can call himself 'I' although he changes in his being as he goes through life, etc.

The *experience of time* (q.v.) is an essential part of this concept. Existence is individually time-bound.

Ego-identity is inseparable from awareness of one's body. It would seem that the face and hands, through which the child first sees, feels and touches other people (the mother) are 'crystallization points in the awareness of ego-identity' (Benedetti, 1964).

It is on this basis (the points mentioned in 1–5 above) that self-image (6) and ego-strength (7) are formed, in the course of personality development within the social context (the process of personalization).

The concepts of self-image and ego-strength are not phenomenologically based; they are global constructs in the area of self-experience and, indirectly, the experience of other people. They presuppose the existence of dimensions 1–5, but unlike these dimensions neither is a fixed or uniform concept; they vary and change throughout life according to mood, environment and performance. These two dimensions seem to a large extent more dependent on culture than dimensions 1–5 (see Hallowell, 1955; Lebra, 1972).

6. Self-image (concept of self, image of one's own personality)

The individual's view of himself, his knowledge of himself, how he feels, sees and understands himself in relation to others, all depend on how he sees himself as viewed and approached by other people at a given moment as well as in the longer perspective of his life and development.[4]

Self-image also includes self-esteem. Anything that does not fit into this concept is easily excluded from one's perception of oneself, a perceptual scotoma.

7. Ego-strength

The concept of ego-strength is very much a global one. Ego-strength may be regarded as the sum of all the dimensions listed under 1–6. It characterizes the totality of an individual in his private being and in his public presence. It embraces in particular the capacity for allo- and autoplastic adaptation (Fenichel, 1971; Hartmann, 1939) and for synthesis (Nunberg, 1939). Federn (1956) has repeatedly pointed out that ego-strength may be a quality of different ego-functions; this is not to be confused with the dimensions discussed here.

In ego-strength we may include: tenacity of purpose, steadfastness in life, assurance and independence (autonomy) in integrating within the personality an individual's own strivings, wishes and drives, the ability to make demands on other people and on the external world and to accept the buffetings of fate and the denial of desires and hopes without too much mortification, the capacity to accept the demands of others without partial or complete surrender. What we call suggestibility or resistance to suggestion is also dependent on ego-strength.

Comments on the above schema. There is no evidence that this schema – which is meant to serve the purposes of classification – actually corresponds to the ontogenesis of ego-experience., As a hypothetical series of dimensions it does, however, receive support from the pathology of severe ego-disturbances. In less severe cases the dimensions are not so clearly placed in sequence, with one depending upon another, but several dimensions may be affected simultaneously in varying degree. In severe disturbances of the lower, basic or central dimensions, the remaining (upper) dimensions are no longer experienced and do not therefore present as disturbances.

By way of example, in severe ego-devitalization, questions of ego-activity, ego-consistency and ego-demarcation, of identity, self-image and ego-strength no longer arise. On the other hand, it is possible for the layers, metaphorically speaking, to disintegrate from the top downwards; ego-strength and self-image may then be individually or globally impaired or disturbed without ego-identity, or the dimensions appearing below it on the list, necessarily being affected. Impairment of ego-consistency is generally associated with impairment of ego-demarcation and ego-vitality (as in delusions of annihilation) but this is not necessarily the case. Ego-identity may be disturbed without overt adverse effects on consistency, demarcation, activity or vitality.

Relationship between this point of view and the ego-psychology of psycho-analysis. This phenomenologically derived view of ego-dimensions does *not* conflict with psycho-analytical theory. The two points of view are on different planes. The concepts discussed here belong to the descriptive, phenomenological plane of observation based on transactions with patients. The schema of suggested dimensions (which has predecessors in Hegel, 1807; Kronfeld, 1922; Gruhle, 1956; Jaspers, 1959; and K. Schneider, 1967) permits us to understand many symptoms of schizophrenia or schizophrenia-like psychoses, but tells us nothing about how the disturbances of the said ego-dimensions arise.

Psycho-analysis, on the other hand, offers no descriptive terminology[5] but only terms relating to genesis: it seeks to explain in causal terms how a condition arises.[6] Psycho-analytical theory with its associated terminology can therefore be applied when we have a careful description which is as free as possible of all interpretations, insofar as this can be obtained.

Psycho-analytical ego-psychology already had a long history in Freud's time (for reviews see Hartmann, 1964b, Laplanche and Pontalis, 1973; Nunberg, 1971; Blanck, G. and R., 1974). However, there is still no agreement as to the nature of the ego. Freud in his early years called it an organization of neurons, later an organization of mental processes with specific links with the id, the super-ego and external reality. Hartmann (1964a, b) has called the ego an apparatus, Rapaport (1967) a structure, Holt[7] a class of functions. Federn (1956) speaks of a connected, continuing cathectic unit. Spitz (1959, 1965) calls the ego an 'organized psychic structure with a multiplicity of systems, apparatuses and functions'. Whatever terms we use and although the ego and its functions appear in Freud's design as 'theoretical constructs' (Bellak, 1973, p. 61) deduced from observation and self-observation, they are not descriptive concepts.

The ego may be regarded as a form of experience or related to experience as a metaphysical construct. This problem was already being tackled by Schilder as early as 1914 and was given particular attention by Federn (1956). Federn (1956) was also one of the first psycho-analysts to refer to the ego-boundary which is so important in the psychopathology of schizophrenia even if it cannot be conceptualized statistically.[8] The relationship between the construct ego and the rest of our mental functions (*Instanzen*) is not uniformly clear. In particular, it is not clearly stated whether ego-regression must be a global process; whether it may affect individual functions only, as Hartmann stresses in the case of ego-weakness; or to what extent ego-regression must parallel instinct regression (Bellak, p. 72).

Among the various groups of factors required for ego-development are inherited ego-qualities, instinctual forces and the influences of the external world (Hartmann, 1964a, p. 336). Hartmann has particularly emphasized that Freud (1937: *Analysis, Terminable and Interminable*) expressly conceded the possibility of 'ego-differences' being determined by heredity. According to Spitz (1965, p. 104) the constituents of the ego include '*innate*, mostly phylogenetically transmitted physiological functions as well as *innate* behaviour patterns' (my italics). Developmentally the ego comes from the id. But the id is a bad mother, a cannibalistic Kali which threatens and may even swallow its own child, thereby making the ego revert to the status of the id (Nunberg, 1971, p. 143 – for theories of ego-development, see p. 43).

There is no general agreement as to which functions may be ascribed to this ego-construct. The ego, which is only partly conscious and which is itself under the control of the super-ego, acts as representative of the reality principle, of the secondary "inward' and 'outward' processes. Inwardly it acts on the id, which is completely unconscious, the seat of the life and death instincts (Eros and Thanatos, libido and mortido, libido and aggression), and facilitates, inhibits or modifies instinctual behaviour. For the id, the ego is thus primarily an 'inhibiting apparatus' (Nunberg, Fenichel). Outwardly, i.e. in the direction of external reality, the ego is a receiving apparatus concerned with perception, apperception, will, intentionality, motility, action, and reality-testing. The defence mechanisms which are so central to the theory of psycho-analysis, are 'localized' in the ego (Freud, 1938, *Gesammelte Werke*, vol. XVII; Freud, A., 1936; Hartmann, 1937/38 in 1964a, b; Rapaport, 1950; Schafer, 1968; for the ego-psychology of Hartmann and Rapaport see also Loch, 1975).

It would seem that, as Hartmann pointed out in 1950 (1964a, b), a complete list of ego-functions has still to be compiled. (For a review of the various registers of ego-functions see Bellak (1973, p. 52).) For twenty years attempts have been made to achieve an assessment of ego-functions in the form of rating scales and scores (see Bellak, 1973, p. 52).

Little is known about modes of ego-functioning in healthy people. According to Hartmann (1964a, p. 351): 'We do not know too much about what form of structural hierarchy of ego-functions is most likely to be found correlated with mental health in a positive way' (see also Vaillant, 1971).

Hartmann (1964a) has repeatedly discussed the question of the ego's energy supply. Has the ego its own sources of energy (which is neither sexual nor aggressive) or has it merely drained sexual and aggressive energy from instinctual drives by virtue of its neutralizing capacity? The question is of importance for the self-cathexis of narcissism in which there is a pathological weakness of ego-functioning due to neutralized sexual and aggressive instinctual energy.

3.3 Constituents, determinants, development

Ego-experience and body-consciousness

Consciousness of one's body is a constituent of ego-experience. Disturbances of bodily sensation – e.g. alteration, alienation, distortion, transformation, devitalization, putrefaction, decay, or swelling – and hypochondriacal fears of a similar nature are inseparable from ego-experience. Many schizophrenic disturbances of ego-experience are expressed predominantly, for example, in a feeling (delusional conviction) that one's face is changing (e.g. 'my face, my nose has become crooked'). On the other hand, physical illnesses may also lead to violent upsets and changes in ego-experience (Schilder, 1914).

Development

The development of ego-consciousness seems to start early, probably in the first year of life. By the second to third year the child has usually acquired an 'ego', the experience of 'I am' (Spitz, 1965, 1972). A child gets to know other people first through his mother, by seeing and recognizing her face and by feeling or grasping with his hands. The act of grasping enables him to become conscious of activity. Herein too lie the roots of ego-demarcation, ego-identity and ego-consistency. The development of ego-consciousness depends on genetically determined factors of maturation of the central nervous system, the perceptual system and the body as a whole; it depends also to a very large extent on the self in relation to and association with others (the process of personification in a micro-and macro-social context – Erikson, 1966; Engel, 1962; Lidz, 1970).

Spitz's studies (1965) are particularly impressive. The decisive figure in the socialization process of ego-development is the 'mothering person'. Not only does she give the child food, warmth and love, and provide the 'optimal frustration' which promotes 'structure (and ego-)-building', but also she is the first person in the external environment to help develop object relations, thus paving the way for 'semantic communication' in his dealings with other people. Other factors which play their part in this process are the conditions in which the child grows up, the physical contact between mother and child, oral and anal freedom or restriction, room to move, the family and its speech, social life with its interactions and goals, and the locality inhabited.

As development proceeds and the social context expands beyond the confines of the family, the child gains experience of life, and patterns are established by so-called identifications through which there can occur an expansion and consolidation of his self-image, complete with consciousness of its role and finally his secure sense of an ego which has been built up and rendered resilient (ego-strength).

Ego-experience, self-experience and culture

Comparative ethnic psychology shows that the demarcation of the individual as a separate being is particularly prominent in European and other Western cultures. Other cultures, e.g. in East and South-east Asia, have not developed such an autonomous, individualistic ego-concept; their members see themselves more as separate and incomplete parts of a family unit (Kimura, 1965, 1967, 1969; Wulff, 1972; group ego, Parin and Morgenthaler, 1964). In the absence of comparative descriptive studies, the effects of this process on psychopathology are not yet clear.

Wulff's observations (1972) on the alleged lack of ego-disturbances in schizophrenics in Vietnam are not convincing. It is quite credible that schizophrenics in Vietnam may not experience and articulate ego-disturbances, as defined in the narrow classical sense of German psychiatry, in the same way as schizophrenics of Western cultures (see his remarks on language). But the fact that schizophrenics there stand out because they do not fit into the complicated sociolinguistic system of interaction and no longer strike the 'right' pattern of behaviour towards their fellows, would still lead one to conclude that they are no longer masters of their own role-identity. In order to feel at home in such a complicated system of communication, they surely must possess the same elementary ego-dimensions as are listed above under 1–5.

In the world of magic, in states of possession (frequently found outside Europe), in mediumistic states and states of trance, in religious and mystical ecstasy, the self is experienced differently and in particular in a less isolated manner than in Western cultures.

3.4 Examination

Ego-consciousness is experienced by self-observation and can be communicated verbally. Pathological changes can be examined partly by questioning and partly by inference from the patient's behaviour, his experiences and his symptoms (see Pathology). Ego-profile scales have also been developed (Bellak, 1973; Semrad *et al.*, 1973).

Components of ego-strength/weakness may also be viewed as the 'neuroticism' of self-rating scales (Eysenck, 1967).

3.5 Pathology

Depersonalization[9]

This term lumps together a very wide variety of disturbed ego-experiences.

The most frequent phenomenon in depersonalization is a feeling of remoteness, of being apparently alienated, unfamiliar, shadowy, lacking life, unreal. An observing ego is still present, experiencing events and noting the changes, mostly unquestioningly. On closer inquiry it appears that corresponding to this alienation from the self (depersonalization) there is also alienation from the human and material world (derealization), though to begin with the patient may feel that one of these two forms of alienation is the more obtrusive. Depersonalization and derealization go together because the ego and its environment are really one. The less a patient takes himself for granted, the more unfamiliar and alien does the world around him become.

On closer inspection, the dimensions listed under 1–5 in Section 3.2 above are seen to be affected in many ways (see below under *Ego-vitality* to *Ego-identity* inclusive).

EXAMPLES

Protocol 1 (Neurotic depression)

'I am more like a shadow now...I'm not aware of myself any more...
everything is remote, pushed far away...as in a fog.' (depersonalization
and derealization).

Protocol 2 (Former schizophrenic)

'I've become uncertain...I have a great inclination to question everything...nothing is natural any more...it can't be taken for granted as it
used to be...
'I feel my life more sensitively than I used to...we live one with another and
yet each is for himself...I am remote from my nearest kin, from my husband
and my children, I live my own life.' This patient showed a loss of the sense
of natural, matter-of-fact living (Blankenburg, 1971), with depersonalization
and derealization in the sense of remoteness and strangeness.

Causal associations. The extent of depersonalization and derealization fluctuates greatly according to the degree of harmony present
in the patient's relationship with others. When relationships are
strained, symptoms of depersonalization may occur or be exacerbated. A warm, sympathetic, caring relationship may, on the other
hand, remove or relieve the sense of alienation. Transient, intermittent
states of depersonalization often occur during psycho-analytical
treatment. It is important that they should be recognized as such, so
as to avoid any suspicion of psychosis, with its attendant anxieties.

Such experiences of alienation are not nosologically specific, i.e.
they are not pathognomonic for any particular illness. They may
occur:

(*a*) In many healthy people in special circumstances, e.g. fatigue,
exhaustion.

(*b*) In adolescence.

(*c*) As a frequent and obtrusive phenomenon in neuroses (neurotic
depression, obsessional neurosis, phobias), especially during life
crises (crises of relationship) and also during psycho-analysis.

(*d*) In all other forms of depression, especially in so-called endogenous depression.

(*e*) In many schizophrenics, especially as premonitory or initial
symptoms, but also during the illness.

(*f*) In toxic psychoses: when under the influence of analgesic or hypnotic drugs, or of hallucinogens; and in other organically based psychoses.

In many psychoses, particularly schizophrenia-like psychoses, we may find one or more of the above-mentioned dimensions particularly affected, to the point of very severe, general ego-disturbance. A whole range of psychotic modes of experience and behaviour may become understandable if we pay closer regard to disturbances of ego-experience.

Ego-vitality

One's sense of being alive may be reduced or lost (see *Depersonalization* above). Severely ill patients are no longer certain that they are in the world, that they are still living.

Ego-vitality is heightened in mania. In rare cases it may lead to genuine delusions of grandeur.

EXAMPLES

Protocol 22 (Schizophrenia)

'That is, so to speak, the key question, whether I exist and whether I am indivisible.' 'Am I still living?' (disturbance of ego-vitality and ego-consistency).

This experience leads to bewilderment and anxiety, to fear of destruction and death. The patient may be benumbed (catatonic stupor) or enter a panic state of motor excitement, running up against obstacles to try and find himself again.

At times the patient hyperventilates, in order to convince himself that he is still alive. In catatonic hyperventilation, the patient forces himself to perform the elementary vital function of breathing so as to assure himself of being able to say 'I am alive'.

Protocol 12 (Schizophrenia)

'It was as if life were outside me, as if it had withered... I was afraid that my soul, that my life would leave me.' This patient was in a profound catatonic stupor.

Protocol 13 (Schizophrenia)

'I am changed, my ego doesn't exist any more.' This deeply perplexed patient could no longer answer simple questions, because the threat to ego-vitality negated all efforts to respond.

Protocol 56 (Endogenous depression)

'I am not alive any more – I already smell like a corpse.' The development of this theme led to delusional experiences (q.v.).

Formation of delusions. Alienation of the self and of the surrounding world can prepare the way for delusions, which include the following types:

Hypochondriacal delusions, delusions of illness, delusions of bodily destruction and of annihilation; delusions of personal destruction, of imminent dissolution; nihilistic delusions of self and the world; delusional interpretations of annihilation as an external threat; delusions of persecution and destruction.

As a psycho-dynamic hypothesis it is conceivable, though the phenomenological evidence is insufficient, that compensation and overcompensation for such experiences of destruction may give rise to delusions of salvation, delusions of improving the world, messianic delusions, etc. If the patient succeeds in building up such delusions, the experience of devitalization will be overcome.

Causal associations. Depressions of every kind, especially severe endogenous depression, may begin with a loss of ego-vitality. The most severe disturbances of ego-vitality are found in schizophrenia and in the schizophrenia-like toxic psychoses associated with psychotomimetic drugs like LSD and mescaline.

Ego-activity

In the less severe stages of disturbance, purposive thought, feeling, perception and motor activity are all inhibited, reduced or delayed. Even small every-day decisions, actions or speech are carried out with difficulty.

Clinically there is slowness to the point of stupor, and whispering, hesitant speech or mutism (see *Basic activity*). In the more severe stages patients lose their normal certainty that they themselves are still actively living and moving, that they are experiencing, perceiving, feeling, thinking, doing, undertaking tasks. This leads to perplexity, bewilderment and retardation to the point of stupor. Bodily sensation is very often severely disturbed; the patients find themselves no longer in tune with their own bodies. In many cases the interpretation is obvious – the patient is trying to break out of this anxiety-provoking loss of activity by making repetitive movements (stereotypies) or repeating words or sentences (verbigeration). This increased striving may, however, change abruptly to catatonic excitement.

There may also be an automatous mimicry of the movements of others (echopraxia) or repetition of sounds or words uttered by others (echolalia). Many patients in this state retain the posture into which they are placed (flexibilitas cerea).[10]

Formation of delusions. The patient, whose ego-demarcation is also often disturbed, feels as if all his experiences and actions were being controlled and distorted by others, and so develops delusions of influence in the domains of motor activity, thought, feeling, perception and speech. Since this influence is mostly experienced as threatening, uncanny and constraining, the experience can become understandably interpreted as a form of persecution (delusions of persecution). Though it occurs more frequently outside European cultures, the notion of possession also belongs to this category.

EXAMPLES

Protocol 120 (Schizophrenia)

'I felt as if I had been paralysed.'

Protocol 22 (Schizophrenia)

The patient made stereotyped circular movements with his arms, at the same time looking at his hands as if spellbound. He did this to show himself that he could still move.

Protocol 16 (Schizophrenia)

'I had no more energy, I was no longer sure I was myself. I was no longer master of my own thoughts and actions; it was as if I were spellbound. In this state I could no longer speak. Then came the fear that I was being overpowered from without, manipulated, persecuted.'

The patient was transfixed in a state of terrible fear (catatonic stupor); from time to time she had to scream loudly.

Protocol 27 (Schizophrenia)

The patient, who often bellowed like an animal in torture, said: 'It isn't I who am screaming; there is something working on my vocal nerves and then a roar comes out of me.'

Protocol 21 (*Schizophrenia*)

'When I see other people or hear them speak, then it can happen that I say the same things and move in the same way and I have this fear that I am the other people.' (Echolalia, echopraxia, uncertain ego-identity.) 'When someone else limps, then I have to walk more slowly.' (Echopraxia, loss of personal identity.)

Causal associations. The most marked disturbances of ego-activity occur in schizophrenics, particularly catatonics. They may feel they are being influenced, though this does not always happen. Such feelings are clearly based on a disturbance of ego-demarcation and ego-consistency (splitting).

Disturbances of ego-activity also occur in schizophrenia-like psychoses of a different kind: toxic psychoses (LSD, mecaline), epileptic psychoses (including twilight states). Severe states of depression can be accompanied by an inhibition of purpose, to the point of stupor, but not usually by feelings of influence.

Ego-consistency

The patients no longer experience themselves as a natural unit, a cohesive whole. They feel inwardly torn (see *Ambivalence*) and split and they are afraid. They may freeze in a catatonic stupor, or become panic-stricken (catatonic excitement). Many feel themselves physically torn asunder by conflicting forces.

This splitting leads to a sense of duplication, with individual parts remaining relatively independent, though there is also a feeling of dissociation. Such experiences of splitting and dissolution are almost always associated with severe disturbances of ego-identity and with bodily disorientation.[11]

Formation of delusions. The delusional interpretation of this schizophrenic existence takes many forms, including delusions of destruction and dissolution; delusions of being torn apart by good and evil powers, e.g. heaven and hell; delusions of destruction applying to the whole world or to the universe (delusions of global or cosmic catastrophe, break-up of the sun, exploding of stars, etc.).[12] When some functions of the self remain relatively independent there may be delusional duplications (ego-duplication) or multiplication (ego-plurality, ego-multiplicity).

EXAMPLES

Protocol 22 (Schizophrenia)

'Everything is completely mixed up...where is my nose, what has happened to my mouth...my right arm? I don't know right from left any more. I don't know exactly where my left leg is. On the right I am a man, on the left a woman. On the right I am my father, at times my mother. Only half of my blood is mine, the rest comes from a man, or a woman....

'Only half my opinion is my own, the other half belongs to other people, to relatives, to voices.

'There is a whirling confusion in my head and in my body...even my stomach and my neck are whirling.'

This patient was very bewildered, in a state of substupor, but could still communicate his experiences.

Protocol 25 (Schizophrenia)

'I have two heads.'

Protocol 34 (Schizophrenia)

'I have been multiplied.' (Plurality)
'I have four heads to carry around.' (Delusion of being a monster)

Protocol 38 (Schizophrenia)

'I am us.' (Multiplication and mingling of ego)

Protocol 37 (Schizophrenia)

'I was afraid of the doves, when they flew up I thought everything was going to explode.' Fear of ego-dissolution and explosion – the patient ran away in a panic.

Protocol 137 (Schizophrenia)

'They've taken my soul away and divided it up.'

Causal associations. Clear-cut disturbances of ego-consistency are to be found in schizophrenia and in schizophrenia-like toxic psychoses.

Ego-demarcation

The patients feel exposed, cast out, defencelessly abandoned to all manner of external influences. They can no longer distinguish between ego and non-ego, between ideas they themselves conceive and ideas that come to them from outside themselves. When this happens their control of reality is lost: they no longer know what is common human reality and they are isolated in an unreal autistic world of their own (alienation).

If this process takes place slowly, patients sometimes gradually withdraw more and more into themselves, encapsulate themselves (autism). In many cases there is a predominant feeling of alienation, of standing apart in time and space: they feel lost and strange, with derealization, difficulty in communication, isolation, mutism in the face of hopelessness and of the impossibility of reaching an understanding with others. The world of their fellow men is no longer their homeland. When this experience is acute and overpowering, it may lead to a rigid state of terror (catatonic stupor), often alternating with catatonic excitement.

Formation of delusions. The feeling of strangeness and unfamiliarity constitutes a delusional mood (*Wahnstimmung*). The patient has no defence against the external influences to which he is exposed (delusion of influence): alien powers influence his thinking, other powers read his thoughts, direct his actions, etc. (cf. *Ego-activity*). Many patients believe that they themselves experience what they see or hear from others (loss of personal identity). Or they think that it is other people who are experiencing or doing what they themselves experience or do (transitivism). Many patients are thus able to form the delusion that it is not they who are sick, but that they are there to help other people who are sick (delusion of altruism, delusion of healing).

The following psycho-dynamic hypotheses are feasible but so far are not based on sound phenomenological evidence. The effort to master such experiences may hypothetically lead to attempts at compensation and overcompensation: when the patient, in one way or another, tries to bridge this sense of alienation and unfamiliarity, he may develop delusions of magical, universal communication, or omnipotence, or of exalted holiness and guidance by God. Isolation and homelessness in the world may find overcompensation in the contents of altruistic delusions: to help others as a healer, to reform or revitalize the world as a Saviour, the Messiah, an Ambassador of God.

Protocol 22 (Schizophrenia)

'My brain is upset. I have to close my eyes or I won't know what is outside and what is inside me. Everything is mixed up within me...' 'There are external voices and internal voices.' The patient felt the internal voices passing through his body.
'I can't get outside any more.' The patient was unable to give his attention to people or things or to distinguish anything in the outside world.
'I don't know if it is winter or summer, I don't know above from below...left from right...'

Protocol 130 (Schizophrenia)

'I don't live anywhere...I exist under my eyes, under my eyelids.' The patient was homeless, isolated, alienated.

Protocol 154 (Depression)

'I have to suffer everything that other patients here in the clinic have to undergo.' (Loss of personal identity)

Protocol 155 (Schizophrenia)

'Just as I am being sent to the bottom, so will many perish.' (Transitivism)

Causal associations. Marked disturbances of ego-demarcation are characteristic of schizophrenia, as well as of schizophrenia-like toxic psychoses, e.g. LSD.

Ego-identity

The uncertainty of being oneself, of knowing oneself to be the same from birth onwards, is encountered in many forms. The less serious disturbances present as feelings of remoteness, distance, unfamiliarity in regard to oneself, depersonalization in the most common sense of the term (see *Depersonalization*). In serious cases the patient loses all assurance of being himself. He no longer knows who he is. This is often accompanied by disturbances of bodily experience and of ego-consistency and ego-vitality.

Formation of delusions. A new identity may appear to take the place of the patient's lost identity, and he believes himself to be someone other than he really is. This delusional transformation of personality, or falsification of identity, would seem mostly to take the form of raising one's status, of improving one's role, except for the delusions of guilt associated with depression. At times there is a delusional belief in sex transformation and, rarely, in metamorphosis into an animal.

Disturbance of ego-identity over time takes place when the patient believes himself to be someone other than he was before,[13] or when he creates for himself a new, delusional life history; for example, the notion that he has lived on earth for thousands of years. This is a form of delusional heredity, which more frequently consists in believing that one's parentage differs from the reality, the change being almost always in the direction of higher rank. The patient is nearly always aware of his real parentage; he lives a kind of double life (Bleuler's 'double registration', 1911), in which both realities are experienced together – the ordinary reality of his fellow men and the reality of his delusion (see *Delusion*). Such delusions of heredity are not usually acted upon in everyday life. Delusional changes that occur on the basis of psycho-organic disorders may, however, be acted upon as if they were real.

EXAMPLES

Protocol 21 (Schizophrenia)

'I am afraid that I am the other people. I know that this is not so, but I still have this fear...I would like to find myself...so that I can find my role in society...an S. can never be an ordinary man, must always be something extra...So I must also be extravagant so that I can feel myself to be my own self. Therefore I cannot act as other ordinary men; therefore I cannot give up the symbols that I have worked out for myself.'

'My face changes according to who I am with.'

Here we find perplexity, catatonic rigidity, slowness in thought and speech, private symbolism, uncertainty of his personal identity and extravagant behaviour arising from a morbid search for this identity.

Protocol 15 (Schizophrenia)

'I didn't know for sure any more that I was I. My relatives had changed too; they did not seem real, they were dressed like people in a play.

'It was like a "salad lettuce" in my thoughts...It was like Calderon's world theatre...like a dream...I could no longer make out what was real and what was imaginary.'

Here there was depersonalization, derealization and disturbed consciousness of reality. The patient's mood was one of forlorn anxiety and bewilderment and he could no longer speak or move (mutism and stupor).

Protocol 16 (Schizophrenia)

'The most uncanny thing was that one didn't know oneself any more, didn't know that one was oneself. One can't control one's action any more, one's thoughts...It is as if I were spellbound...at the same time one gets more and more fearful, one seems to be overpowered, manipulated from outside ...my life was in pieces.'

The patient was rigid with fear; he was stuporose, had to cry out, could not speak.

Protocol 17 (Schizophrenia)

'I felt as if I myself were an old woman, as if I had changed into my mother and my mother into me. Fear made my thoughts confused.'

Protocol 22 (Schizophrenia)

'My skin is different, I have cowhide on my nose and also elsewhere on my body.'

(Why are you so stiff?) 'Because I don't know what to do, who I am. I'm bored and at the same time frightened of going out.'

(When addressed by his own name.) 'Werner, yes, if you call me that, now I know again who I am.'

Protocol 23 (Schizophrenia)

The patient kept on repeating: 'I am a man', as though reassuring himself in the face of threatened ego-identity.

Protocol 24 (Schizophrenia)

He repeated the phrase, 'I am who I am', thereby reassuring himself of his identity.

Protocol 34 (Schizophrenia)

'I am an animal...I have four heads to carry around...I am in the family way and I will bring an animal into the world...I have been sent here as the Blessed Lady of God, I am the Devil.'
The patient exhibited delusions of pregnancy by an animal, delusions of transformation, dissolution and guilt.

Protocol 35 (Schizophrenia)

'My skeleton has changed, I have a crooked hand, that is how I know my body.'
'...as a man I am Swiss, as a woman Argentinian.'

Protocol 37 (Schizophrenia)

'My flesh is not like the flesh of other men.'

Protocol 129 (Schizophrenia)

'Probably I don't belong in this world at all...I am not as other men...why should I have a name?'

Protocol 27 (Schizophrenia-like psychosis in an epileptic)

'I am a Professor of Veterinary Medicine, Director of the Institution, and I am here to make hebephrenia. I am a master builder, I am the head master builder, the Canton's building inspector...'
Psycho-dynamically this delusion could be regarded as a compensation for feelings of inferiority in a man of low intelligence.

Protocol 151 (Pick's disease)

This patient, who had undergone severe psycho-organic changes, believed himself to be President of the Confederation, and he travelled without a ticket to his 'seat of office'.

Causal associations. These are found (*a*) most frequently in schizophrenia; (*b*) in severe depressions, e.g. 'I am the Devil himself'; (*c*) in organically based psychoses (chronic organic psychosyndrome).

Self-image

The way in which an individual sees himself, what he thinks of himself, the idea he has of his own personality – all these can undergo many different fluctuations and changes without there being any impairment of ego-consciousness in the sense of 1–5 in section 3.2 above.

The extent to which this view of oneself is shared by other people, the extent to which it is inadequate or distorted, pitched too low or too high, can be subject to great variation.

Change in personality.

The feeling that one's personality, one's whole being, is changed can occur during the course of life, especially if there is misfortune or suffering attributable to a blow of fate.

Such changes are experienced with varying force, depending on the degree of introspection. During puberty and at the commencement of adolescence one may be very much aware of a change in personality, especially when leaving the narrow circle of the family. In this period of crisis many vulnerable individuals (those with weak egos) suffer a fundamental shattering of the personality (a so-called crisis of adolescence) with feelings of estrangement (depersonalization); this may occur spontaneously, or under the added stress of changes in environment and consequent role, e.g. leaving home, military service, apprenticeship, engagement, marriage, parenthood. At times this may develop into the severely disturbed ego-experience of schizophrenia which in males first manifests itself around the age of 17.

Personality changes may also be experienced in cases of long and severe illness (in particular terminal illnesses), of mutilation or maiming (the mutilation psyche), of long spells in prison or concentration camp, or as a result of war experiences.

Obsessions

Many impulses or inclinations towards certain actions, thoughts or ideas are for no reason firmly rejected by the conscience (*conscientia*

– consciousness and conscience), or after rational consideration are rejected as unethical, amoral, stupid, unreasonable. They are regarded by the personality as not in keeping with its self-image and are repelled. They may then seem to be alien, 'not really me', 'undesirable'. The affected individual is then invaded by these impulses and fears (see *Obsessions and Phobias*). In so-called obsessional neurosis they are alien to the personality but they are not imposed from without. While schizophrenics may experience genuine obsessions in this narrow sense, they also experience every transitional form up to complete subjugation to external control.

Self-esteem

Self-esteem is closely associated with self-image. It varies between exaggerated feelings of self-esteem (in the opinion of others) and feelings of inferiority. Both may refer to the individual's life as a whole, or, more commonly, apply only to intellectual attainment or to physical appearance. Both may be innate character traits, in which case they are usually permanent or at least long-lasting; or they may be part of a psychosis, when they are usually episodic.

Character traits include self-satisfaction, conceit and arrogance, or lack of self-confidence, timidity and shyness. In mania self-esteem is morbidly heightened and more extensive; in depression, there is self-denigration.

Ego-strength

It is intrinsic to this global concept that its pathology cannot be concisely specified. When considering an individual's various modes of experience and behaviour, all we can reasonably do is to bear in mind this aspect of existence, which closely affects man's ability to be free, to be himself.

Those individuals with weak egos are unable to develop their own selves sufficiently. To a large extent their lives are modelled on those of other people, e.g. their teachers. In the effort to behave according to the norm, their individualities are suppressed and stunted, or may break out in perverted forms.

We should mention here the various notions of degeneration and the subjugation of the self. A few key terms point the way: suggestibility, dependence; infantilism with its lack of self-reliance in feeling, will, thought and action; hysterical breakdown; restricted freedom of action due to obsessions and phobias; the various disturbances which occur in the sexual sphere and which manifest themselves in perversions; addictive degeneration.

The most severe dissolution of individuality occurs in schizophrenia (see section 3.5, *Ego-vitality* to *Ego-identity*). In manic elation the individual's feet are no longer on the ground, e.g. a manic patient said: 'I have too much air under my feet'. In melancholic depression, by contrast, the dominant feeling is the nothingness of everything connected with the self. For the psycho-organic patient with an amnestic syndrome, existence loses its temporal order – there is no longer a sequence of past, present and future.

The following (unabridged) first interview portrays the involvement of the various ego-dimensions discussed above and may serve to summarize the pathology of ego-consciousness presented in this chapter. In order to carry out a hermeneutic analysis, we must have before us the text of such terse statements by the patient, which often resemble a cry for help. It is best to have the material taken down by a stenographer, with notes on non-verbal behaviour. Recording and video machines sometimes make such patients more disturbed: they are in any case liable to form delusions and their anxiety and perplexity render them more aware of what is going on around them. It may be added that the following lay-out separates the patient's statements from the observations and analysis: the commentary has been kept to a minimum for reasons of space.

Protocol 179 (Schizophrenia of recent onset, first attack)

Protocol	Commentary
(The patient was a young man, slim, tall and dark, who kept holding his head and talking in monologues.)	
I can't see my way out any more...	Disturbance of reality, of reality orientation. Loss of perspective.
In time...	Disturbance of his own sense of time.

Day and night (repeated several times)	Day and night repeated in incantation as milestones of orientation.
Whether I am living in a primaeval forest like primitive man...	Isolation, alienation, no pedigree, no family which would give him an identity of origin.
(Smells and sniffs at the backs of his hands)	Sniffing, an archaic searching behaviour, seeking himself, looking for assurance because his identity and his vitality are threatened (? smells like a corpse)
I feel as if I weren't here, everything is lost...	Ego-vitality threatened (Jaspers, consciousness of existence) His own destruction corresponds to ideas of world destruction.
I wonder at it, where a man comes from...	Questioning his identity of origin.
I'm chasing after myself too much...	Expresses his puzzled groping after himself, his efforts to find himself (vitality, activity, consistency).
(Looks wonderingly at his hands)	Observing his threatened ego-activity and ego-vitality (? ego-identity).
Very likely I am still alive...	Threat to ego-vitality.
I believe at all events that I am still alive	Reassuring himself in the face of threatened ego-vitality.
Yes, I'm still alive...	Reassuring himself in the face of threatened ego-vitality
I'm afraid of reality...	Fear of reality, i.e. of ego-destruction.
(Moves his index finger along the edge of the table)	Tactile and spatial attempt at orientation, at finding himself.
I keep going further backwards...	Brooding on his identity of origin.
In the end I can't make out any more if that is real or not...	Brooding, losing consciousness of experience and of reality.
I didn't know any more whether I existed; I kept looking in the mirror...	Loss of ego-identity, reassures himself by looking in the mirror. The face is the special symbol of ego-identity.
I have no faith in myself...	Ego-weakness, uncertainty of identity.

I couldn't fit myself into any pigeon-hole any more...

Loss of role-awareness (self-image).

I watch other people too closely; I look at what they do...

Orientation; aware of his own weakness, he holds on to the *alter ego*, the non-ego.

I don't think I could hold my own...

Ego-weakness, weak standing, threat to existence.

I have the 'big drum', I am the best, so then I must hold my own...

Overplaying his own weakness calls for an effort to hold his own.

I try to wear a mask around me, a kind of support...

Recognizes this false overplaying as an attempt to gain a new support.

Then again I want to help everyone (shakes his head in bewilderment)

Living for others improves his experience of himself.

(Clasps his head) Something is there, I'm giving myself cramps...
I will hold my own...
I will be represented everywhere...join in the conversation everywhere...I talk too much...

'His head is empty.' Bewilderment. Tries frantically to clarify events, to hold his own, to exert influence on others, to take part in decisions.

I listen to everything that other people say, I am then diverted...I want to take what they say into my own brain...

His own ego-consciousness being threatened, he is oriented towards the non-ego. Seeking support.

A woman said: 'Now we've got two pansies here'...

Probably an auditory hallucination. His fear makes him hear 'his theme', from a woman.

Then I shrank into myself. I thought I was a pansy...

He has the idea of himself as a homosexual: uncertainty of sexual orientation as part of ego identity.

When I came back from holiday everything was different.

Derealization.

They had been talking about me. The others didn't want to know me any more...

Delusion of reference, (?) voices, isolation, sense of alienation and depersonalization.

I don't believe in myself any more...

Summarizes his loss of ego-consciousness.

Something has mixed me up...

Orientation to himself and to the world around uncertain. Disturbed thinking.

I must interest myself in
everything...
Everything has got to follow me
in the dance
I must be the greatest...

In delusions of reference
everything is significant.
Everything revolves around him.

Frantic desire for power as he
experiences his own lack
thereof.

I let myself be influenced by
others...
Something is controlling me or
am I controlling myself...
Lately I have had the feeling that
something is confusing my
brain;
I want to find out something but
what?...

In his own lack of power he feels
the influence of others.
Experience of being controlled
from without, vacillating.
The threat to his ego makes him
anxious, removes his sense of
perspective, makes it impossible
for him to think clearly
concerning the 'something' that
he is looking for – see below.

(How long has this been going
on?)
For about two weeks, but I don't
know, I haven't slept for a long
time and it is now July – or
have I lost my memory?...
Or someone will find out...

Loss of sense of time.
Life is no longer set in time.

'Someone' is an expression of the
lost feeling of his own self.

What I am and where I come
from, I myself want to know
where I come from. Perhaps
from another world? Surely not.

He is searching for ego-identity.
Identity of origin. Not
'someone' – he himself. Identity
of origin. Alienation. The fate of
Kaspar-Hauser.

But perhaps they want to know
whether my mother is a
whore...

Origin on mother's side; if
mother had been a whore, then
anyone could be father, so that
his parentage cannot be settled.

Perhaps I am afraid of my
parentage, I am afraid I was
abandoned on the doorstep, a
foundling...
I am afraid that there is no one
any more who can console me,
console me for what? (Laughs)

His maternal descent is not clear.
He has lost his identity of
origin.Kaspar-Hauser-foundling.

Isolation, alienation. Fear,
looking for help. Rejects his
fears (seems then to be
parathymic).

I simply watch other people too much	He talks to himself: he sets too much store by other people.
I have doubts about myself...	Summarizes his threatened ego.
I make myself confused...	Bewilderment.
Something is in my head but I don't know what – perhaps too much studying...	Tries to pull himself together.
Or is it something stronger than me (laughs)...	In his own state of impotence, he is threatened by the superior power of others.
Am I from another planet?	The theme of his origin, isolation.
Something is trying to make me confused...	Vacillates between the assumption of an alien influence
Either it is I myself or something else.	destroying his consistency and the experience of himself
I think (laughs) it is I myself.	changing, something that is not controlled by outsiders.

3.6   Psycho-analytical ego-pathology of the psychoses

As we have already indicated, psycho-analysis seeks to provide not a description but a genetic, psycho-dynamic explanation of processes. Every such interpretation should, of course, be made 'against the guiding line of experience' (Freud, 1931, in the Foreword to Nunberg, 1959), if psycho-analysis is not to cut itself off completely from demonstrable facts.

The following short account of psycho-analytical ego-pathology takes the form of a review of the literature. No opinion is expressed on the value of the various theories. It is to be hoped, however, that the different points of view mean approximately something similar, even if they are expressed in very different terms. The dimensions arrived at phenomenologically could provide a stimulus to further differentiation in the psycho-analytical theory of psychosis, while at the same time psycho-analytical ego-psychology could lend further depth to non-interpretative observation. A third approach to research is offered by the empirical statistical method (see Bellak, 1973, with his ego-profile scale; and Semrad and his co-workers, 1973).

Freud himself did not develop a systematic theory of psychosis (see Hartmann, 1964a, p. 375). After his early work on defensive neuropsychoses and on the Schreber case, his main interest lay more in the neuroses and the perversions. However, many indications of his thinking are to be found scattered throughout his work (see also p. 18).

According to Freud (1924a), psychosis occurs when the ego is too weak to mediate between the claims of the id and the demands of the external world. The ego capitulates and regresses to a narcissistic level (Freud, 1911), denying reality and projecting a different version of the external world. A delusion is therefore an attempt at reconstruction produced by the ego as a form of self-defence. According to Freud, the ego can 'deform itself', 'submit to encroachments', 'divide itself' (Freud, 1924b, p. 391); it can be split, as a result of a 'rift from within'[14] (Freud, 1938, p. 60); ego-weakness may also result from organic and hereditary causes (Freud, 1937, *Analysis Terminable and Interminable*, see *Gesammelte Werke*).

Freud's successors have retained his basic hypotheses. The main defence mechanism in psychosis remains a regression of the ego. Schizophrenia is a disturbance of ego-structure and ego-functioning, a sickness of the ego. There are many formulations of this ego-sickness, all sounding much the same; dissolution of the ego, structural ego-deficit, disturbance of ego-boundaries, of ego-identity, disintegration of ideal egos (Schilder, 1925), archaic ego-sickness (Ammon, 1973), egopathy (Kisker, 1964, 1968), shattering of the ego and attempt to regain assurance (Sullivan, 1962), ego-defect (Freeman *et al.*, 1965). The views of Nunberg and Fenichel are given below as examples. Federn and Hartmann introduced new points of view concerning schizophrenia.[15]

Nunberg (1939, 1971) has discussed psychosis in relation to the splitting of the synthesizing function of the ego. Putting particular emphasis on the synthetic function of the ego (Nunberg, 1971) he regards psychosis as a 'failure in ego-synthesis' (p. 181). In paranoid schizophrenia 'the synthetic function of the ego knows no limitations; everything is *indiscriminately* mixed and melted together; it is systematized and eventually results in delusional ideas' (p. 181).[16]

Paralogical thought connections and delusions become an expression of the tendency of the ego to rationalize, serving to fill the 'gaps caused by the splitting of the ego' (p. 179). Hallucinations are manifestations of a further ego-disturbance, that of ego-perception (p. 324). Finally, Nunberg goes so far as to assert that 'the overt symptoms represent a *strident* attempt at restitution or cure'.[16]

Fenichel (1946, 1971) sees psychosis as a regressive breakdown of the ego and, like Nunberg, adheres closely to Freud. For him also the psychotic ego is too weak to cope with the demands of the id. Its break with reality, which limits its instinctual freedom (1971, p. 439), means the same thing as regression to narcissism, object loss, withdrawal from the external world, breakdown of the ego (1971, p. 415). Schizophrenic symptoms are partly a direct expression of a regressive breakdown of the ego and partly a state of 'primitivization', e.g. ideas of the end of the world, physical sensations, depersonalization, catatonic symptoms; other symptoms represent various attempts at restitution, e.g. hallucinations and delusions (1971, p. 417); the hallucinations are 'substitutes for perceptions' (1971, p. 425).

Federn (1956), in developing the notion of psychosis in terms of an overthrow of the ego and a disturbance of ego-boundaries, brought essentially new points of view to bear on the ego-psychology of the psychoses, which for him comprise 'all ego-diseases' (p. 205). Schizophrenic psychoses become manifestations of the defeat of the ego. The essential difference between Federn's ideas and Freud's concept of psychoses as attempts at restitution, i.e. as a form of defence, is as follows: 'The psychosis itself is not a defence, but a defeat of the ego' (p. 175). The schizophrenic process consists in loss of cathexis of the mental and bodily ego-boundaries.[17] It is only as protection (defence) against this that the ego regresses to earlier stages (p. 177). Like Freud in 1937, Federn also concedes the possibility of organically based ego-weaknesses (p. 180).

Federn expressly emphasizes that all ego-functions are not necessarily affected in the same degree of severity. 'The psychotic process does not proceed simultaneously in the totality of the ego-relations and of the ego-boundaries' (p. 130). 'Loss of reality is the consequence, not the cause, of the basic psychotic deficiency' (p. 148). Hypochondriacal complaints and somatic distortions stem from the withdrawal of ego-cathexis from the affected organs (p. 150). Hallucinations and delusions are the consequence of damage to the ego and not attempts at restitution. Ego-weakness (which must always be considered in relation to specific ego-functions) leads to disturbances of perception and of thought. Weakening of the ego-boundary leads to confusion between the real and the non-real, to an invasion by the non-ego. As a protection against this invasion of false realities from the unconscious, the ego regresses to earlier stages.

A general ego-weakness and a total depletion of energy leads to a complete breakdown of the ego in all its functions.

Psycho-analytical writers whose points of view reflect a somewhat more genuine contact with patients do not put so much stress on libidinous ego-inflation, on the omnipotence and megalomania of the narcissistic ego. They are also less inclined to accept latent homosexuality as a motive for the formation of schizophrenic delusions (Freud, 1911). Some authors, of course, draw ego-cosmically (Federn, 1956) on their own imaginative reality.

We are indebted to Hartmann (1964a) for fundamental contributions to psycho-analytical ego-psychology. He has stressed the notion of psychosis in terms of regression and disintegration of a weak ego that is incapable of neutralization. His most important work on the ego-psychopathology of schizophrenia dates from 1953 (*Contribution to the Metapsychology of Schizophrenia*). Hartmann is concerned not so much with explaining different psychopathological phenomena as with defining more precisely the central ego-disturbance. 'The ego that reacts pathologically (to reality) is very likely already a disturbed ego, but we know little about the specific nature of this vulnerability' (p. 376).

Hartmann assumes that there is an anomaly in the primary autonomy of the ego, i.e. an anomaly that is independent of the id and of the external world, which could be hereditary (p. 395).

What the schizophrenic most obviously lacks is the organized, ego-integrated stability of adequate defence mechanisms. The ailing ego is left predominantly with primitive defences, e.g. turning against the self, reversal into its opposite, projection, detachment of libido (p. 377). According to Hartmann weakness of the ego means, above all, impaired ability to neutralize libidinous energy in the sense of depriving it of sexuality and aggression (p. 384).

With regard to Freud's (1924a) observations on the difference between neurosis and psychosis, Hartmann also asserts that when the ego withdraws from reality into psychosis, it acts in the service of the id. The ailing ego cannot solve its instinctual problems other than by a withdrawal from reality. This may be because the demands of the id are absolutely overpowering, or because the ego is relatively too weak to cope with an instinctual demand which in itself is not overwhelmingly strong (p. 376).

As a defence against the demands of the id, which it cannot

overcome, the ego regresses to a narcissistic stage,[18] which accounts
for a whole series of symptoms: disturbances of thought, speech and
affect. Hartmann tries to define the process of narcissistic regression:
the libido, in retreat from the external world, forms a cathexis with
the self, not the ego, a view which is in agreement with Freud (1911).
As a consequence of the ego's poor ability to neutralize, however,
the submersion of the self and of ego-functions takes place through
the medium of non-neutralized libido. Consequently narcissistic
self-cathexis is sexualized, which may be seen in a megalomanic
overestimation of the self (p. 384).

Hartmann sees the disintegration of the ego as a consequence of
the (regressive) object loss and sexualization of the self (p. 385); or
of its submersion by non-neutralized aggressive drives which are
directed against the self (p. 388); or, through defects in the structure
of the super-ego, of a violent breaking out against the external world
(p. 386).

Because the ego lacks neutralized energy, there occurs a de-
differentiation of the ego (p. 391) which is therefore unable to sustain
relationships with inner and outer reality.

Winkler (1954, 1971), Winkler and Wieser (1959): To the existing
mechanisms of defence (projection, subject/object reversal, external-
ization of the super-ego, denial of reality) Winkler added two defence
mechanisms of the ego that are 'specific to schizophrenia' (1954, p.
235): anachoresis of the ego (1954) and mythification of the ego
(Winkler *et al.*, 1959).

Anachoresis of the ego refers to the withdrawal of the ego from
incompatible contents of consciousness, i.e. from commands of the
id that are unacceptable to the super-ego. A splitting-off therefore
takes place (p. 240) (cf. E. Bleuler, 1911; and Freud, 1938). Impulses
from the id remain in consciousness, their strength and content
unchanged but with their ego-quality impaired (p. 235). The loss of
ego-quality brings with it a gain in the form of a shedding of guilt.
The consequences of ego-anachoresis are the familiar symptoms of
alienation, alien influences affecting thought, etc. 'The schizophrenic
can, by means of anachoresis, shrug off on to the external world
anything that is burdensome to him' (p. 236).

In many cases ego-anachoresis alone is clearly not enough 'to rid
the ego of certain experiences' (1954, p. 240). The ego can then

withdraw into a mythical abstraction in order to remove the self from feelings of guilt. 'The ego withdraws from a personal existence into a collective mythical existence' (1959, p. 78, cf. Jung, 1952).

Working in child analytical psychology Mahler (1951–72, 1958, 1968, 1972) has drawn up a differentiated scale of identity development of the ego which, as in Hartmann's theory, is constructed within an undifferentiated matrix from which develop both the ego and the id: Freud's primary narcissistic stage is divided into an autistic (omnipotent, objectless) and a symbiotic phase. The third phase is that of separation–individuation. Disturbances in the symbiotic phase lead to (autistic) childhood psychoses; disturbances in the third phase lead to borderline illnesses.

Following Hartmann's differentiation into ego, self and self-representations, Jacobson (1964), like Balint (1952), has discarded Freud's concept of primary narcissism and masochism and has interpreted secondary narcissism in terms of the cathexis of self-representation with libido and aggression (cf. Hartmann's ideas about the ego's powers of neutralization). In her concept of psychosis she follows the usual assumptions of regression: the psychotic patient returns regressively to an undifferentiated state of self- and object-representation, which leads to a loss of identity. Narcissistic neuroses and borderline illnesses represent the expression of narcissistic identifications.

Kernberg (1967, 1970, 1972) views psychopathological symptoms as the expression of disturbances in the internalization of object relations, leading to a breakdown of ego-integration. He has proposed a four-stage scale of development and relates the different psychiatric disorders, in particular borderline disturbances, to the different stages of development.

(1) First comes the primarily narcissistic, autistic, undifferentiated stage, in which no distinction is made between self-representation and object-representation, neither of which is internalized into an ego-core. If reality relationships are lacking, failure of development beyond this stage leads to a psychosis; if reality relationships are present, a severely autistic and affectless personality is the result.

(2) The next stage is the development of the primary intrapsychic structure by consolidation of the undifferentiated self-object. At this stage there is a danger of extreme polarization into 'all good

self-object' and 'all bad self-object', of failure to achieve a distinction between self and non-self, and of weakness in ego-boundary, 'ego-dissolution', etc. (schizophrenia).

(3) 'Normal splitting' maintains a good relationship with the mother, in spite of frustration (love is not too much contaminated by hatred). In pathological splitting (borderline personalities, etc.) we get alternatives of 'only good' or 'only bad'. The self-image is not sufficiently distinguished from the object-image.

(4) The fourth stage comprises an integration of all good and all bad self- and object-images into one concept of self and object. Following Freud, regression in neurosis is regarded as a form of defence.

Kohut (1971) advances the notion of 'narcissistic personality disturbances', to be distinguished from transference and borderline states. There are two lines of development leading from auto-eroticism through narcissism to object love and a higher and altered form of narcissism. Kohut's concepts deviate at times strongly from those of psycho-analytical ego-psychology. Even more strongly than Kernberg he uses concepts to underpin psychotherapeutic experience with special personalities.

G. and R. Blanck (1974) distinguish even more sharply between the four basic forms of ego-modification (ego-defect, ego-deviation, ego-distortion, ego-regression) and have developed special techniques of ego-psychotherapy.

3.7 Indications for further research

Dimensions 1–5 (and the more global and less clear-cut dimensions 6 and 7) are constructs, like everything which we comprehend and to which we give a name. The overlapping that is present in our proposed classification does not constitute an argument against it. The fact that disturbances in these dimensions are found in aetiologically different illnesses requiring psychiatric treatment shows that the ego-disturbances in question are aetiologically non-specific or, at most, typical of schizophrenia-like psychoses of different aetiology. Further investigations must aim at an increase in documented material on such patient experiences and at the uniform recording, collecting and documentation, by means of questionnaires, for

Table 1. *Pathology of ego-consciousness*

| Dimension | Catatonic symptoms | | | | Alienation | | Delusion | Secondary delusion | Causative factors |
	Anxiety	Stupor	Excitement	Other	Depersonalization	Derealization			
Ego-vitality	+	+		Hyperventilation	+	(+)	Delusion of destruction Hypochondriacal delusion Nihilistic delusion Delusion of persecution	? Messianic delusion ? Delusion of reforming the world Delusion of reference	Depression Schizophrenia Toxic psychoses
Ego-activity	+	+	(+)	Stereotypy Verbigeration Echopraxia Echolalia Flexibilitas cerea	(+)		Alien influence Persecution	? Divine guidance	Possession Schizophrenia Toxic psychoses Depression
Ego-consistency	+	+	(+)		(+)		Destruction Torn asunder End of the world Monster delusion Multiplication	? Delusion of pregnancy ? Delusion of birth	Schizophrenia Toxic psychoses
Ego-demarcation	+	(+)	(+)		(+)	(+)	Alien influence Loss of personal identity Transitivism	? Omnipotence ? Telepathy ? Altruistic delusion	Schizophrenia Toxic psychoses
Ego-identity	+	(+)			+	+	Delusion of change Delusion of origin		Schizophrenia Toxic psychoses

self-rating or for rating by others, which alone can form the basis for multivariate statistical analysis. Only then will it be possible to determine whether the dimensions proposed receive statistical support (Cluster).

In the light of this ego-pathology the concept of the so-called borderline cases (E. Bleuler, 1911, latent schizophrenia) must be re-examined. We must also examine what prognostic use may be made of this approach and what therapeutic indications may result from it.

4

CONSCIOUSNESS OF EXPERIENCE, REALITY TESTING
(*Erfahrungsbewußtsein* and *Realitätsbewußtsein*)

This is *one* capacity of the conscious man, it is not his 'own' consciousness.

4.1 Definition

Consciousness of experience is knowledge of the modality in which every experience occurs – knowledge that comes to us simultaneously with the experience itself. Reality testing[1] provides the associated knowledge that what is perceived is real.[2]

4.2 Function

It is basic to our existence that we are open to experience; in our behaviour we experience, perceive, understand and proceed accordingly. The modality of every experience[3] is known to us and we have many such modalities. It is on this that the significance of a particular experience depends, a significance that varies according to our history and present situation, and this is what makes the experience relevant to our action.

Phenomenologically it is clearly an irreducible ability of a lucid, self-conscious individual that out of all his manifold modes of experience he should know the modality in which a particular experience occurs. We 'know', we are at a given moment certain, that, for example, we perceive something and can distinguish it from an image, however graphic and living a representation that image may be (see Table 2, p. 144). Similarly we know the modes by which we receive the many other kinds of experience: we have experience of the self (see ego-consciousness and its various dimensions), perception, hallucination, pseudo-hallucination, fantasy, vision, imagery, memory, thought, ideation, imagination, suspicion, sensing, intuition, dream and ecstasy, as well as the experience of mood and

77

feeling, of wishes, drives, hopes and expectations. Experience is thus accompanied by knowledge as to whether the particular experience is ours alone or to what extent it can be shared with others.

In all sensory perception the 'certainty of reality' (Jaspers) is, in general, 'simply given to us'.[4] It is not a question of experiencing that we perceive something and later passing judgement on it. According to Kloos (1938) reality judgements are implicit. We can perceive things that have the character of objects and at the same time know that these things, although presented to us through the sensorium, are not really there. We can see something physically and yet know that what we see is not presented to us in the modality of sight but is, for example, a vision or an hallucination. It cannot for that reason be regarded as less real. Perceptions, genuine hallucinations, pseudo-hallucinations, delusions, are all realities for those who experience them and whose actions are determined by them, but they are experienced through different modalities.

There is, however, another way of determining what is real. If we have doubts about a perceptual experience because, for example, it is unclear, very unusual or striking in some way, then we can test whether our experience is correct by means of what Jaspers (1959) calls a secondary reality judgement and Kloos (1938) refers to as an explicit reality judgement. *This secondary reality control is achieved by:*

(*a*) Repeating the experience, while paying meticulous attention, with heightened attentiveness, to the sensory modality involved, in so far as it is possible to achieve the same effect again. This is more easily done with visual than with auditory experiences. The more physical the experience, e.g. bodily feelings, the more difficult it is to test. The distinction between errors of bodily sensation and bodily hallucinosis is an arbitrary one.

(*b*) Employing other sensory qualities, e.g. gazing steadily, testing by touch.

(*c*) Testing in the light of previous experience. Asking such questions as: Have I ever experienced anything like this before? In the light of my experience, can this really be?

(*d*) Using the criterion of common sense, of reality in the sense of what normal people in a given cultural group can accept without difficulty. This social criterion involves other people.

4.3 Foundations

The foundations have all been listed under *Consciousness*. They include functioning of the sensory organs, attention, memory and remembering, thought, etc. These are some of the prerequisites of the complex components of such operations. From the neurophysiological standpoint, the development of reality testing goes hand in hand with that of ego-consciousness, representing the interaction of afferent stimuli and efferent behaviour.

4.4 Examination

The methods of examination comprise self-examination and observation of others, conversation and observation of behaviour.

4.5 Pathology

In special circumstances

In states of reduced wakefulness, fatigue, sensory isolation, under the affective stress of life crises and conflicts, or when the field of consciousness is narrowed in states of tense and heightened attentiveness, then consciousness of experience may disappear or become uncertain. It may no longer be possible to distinguish clearly between sensory perceptions and dream, fantasy, illusion or vision. Familiar surroundings may seem unreal.

Altered states of consciousness

Reality testing may be completely suspended (acute exogenous reaction). The patient can have vivid hallucinations which he usually no longer recognizes as such, taking them for perceptual experiences, e.g. delirium. Under the influence of hallucinogens, or in experimental situations, hallucinations can often still be recognized as such.[5]

Dementia

In dementia, reality control may be absent, leaving the way open to paranoid hallucinatory psychoses.

Disturbances of ego-consciousness

In disturbances of ego-consciousness (q.v.) consciousness of experience and reality testing may be absent or uncertain. The patient is no longer sure of the modality of his experiences; he can no longer distinguish between thoughts, words that he hears ('voices'), fantasies, feelings, bodily sensations and images. Thoughts are 'felt' or 'heard'; words are felt as pains in his brain – 'Every word is a pain in my brain'. The patient may ask: 'Am I really hearing this, or is it perhaps another experience that is like hearing, for which there is no precise name in our everyday language?'

It is as if to the patient everyday experiences are no longer self-evident.[6]

EXAMPLES

Protocol 93 (Schizophrenia)

'I have been driven into a development that makes me ill. I have become schizophrenic, that is to say, I am no longer properly responsible in my judgement and I have lost my natural feelings.'

Protocol 148 (Schizophrenia)

'Things aren't as self-evident as they used to be. I am a bit unsure, I have the feeling I may be ill, but not physically... A funny feeling, I thought things that otherwise I wouldn't think. Things aren't natural any more, they aren't quite normal, they are funny... And I'm anxious too, I'm more sensitive... I have a great inclination to question everything... I have become uncertain... I'm no longer as spontaneous in my feelings... I feel my life more sensitively than I used to...'

Protocol 91 (Schizophrenia)

'Reality has changed. I can see things like other people but there is a filter in my brain (points to his temples) which controls what comes in and what does not. Reality doesn't correspond to mankind any more – the transition in the mind is not complete.'

The modalities of experience change in a strange way. Noises change in the head to words; words become 'thoughts in the head'. What is seen can simultaneously be known as not really there, or may seem to be presented through some intermediary – 'like a film', 'like a transparency'.

Protocol 92 (Schizophrenia)

The patient became disturbed by various real noises, even by the twittering of birds. 'In my head I hear words in these noises and they are directed at me, in the same rhythm as the noise.' The content of these words was a commentary on what she was thinking at the time.

She 'saw' flowers, deer, hares, a gigantic face, but at the same time knew that these were not really there. Then a woman appeared before her 'as if in a transparency, with a computer instead of a face' (cf. ego-identity and face).

Sometimes the patient complains of hearing something and, at the same time, 'having it in the head'.

Protocol 88 (Schizophrenia)

The patient 'heard' many 'voices' and said of them: 'It is not like proper hearing, I simply have voices in my head'.

In severe disturbances of ego-experience several dimensions are often involved simultaneously, though the degree of involvement may vary and one or another may temporarily predominate. When all differentiation of experience, and all reality testing, disappear and the patient himself notices this, he may describe his distraught existence by telling us 'I am complete chaos' (*Protocol 129*).

Disturbance of ego-vitality (and at the same time of other dimensions)
Protocol 22 (Schizophrenia)
'I don't know whether I am alive or whether I am dead...' Here there were 'external voices' (the voice of someone conversing with him) and 'internal voices'. 'They come from me myself and I feel them pass through my body...Only half my thoughts are my own, the rest belong to other people, to voices.'

Disturbance of ego-activity

Is it my own experience, or is it 'being done' to me, 'administered', 'suggested', 'as if someone was influencing me'? (*Protocol 5*).

Protocol 20 (Schizophrenia)

'I have difficulty in making out what were real voices, noises, and what I imagined. I started asking myself in despair: What is real, then? I wondered if someone had suggested it to me, or if perhaps it had really happened that I heard things which didn't exist.... I couldn't separate what was real any more from what was coming out of me – that was terrible; it was as if my world was ending, there was just too much coming in on me.' This gave rise to a feeling of being overpowered (a persecutory delusion).

Disturbance of ego-consistency

The patient is concerned about where his qualitatively uncertain experiences come from. He asks whether his experiences of thinking, hearing or being addressed are situated in his head, or come out of his body 'like a current'. 'Do I hear with my heart, from my stomach, from my belly?'

Protocol 31 (Schizophrenia)

This female patient had 'voices in my inner heart'.

Protocol 136 (Schizophrenia)

'What horrible things are being said to me right in the middle of my head.'

Disturbance of ego-demarcation

Does the experience come from outside my body? Are the voices, images, bodily sensations, pains, thoughts 'administered to me from outside'? Are my feelings and thoughts known to others, 'read off' by them, heard by them?

EXAMPLE

See *Protocol 22* (p. 81).

Protocol 32 (Schizophrenia)

'Voices plague me in my head. At night the voices leave my head and then speak against me from outside.'

Disturbance of ego-identity

The patient is uncertain whether he is undergoing his own experiences or those of other people (*apersonalization*); he can also ask whether other people have his experiences (*transitivism*).

EXAMPLE

Protocol 3 (*Schizophrenia*)

This patient claimed she could read other people's thoughts. 'I even have to share the dreams of those who sleep in the same room with me.'

4.6   Therapeutic indications

Isolation and an inability to communicate, to speak freely with others about one's own and about shared experiences, can provoke uncertainty or cause loss of consciousness of experience and of reality testing. It therefore helps the patient if we speak with him, associate with him, question him, let him speak, and also share a common task (e.g. in occupational therapy, group gymnastics, movement therapy). Even those patients with clouded consciousness obtain support from such participation, and their hallucinations may decrease or disappear. Even delusions of reference in dements can, for example, disappear if the patient is assimilated into a secure community atmosphere. Active association and conversation is particularly important for patients whose ego-consciousness is disturbed. Although seriously and acutely ill patients are sometimes no longer capable of exclusively verbal contact, conversation, a walk, a game with a ball or communal exercise can increase ego-consciousness and help the patient recover some grasp of his experiences and of reality. In the most severe cases of overwhelming chaos with prominent psychotic features (hallucinations, delusions, severe anxiety) neuroleptic drugs may be required in order to make such 'communal activity' possible (Bleuler, 1969).

ORIENTATION

5.1 Definition

Not being lost; knowing where one is; being aware of one's setting in time and place, and of the realities of one's person and situation.

5.2 Function

Orientation enables man to grasp the actualities of his current temporal, spatial, geographical and biographical setting and to make himself at home in it. Orientation is thus a prerequisite for adaptation and practical living in general. The distinction between a relatively stable, *practical* orientation, which is reflected in behaviour, and a more labile, *theoretical* orientation is important when assessing functional deficits.

Orientation in time

This entails knowledge of the date, day of the week, time of day, month, year and season. Practical awareness of the time of day and season of the year is relatively stable. Reference points for orientation in time are fluid and demand constant checking. Unlike orientation in space, orientation in time is labile and easily disturbed.

Orientation in space

This comprises knowledge of current location in its geographical setting. Orientation in place is fairly stable with regard to familiar places, e.g. home, row of houses, block of flats, but in new surroundings it has to be acquired and is at first more labile. (Note: This is not to be confused with spatial orientation which refers to geometric space (see *Agnosias*).)

Orientation for person

(autopsychic orientation) covers knowledge of who and what one is (including birthday, place of birth, parentage, name, profession, role at different ages, role in social context) preserving an uninterrupted view of an individual's own past and present. Autopsychic orientation in the broad sense means having a picture of oneself and is thus closely associated with the forms of orientation already mentioned.

Situational orientation

This refers to an individual's grasp (apprehension) of his current situation and its significance for and connection with his own person. Situational orientation thus means, for example, knowing that one is a patient in a hospital, recognizing that one is being examined, that there is a doctor or a nursing sister present, etc. It also means knowing why we are in a given place and what is our relationship to the other people who are there. To this extent situational orientation is closely connected with orientation in place and time and with personal orientation. It is, however, a much more complex process. Situational orientation requires that one sees oneself in relation to a biographical setting. As such it calls for the ability to grasp, understand and interpret an actual situation in the context of an individual life history.

5.3   Prerequisites

These include intact consciousness and sensorium (sensory perception); attention or set; a certain degree of intelligence so that there can be alert apprehension and grasp, especially in respect of situational orientation and understanding; memory capacity and a sense of time. In severe intellectual defect and severe disturbances of memory, orientation is impaired even when consciousness is clear. Situational orientation also calls for the capacity of self-observation (see above).

5.4　Examination

Since the syndrome of disturbed orientation is so important for diagnosis and consequently for treatment, it is essential to be particularly careful in the assessment of each patient in this regard. The examiner cannot always rely on responses to direct questioning but must also take account of what comes to light in conversation and in observation of behaviour. Different components of orientation like time and place are not always disturbed to the same degree and particular deficits carry different diagnostic significance. Moreover, orientation, like most psychopathological symptoms, may fluctuate according to the patient's situation and surroundings. A good conversational relationship with the patient can thus do more to improve his general orientation than an attitude which keeps him at a distance.

5.5　Pathology

Uncertainty and fluctuation in orientation

Here orientation is not completely absent but is uncertain and inconstant. Orientation in time is usually first to suffer, then situational orientation, and lastly orientation in place and in person.

Loss of orientation, disorientation

Loss of orientation does not necessarily occur in all areas simultaneously and to the same degree. Temporal and situational orientation are generally the first to be affected, then orientation in place and lastly autopsychic orientation. It is also important to distinguish between practical orientation, as shown by the patient's behaviour, and abstract orientation, demonstrated by the response to questioning.

Disorientation in time

The loss of all practical knowledge of the time of day and season of the year is more serious than a failure to identify the date or day of the week. The disturbance is severe when the patient no longer recalls the month, even approximately, the season of the year, or the year itself. Disorientation in time may occur even in states of slightly impaired consciousness and in many less severe memory disorders.

Disorientation in place

Disorientation in place may fluctuate: for example, a senile dement may know by day that he is in hospital, and so become unhappy, but fail to identify the place and the name of the hospital; at night, however, he may think himself to be at home, or to be lost, so that he anxiously looks for the way home. The difference between practical and abstract orientation is often striking: for example, a patient may be perfectly at home when walking in the clinic grounds, but on being questioned may know nothing at all about the building in which he is housed, its geographical location or even the name of the relevant town. Theoretical disorientation is of less significance than practical. Disorientation in place should be assessed very differently according to the familiarity or strangeness of the place in which the patient is situated: that is to say, practical disorientation in his own home counts for far more than the same symptoms in the unfamiliar surroundings of the hospital, especially when these are quite new to the patient.

Personal disorientation

Brief spells of autopsychic uncertainty or disorientation may occur when emerging from a state of disturbed consciousness, in rare cases when awakening from deep sleep: they are usually quickly corrected, in a matter of seconds. When such personal disorientation lasts for a long time it is ominous: the patient no longer knows who he is. For example, an elderly woman, who was in a confused, arterio-sclerotic state, did not know that she was Mrs N. N. and had five children and several grandchildren; she gave her maiden name.

Severe personal disorientation of this kind is almost always associated with other qualitative disturbances in orientation.

Situational disorientation

Brief spells may occur when emerging from states of disturbed consciousness, and more rarely from deep sleep, especially in unfamiliar surroundings. If the disorientation persists, though it may vary in intensity, it is a sign of severe disturbance, usually of an organic nature.

False orientation

When orientation is uncertain or lacking, confabulated orientation may take its place. For example, an inpatient with arteriosclerotic dementia thought he was at home. A drunkard in detention claimed that he was at his place of work. A senile dement thought in summertime that it was already winter. An elderly dement talked of himself as a little boy who had to cross the street to buy something for his grandmother.

Such confabulation is fleeting and changeable, which serves to distinguish it from delusional thinking. In general, it is of no therapeutic significance.

Delusional misorientation and 'double registration'

Misorientations occur in delusion and particularly in the syndrome of hallucinatory paranoia. For example, misorientation in place and situation: a depressive patient, plagued by feelings of guilt, thought he was in prison, mistook his fellow-workers for detectives, thought his clinical examination was a judicial trial.

For autopsychic misorientation and delusional change of identity, see *Ego-consciousness* and *Delusion*.

5.6   Causal associations of disturbed orientation

Disorientation is a very important symptom in psychopathology. When it is acute and transient, it points to a disturbance of consciousness that has an organic and cerebral basis, and to psychosis. If persistent, it points to advanced cerebral damage. More rarely, disturbances of orientation are an expression of hysterical psychogenic states (e.g. hysterical twilight state) or delusional and hallucinatory misidentification of self and situation.

Disorientation may occur in all disturbed states of consciousness, i.e. in the acute exogenous reaction type, in organic psychoses and in psychogenic states, e.g. an hysterical twilight state. These also include disturbances of orientation occurring in severe affective states, e.g. states of overpowering anxiety and panic.

In the amnestic or psycho-organic syndrome, disorientation may occur as either a transient or a persistent state.

6

EXPERIENCE OF TIME

6.1 Concepts

Experience of time in the narrow sense

This is an awareness of time as a biographically coherent, direct continuum of past, present and future (ego-time). Time experienced in this way, which gives one a sense of one's own continuity and puts existence into a temporal framework, is not a steady flow but is a developmental experience with a tempo which varies with each individual.

Timing, sense of time

This refers to perception of the duration of events, or the discrimination between the duration of two or more events. It also implies the assessment of objective time. Such objective time runs its course steadily and inevitably, beyond individual control. It is governed essentially by external markers – hours, days, seasons of the year. Such a sense of time is constructed on the basis of experience of time.

6.2 Function

A sense of time makes it possible to develop an orientation in time (q.v.) and is thus of great importance for orientation as a whole. The experience of time as an experience of our own development is a component part of our consciousness of ourselves: the experience of the continuity of the ego in the face of changes in ourselves and in the world about us, in spatial and social situations and our own roles within them. Experience of time is thus part of our experience of ourselves and our identity. Without experience of time there can be no intentionality.

6.3   Foundations

Sense of time is a construct covering our perception of the passage of time. Its foundations are vigilance; consciousness; memory functions, which make it possible to experience the passage of time as a sequential flow; and intelligence, which makes it possible to grasp the concept of time. The experience of time is further governed by the total state of the organism, including such factors as metabolism, body temperature, circadian rhythm, mood, motivation, activity, etc. These belong together and form part of the whole afferent complex.

In our culture experience of time and sense of time develop around the eighth year. Our judgement of time becomes more stable with age. Elderly people estimate a given period of time as shorter than do the young. Men have a more accurate and stable sense of time than women.

The more active a person is, the fuller his life, the more quickly time seems to pass (cf. 'pastime' – *Kurzweil*, literally 'short time'). By contrast, an overestimate of the passage of time (boredom – *Langweil*, literally 'long time') is associated with low motivation for what one is doing, poverty of experience and poor motivation for future activity when nothing is happening at present. When there are heavy demands on a person's time because of a pressure of events, the passage of time is overestimated. In retrospect these relationships are reversed.

6.4   Examination

The patient's estimation of time can be tested by asking him to assess given periods of time by means of a subjective-numerical scale (seconds, minutes). Such measurements have so far proved to be of little importance in clinical psychiatry.

The patient's experience of time can be judged during conversation with him.

6.5   Pathology

Acceleration of time. (*The experience of time being snatched away*)

Here time seems to pass more quickly, to rush by.

Causal associations. This phenomenon is encountered as a reaction to catastrophe, e.g. the experience of being involved in a crash; at the start of epileptic attacks (aura); under the influence of psychotropic substances (mescaline, psilocybin, LSD, amphetamine, scopolamine); in manic euphoria.

Slowing-down of time. (*Time is stretched out until it is at a standstill*)

Time passes more slowly than usual, finally seeming to stand still, e.g. 'time doesn't move any more', 'everything is at a standstill'.

Causal associations. This phenomenon is encountered most frequently in severe states of depression, particularly in so-called endogenous depression, in the schizophrenias, in ecstatic states, in convulsive conditions and under the influence of certain drugs, e.g. neuroleptics, LSD, quinine, nitrous oxide.

Loss of temporal reality

Here there is no sense of temporal continuity. 'Life seems to exist only in the present; it is divorced from the past and from the future' (Beringer, 1927). A depressive patient said: 'There is no time any more'. Existence appears to be frozen in an eternally present torment. There is a 'timeless vacuum'. A lack of awareness of progress in one's own personal history is often accompanied by the feeling of unreality (depersonalization) and by other alienation experiences (derealization). The feeling of discontinuity is also part of this loss of temporal reality: time races on, stands still, can even seem to go backwards, or to be absent for varying periods.

Causal associations. This occurs in dreams, in states of clouded consciousness (the acute exogenous reaction type), in severe amnestic psychosyndromes (Korsakoff's syndrome), in severe exhaustion, in severe depression, under the influence of hallucinogens, and sometimes in schizophrenics with marked derealization and depersonalization.

Disturbance of the categories of time

The relationship between past, present and future are distorted. One
or more of these dimensions may disappear. There may be, for
example, loss of time, loss of the past, inability to see the future,
confusion between the past and the present and reversion to the past.
Ecmnesia: Here the past is experienced as the present, i.e. the
patient lives in the distant past, believing it to be the present.
Causal associations. The disturbance is associated with severe
oligophrenia, with dreams, with acute exogenous reaction type
(confusion – *Umdämmerung* – delirium). Ecmnesia can occur in
severe amnestic psychosyndromes (Korsakoff's syndrome). As an
example, a senile dement stated that he had just come back from the
first errand he had to undertake for his mother; he had no idea of
his actual age and his dementia prevented him from correcting his
statements in the light of circumstances.

Other conditions include the influence of hallucinogens, psychogenic emergencies, and sometimes schizophrenia in which delusional
memories predominate.

EXAMPLE

Protocol 145

A schizophrenic of about forty stated that he had lived for two thousand years
in an underground clinic in a lake.

In melancholia the past may be endowed with an excessively
guilt-laden emphasis and the future may appear to be a dark vacuum.

MEMORY (MNESTIC FUNCTIONS)

7.1 Definition

Mnestic functions enable us to retain our experiences, to register and not forget them, to recall and retrieve them, to ecphorize.

The distinction between memory (*Gedächtnis*) as storage, and remembering (*Erinnerung*) as retrieving what has been stored in our memory is neither linguistically nor etymologically justifiable; *Gedächtnis* means 'thinking of something' (cf. *gedacht*, thought, *gedenken*, to think of, to have in mind) and is generally used intransitively in a purely substantive way – to have something in our memory (*etwas im Gedächtnis zu haben*); in the expression 'to call to mind' (*ins Gedächtnis rufen*) it is used both transitively (to call to someone else's mind – to remind someone of) and intransitively (to call to one's own mind, to remember). Remembering (*erinnern, sich erinnern*) means 'reminding oneself' (i.e. the intransitive form): having something 'in one's thoughts' – thinking of it, remembering it. In the transitive form it means 'causing someone else to think of something', reminding someone else of something.

7.2 Function

Memory, the ability to retain and recall earlier experiences, is of fundamental importance in our lives. It is *not a unitary function* but, theoretically analysed, consists of a series of different operations: perception, experience, practice, learning, recall, making the past live in the present, recognition, comparison, combination, re-learning, etc.

Without memory we cannot recognize what we perceive. There are thus different areas of memory – visual, tactile, verbal, etc. – which may at times be subject to independent impairment. *Without memory there can be no learning*, and the more interest we have in a subject, the more easily we learn by motivated participation. Furthermore, learning is the basis of a very wide variety of accomplishments, not only practical abilities but also capacity for new, inventive, artistic and creative activities (for the literature see Bilodeau, 1966).

All our experiences are present in our memories – whether formed or not – and may be retrieved. It is memory which makes possible man's sense of historical continuity. What has happened is given shape and condensed in memory in a way which is biographically valid for the individual but which is also stamped by social and cultural factors: what has happened has a lasting influence upon our present, in which it becomes incorporated, as well as upon our future.

There is a difference between a routine memory of insignificant, meaningless material and a logical memory which retains at our disposal the essential content of experience. Whenever there is meaning and significance in what we record, and when it also appeals to us emotionally, then the process of learning is much improved.

Memory and affect. When something is repugnant or offensive to us, injures us, or makes us unwell, we forget it more quickly than something which has struck as as pleasant, although not as quickly as something that is neutral and of no account. What is pleasant stays longest in our memory; childhood and youth, for example, may become increasingly attractive. It is not yet clear how far *forgetting*, as opposed to failing to remember, is a more active process with a definite function which involves organization, repression, new impressions and affective adjustment. Activity, sympathy, interest, enthusiasm, pleasure all make remembering easier. Fatigue, apathy and depression render it more difficult.

Labile and stable memory. For about one hour after being registered, the memory of an experience is labile and is easily extinguished, e.g. by new impressions, stress, electro-shock. This is labile memory. What is present after this time remains for years, or even for life.

7.3 Foundations

From the psychological point of view memory, in the sense of retaining experience, and remembering, in the sense of having our earlier experiences automatically at our disposal, consists of a vast number of cognitive functions that depend on the state of our consciousness, on adjustment, attention, motivation and interest and on the organization of the material in question. It is thus not surprising that, anatomically and physiologically speaking, they are not circumscribed, localized cerebral processes but are based on the functioning of the cerebrum as a whole, with many pathways and centres and with separate specialized and crucial functional foci particularly in the limbic system and its bi-temporal connections.

The hypothesis that experience is stored in the form of traces (engrams) has so far been neither confirmed nor confuted.

7.4 Examination

Memory can be tested only by reviving memories, by remembering in free conversation, or by the use of tests. For practical clinical purposes it may usefully be divided into: (*a*) recent memory (ability to take things in) which covers a time span of about 30 to 60 minutes, is labile and can be easily disturbed;[1] (*b*) long-term memory, involving more remote experiences, and tending to be stable.

7.5 Pathology of memory

General (diffuse) disturbances of memory (hypomnesias, amnesias, dysmnesias)

In the organic or amnestic psychosyndrome, where diffuse damage of the most varied kinds affects the whole brain, short-term memory is the first to suffer, long-term memory remaining longer unimpaired. Remembering becomes imprecise. What is remembered is confused and finally memory completely disappears.

In the so-called Korsakoff Syndrome gaps in memory are filled by confabulations. These are, as it were, pressed into being in order to replace lost memories. Functionally their purpose appears to be to restore continuity, though to the patient they are real memories.

'Poor memory' is a very frequent complaint in patients suffering from every type of depression. We cannot write off this weakness of memory as a consequence of depressive feelings of inadequacy, since the act of remembering, of calling to mind, presents real difficulties to patients in this state.

In severe disturbances of memory the patient loses all coherent sense of his own chronological and biographical development and with it all knowledge of the stage of development he has reached and of the biographical context of his present state.

EXAMPLES

Protocol 175 (Brain damage due to hanging)

A 23-year-old man made an almost fatal attempt to hang himself and recovered consciousness only after a coma lasting several days. A year later he could not recall the incident and its effects; in addition he was unaware of his profession, his marriage and child, his age, his father's death, the site of his home and his own whereabouts. He recognized only his mother and let her look after him as if he were a little boy.

Protocol 176 (Post-traumatic, amnestic psychosyndrome)

This 42-year-old builder's draughtsman fell from some scaffolding and was in a deep coma for weeks, after which he was completely disoriented, incontinent and unable to feed or dress himself. A year after his fall he did not recognize his wife and child, did not know that he was married and a father, but believed himself to be at home with his parents. He recognized his mother, but no one in the ward where he is being cared for. He retained no memory of his father's death.

In less severe cases early memories are still good, though the more recent past can no longer be recalled and fresh events, proposals and plans can no longer be retained.

EXAMPLE

Protocol 177 (Senile dementia)

This 78-year-old woman no longer knew where she was, could not find her way home when she went out, constantly mislaid her household things and purse, no longer knew her age, the date, the year or the season, the name of the doctor, or any numbers which were repeated to her. Nonetheless, in relaxed conversation she was still able to talk quite coherently about her youth.

Circumscribed amnesias and hypomnesias

These are gaps in memory which are limited in content or in time. Such lacunae or insular amnesias may be total or partial. If such an amnesia occurs, for example in a case of cranial injury associated with *commotio cerebri*, then we get what are called (*a*) *simple amnesia* for the accident causing the injury; (*b*) *retrograde amnesia* for the time immediately before the accident; (*c*) *anterograde amnesia* for the time immediately after the accident (Fig. 6).

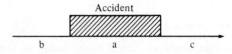

Fig. 6. Circumscribed amnesias: *commotio cerebri*.

The following factors can underlie such amnesias:

Organic. Examples are to be found in *commotio cerebri* and states of intoxication like pathological drunkenness. Amnesia occurs in all forms of organic clouding of consciousness.

Psychogenic. In affectively toned hysterical states, such as extreme fear, anxiety, panic, rage or despair, there is usually a psychogenic narrowing of consciousness followed by partial amnesia. Psychogenic amnesias also occur when memories are denied because of affective needs: what is painful is repressed and split off.

Hypermnesia

Hypermnesia, or heightened memory power, occurs sometimes in states of fever. It may be induced by drugs, or it may occur in experiences of disaster, e.g. an air crash, and in the aura preceding epileptic attacks.

Falsifications of memory (paramnesias)

These are retrospective falsifications of remembered material.

Falsification in derealization and delusion includes so-called delusional memory, the alteration of remembered material to fit in with the delusion and the apparent memories which crop up in delusions but which correspond to no real past experience.

Pseudological memories are pseudo-biographical accounts arising from an affective need, e.g. justification or making excuses, telling tales, boasting, making oneself interesting. In the end this tendency merges into frank lying.

Confabulations refer to pseudo-memories in the amnestic psychosyndrome.

Claims of familiarity or strangeness. Paramnesias also include false recognition, false familiarity, claims of familiarity or, rarely, of strangeness (*déjà vu, déjà vécu, jamais vu, jamais vécu*). The patient is convinced that he has, or has not, seen something, or heard it, or experienced it.

Such falsifications of memory with claims of familiarity or strangeness occur at times in epilepsy, as well as in other circumstances. On the whole they are rare.

EXAMPLE

Protocol 167 (*Epilepsy*)

See p. 136.

8

ATTENTION AND CONCENTRATION

8.1 Definition

Attention means the active or passive focusing of consciousness on an experience; concentration means maintaining this focus.

8.2 Function

Attention enables us to differentiate our experience, perception and thinking. It plays an important part in man's interaction with his environment. Attention thus belongs to the basic functions of existence, enabling the individual to pay heed to his surroundings. Attention and apprehension together must sift everything that comes from the external world about us, weigh it up and estimate its significance. Everything that impinges on the sensorium has to be classified according to whether it is important or trivial, significant or meaningless, dangerous or harmless.

While active application, the fixation and maintenance of attention, is described as *active* attention and concentration, being captivated or fascinated by an experience is called *passive* attention, fixation or *fascination*. When attention is very intense, its range and flexibility may be reduced. A patient who is fascinated by his hallucinatory experience is unable to bring attention to bear upon his surroundings.

8.3 Prerequisites

In order to be attentive, it is necessary to be awake and in a state of unclouded consciousness. This calls for intact functioning of all aspects of cerebration and for an intact sensorium.

The ability to direct one's attention and to achieve attentiveness is also governed by total previous experience, by intelligence and also by mood which plays an important part in determining the object on which attention is directed; for example, a person in a state of grief and sorrow may withdraw into himself and pay no more attention to the surroundings. A patient with delusions of persecution, whose mood is one of suspicion and alarm, may pay more intensive regard to possible signs of persecution.

8.4 Examination

In clinical psychiatry attention and concentration are examined by observing the patient's behaviour, both verbal and non-verbal. Attention and concentration may be described in terms of their intensity, range, persistence, and flexibility or elasticity.

8.5 Pathology of attention

It is possible to pick out certain pathological components (by synthetic analysis, for didactic purposes).

Lack of attention and disturbance of concentration

This signifies an inability to direct attention to an object, to focus on it in an organized way, disturbance of the ability to fixate attention, to maintain persistent application to a given activity, object or experience. There is marked distractibility. Very severe distraction and complete lack of attention are called aprosexia, which is encountered, for example, in confused states.

Narrowing of attention

There is a considerable spectrum ranging from broad, wide-awake attention bestowed on many things to narrow concentration on a few. This narrowing is encountered in the passive attention of hallucinations, e.g. hearing voices, in severe delusional experiences, under strong affective influences, e.g. depression, sorrow, worry, fright, anxiety. In all these states the field of attention is narrowed.

Fluctuation in attention and concentration

Fluctuations in the duration of attention may be related to interest, to personal involvement in the matter in question. Anything that concerns the patient, that touches him or arouses his sense of involvement, will make his attention last longer. When talking with the patient and forming an opinion of his capacity for attention and concentration, it is very important to bear in mind that the relationship between two partners in a dialogue plays a large part in determining attentiveness.

A manic patient, full of ideas, thoughts and drives, has difficulty in fixing his attention on something specific and in keeping it there (fluctuating attention, distractibility, poor concentration).

8.6   Causal associations of disturbances of attention and concentration

Disturbances of attention and concentration are in no way specific to or even typical of any particular mental disorder. They are of little pathognomonic significance. Attentiveness suffers in many everyday situations of conflict, in neurotic disorders, in various affective states caused by worry, sorrow, vexation, and particularly in all kinds of anxiety. Disturbances of this kind are found in fatigue and under the influences of depressants, alcohol and various drugs. Stimulants, e.g. amphetamine, may heighten attentiveness briefly by raising levels of activity. Attention is disturbed in all mental disorders associated with diffuse cerebral damage (the organic psychosyndrome). Attention is reduced or obliterated in all acute exogenous disturbances (exogenous reaction type), and in clouding of consciousness. But even when consciousness is clear, attention may be disturbed; in affective states, e.g. melancholia and mania, the patient is unable to attend to anything or to concentrate.

In schizophrenia attention and concentration vary. In an acute schizophrenic episode of dramatic onset, active attention is almost impossible and the patient accordingly pays no heed to his surroundings. Many patients are fixated on their own inner experiences; they may be fascinated, spellbound by, for example, hallucinations or delusions, often by impending doom. In chronic schizophrenia attention is often not overtly disturbed, so long as the theme of the patient's delusions is not touched upon. Many paranoid patients, particularly those with delusions of influence or of persecution, experience the world as directly hostile to them: their attention is then heightened, as they are always on the alert, searching their surroundings for suspicious signs.

8.7 Attention and sensory illusions

Sensory illusions (hypnoid hallucinations) may occur in states of severely reduced attention, in fatigue, or when falling asleep. However, hallucinations, and in particular illusions, may also occur when attention is heightened or overstrained. Thus a child who has to go, alone and fearful, through a wood at night, can become so tense and over-alert that a bush, for example, becomes for him a lurking figure and the rustling of trees can become the steps of pursuers catching up on him (illusionary misinterpretation).

9

THOUGHT, LANGUAGE, SPEECH

9.1 Definition

Thinking means a state of readiness to question, perceive, grasp, describe, interpret, to see causal and explanatory connections, to consider, decide and make judgements preparatory to appropriate action, in short, it means organizing all the data we are given, both material and immaterial, concerning ourselves and our world.

Language is thinking in signs or symbols and as such contributes to the organizing function of thought.

In speech, and writing, we communicate what is formulated in symbols, either as factual communications or as an expression of the current mood or intention of the speaker.

9.2 Function

Thinking in the sense defined above comprises concentration (keeping one's attention fixed on something), reflection (occupying oneself with something), knowing and recognizing, organizing and connecting according to logical categories – sameness, similarity, difference, significance, consequence, cause – and according to affective factors (mood, desires, tendencies, drives, aims, motivation), combining, considering, judging, deciding, preparing for action (for details see section on the psychology of thinking).

Thinking passes through different developmental stages, from the more amorphous, less structured modes of thought that are not, or are only slightly, subject to logical laws, are more dependent on mood and often also more graphic and pictorial, to the less graphic, more abstract and more conceptual forms of thought.

A man's thinking, judgement, critical ability, insight (reflective self-judgement), his ability to keep to the point and not be affected by mood – all these capacities (their nature, tempo, richness of content, agility and the extent to which they are pictorial) tell us not only about his ability to think in the sense of rational, logical categorization (intelligence) but also about his current mood and his essential being (see Robinson, 1972).

For this reason disorders of thought cannot be viewed in isolation, but must be seen as an expression of the whole man's total state. Language is the medium and expression of thought. In the absence of speech it is difficult to form any idea of a man's way of thinking. Such understanding is acquired essentially in conversation.

9.3   Foundations and determinants

Psychological and physiological foundations

Vigilance, lucidity of consciousness and ego-consciousness, intelligence, memory and affect are the most important psychological determinants of thought. Intact functioning of the total brain is the essential prerequisite. For the understanding and expression of language in speech, writing and reading, the basic requirement is the functioning of certain cerebral regions (see *Neurophysiology*). For speech we need, apart from ability to think and linguistic ability, an intact motor co-ordination of the whole apparatus of speech, i.e. respiratory organs, vocal cords, phonation area, pharynx, mouth, teeth and lips.

Social and cultural determinants

The symbols of language, and therefore of thinking, are governed or normalized by social and cultural factors. They are fashioned and acquired in the course of an individual's development in a given micro- and macro-sociological setting, undergoing further modifications according to his life history, experience and mood. (For the development of thinking see in particular Piaget, 1967, 1973.)

9.4   Examination

Examination of a patient's thought and speech is best carried out in the course of conversation and by observation of behaviour. The context in which recognizable thought disorders occur determines essentially how one views and understands them (for further details see Kind, 1973; for tests of thought disorder see *Test Psychology*).

9.5 Pathology

The following isolated concepts should be regarded as aids to description and classification. They do not constitute a basis on which to dissect a patient into separate functions, as this would prevent us from seeing his existence as a process which invariably includes the final product, i.e. what the patient has become. The concepts put forward can, if used properly, enable us to understand the patient better, to come closer to him; that is the foundation of therapy.

Formal thought disturbances

This term covers some common disturbances of thought processes. They are nosologically non-specific. Observing them enables us to assess more clearly the patient's true state of mind.

Inhibition of thought

There seems to be a brake on all thinking which, with speaking, proceeds irregularly, haltingly and laboriously, as if there were a resistance that had to be overcome. This impeding of the tempo, content and purposiveness of thought processes cannot be overcome even if the patient makes obvious efforts to do so. Clinically such inhibition of thought appears as difficulty in, or even loss of, verbal communication. It can be a consequence of general lack of drive (lack of productivity, lack of ideas, emptiness of thought) or it may be based on affective (depressive) resistances (anxiety, guilt), either real or delusional.

Causal associations. Disturbance of thought occurs in association with the psycho-organic syndrome, clouding of consciousness, depression of various kinds, schizophrenia.

EXAMPLES

Protocol 101 (Schizophrenia)

'I couldn't settle anything any more. My thoughts went round in circles and would then suddenly break off, and then begin at the beginning again. So I could never come to any conclusion.'

Protocol 100 (Schizophrenia)

'The worst thing is thinking. I can't make any headway any more with thinking. My thoughts go round in circles and sometimes I have the feeling that I have no thoughts any more...and no memory either...and I can't concentrate on anything.'

Perseveration of thought

Here thinking is 'rooted to the spot'. The same thought, or the same few thoughts, circulate in the patient's head, constantly pressing upon him, without leading to any development or conclusion. This may be described as circles of thought, depressive brooding, melancholy rumination, meditation.

Causal associations. Perseveration of thought often occurs when an individual is on the point of falling asleep, in insomnia associated with worry, in depressive reactions of all kinds, and also in the psycho-organic syndrome. Most obsessional thoughts (p. 223) are also perseverating.

(N.B. Narrowing of thought (see p. 108) is not the same as perseveration.)

Thought blocking

Here there is a sudden break in the thought process. The patient stops in the middle of talking, is silent, loses the thread, sometimes taking up the conversation again on a different subject. Blocks occur in states of unclouded consciousness and should not be confused with the interruption of the flow of thought that occurs in brief loss of consciousness (absence). Thought blocking may occur also in moments of sudden and complete bewilderment, in states of terror and when there is a feeling of inner emptiness. In schizophrenia there is also an active blocking due to negativism.

Break in thought

Here the patient himself experiences the sudden interruption of his flow of thought. Breaks in thought are, like blocking, recognisable by the sudden halting of speech.

Deceleration of thought

This refers to a slowing down of thought processes that is generally continuous. It can be recognised by the sticky, viscous and torpid nature of the patient's speech and reactions. Inhibited thinking is often also slow.

Deceleration of thought is found in states of clouded consciousness, in somnolence, in retarded depression, in the psycho-organic syndrome, in severely afflicted and distressed schizophrenics. Speech is also slowed down (bradyphasia).

EXAMPLE

Protocol 94 (Schizophrenia)

This patient noticed that his thinking was impeded and blamed this on alien influences: 'I am being made weary in my thinking.'

Acceleration of thought: flight of ideas

Thought and speech are speeded up. When there is flight of ideas, thinking is no longer directed towards an end, but keeps changing or losing its goal. Thoughts are constantly diverted by the intervention of new ideas. In contrast to confused, incoherent thinking, it is usually possible to follow the superficial and fleeting association of ideas. (See also *Tachyphasia* and *Logorrhoea*.) The patient himself can experience his flight of ideas as pressure of thoughts or flight of thoughts. Sometimes he uses this as a means of escaping or parrying questions.

EXAMPLE

Protocol 131 (Schizophrenia)

A young patient lamented despairingly: 'My thinking is in disarray, I have a flight of ideas...I can't think any more...I am falling to pieces.'

Narrowing of thought

This is characterized by a restriction of the range of content of thought, by poverty of thematic material, a fixation on a few ideas and a reduction in mental agility. The narrowed thinking lacks perspective, fails to cover different points of view. In conversation the patient finds it difficult to move from one topic to another. He can himself experience the restriction as being unable to get away from certain thoughts, as thinking in circles or brooding.

EXAMPLE

Protocol 113 (Depression)

The patient's thoughts kept circling round bodily decay and putrefaction. Unable to sleep at night, she constantly brooded on her misery: 'My thoughts can't get anywhere. It is as if they were standing still.'

Circumstantial thinking

Here the patient loses himself verbosely and pedantically in trifling details and does not pursue a particular goal. Incidental trivialities cannot be left alone.

EXAMPLE

Protocol 63 (Schizophrenia)

The patient, a young woman, was bewildered and could hardly speak. She felt her own inability to think. 'Perhaps...I don't know...once it was so, once so...I can't judge that, anything, just for that reason....'

Circumstantial thinking can be a consequence of defective powers of abstraction, or of an inability to drop what is not important even when it is intellectually recognized as trivial (pedantry, anancasmus).

Unclear thinking

Unable to stress what is important, the patient cannot distinguish between foreground and background. Main theme and incidental theme are not therefore organized towards any goal of thinking. Without being accelerated, thinking may be volatile and unclear, in the sense that it lacks intelligibility.

Paralogical thinking

Here patients mix heterogeneous topics (contamination), telescope several ideas and images which are not exactly contradictory (compression), replace familiar concepts by all manner of other concepts (substitution), or slip from the main line of thought to a side-track (side-tracking of thought), lose logical coherence, or make sudden leaps in thought (see *Incoherence*). Thinking may be curiously stiff, rigid, one-track, unempathic and at times confused, corresponding to rigidity of affect).

EXAMPLES

Protocol 115 (Schizophrenia)

'I have read the Bible too. I always get it mixed up, because I speak perfect French.'

Protocol 136 (Schizophrenia)

This man, who knew that he was ill, wrote in an essay on 'The problematics of death':
'Now he sees corpses again
they are like
No, Lord, but – that was to cheat death
Yes, a cry
Ei, ei – they also believe in Christ.'
One of his poems had the title 'Comforting mercy and counsel';
'One should bathe
not be bathetic
bathe, and by and by.'
He recognized his thought disturbance as an expression of his disturbed ego-identity and his loss of self. This was expressed in his 'Prayer':
'Clarity, I long for you
return
saturate my thoughts
tell me who I am
and stay in my songs,
lead me back to myself
clarity come
and be my good fortune.'

Incoherent (confused) thinking

The patient's thinking, and with it his speech, no longer has any logical or affectively appropriate coherence; it consists of an apparently haphazard muddle of broken fragments of thought (*dissociated thinking*). Incoherent thinking may be associated with changes in the speed of thought in the direction of either acceleration or retardation.

Sentence construction is disturbed (paragrammatism, parasyntax), sometimes to such an extent that speech consists of unintelligible, empty words or mixtures of syllables (schizophasia, fragmented speech). On the other hand, there is also a form of confused thinking in which the patient's sentences are syntactically correct but the content of his speech makes no recognizable sense to normal people.

EXAMPLE

Protocol 19 (Schizophrenia)

'I have heard I am Elizabeth. Very likely they have heard how they remove the brain.... They want to try and stop the end of the world for me...to counter-head thoughts...heavens, wind and weather and that people get into another mood, that I call segmenting. I saw the murder, I should have induced hypnosis, that comes from the one who calls himself Emperor...One sees that one's body is violated...I saw how they removed my brain, it was like a white cloud that came out of the brain when they took away my brain. Also I then saw a little cherub, he gave me back my brain again in heaven. Hundreds of snakes have bored through me, into my head, into my body, into my neck. My neck is hurting. The snakes have eaten my brain. It is as if they wanted to make me stupid, but the good Powers helped me and healed the wounds again. One of the snakes was gigantically big, it was a boa, it is in my neck and has torn a piece out of it....' 'The world used to consist of blue-eyed people and how brains work. Those with blue eyes work differently in their brains from those with brown, and then come the yellow, the Chinese...'

'Goodness, one can live well, and create, but one goes to pieces. It is like sequestration which the dear God then heals with ointment, bandages, and machines put into the heart.'

Fragmented thinking in states of unclouded consciousness is also called confusion (*Verworrenheit*) and serves to distinguish this state from the state of unclear, disjointed thinking that is associated with clouded consciousness and memory disturbance in the psycho-organic syndrome (*Verwirrtheit*).

Thought disorders associated with disturbances of ego-experience

Characteristic thought disorders are found predominantly in disturbances of ego-activity and ego-demarcation (q.v.) in schizophrenics.

Thought spreading

The patient complains that others know his thoughts and can read them (thought reading), and that his thoughts no longer belong to himself.

Thought withdrawal (*thought expropriation*)

Patients feel that their thoughts are being taken away, withdrawn from them.

Thought prompting, thought directing

The patient feels that his thoughts are being created, guided, steered, prompted, pressed upon him by other people.

The above disturbances often occur simultaneously.

EXAMPLE

Protocol 62 (Schizophrenia)

'My energy for thinking has declined...The vitality of the dead influences me...Paragraphic schooling...' The patient feels that others are experiencing his thoughts, reading his thoughts, that they are taking his thoughts away from him and giving him strange thoughts which are not his own. Other people can also influence his feelings, his will, his actions.

Aphasias

Aphasias are speech disorders resulting from localized cerebral lesions of the dominant hemisphere (the left hemisphere in right-handed people). There are several clinical forms of aphasia which vary according to the area affected. Expressive (motor) aphasia (Broca's aphasia) is the result of injury to Broca's area of the brain. Sensory aphasia is the result of injury to the posterior parts of the temporal convolution, the connections to the parietal and occipital lobes.

Only a few key words are given here. (For details see *Neuropsychology*.)

Expressive (so-called motor) aphasia (Broca)

In Broca's aphasia, which in its pure form is not very common, the patient can understand what is spoken or read to him, but he cannot himself speak. He is mute or his words are garbled, *paraphasias* of letters and syllables. Stereotyped repetition of syllables is frequent. The patient has an inner picture of the word and can state the number of syllables it has. Words are often also slightly misunderstood, or wrongly used.

Sensory aphasia (Wernicke)

This is a form of speech disorder that may amount to word deafness. The patient has no inner picture of the word. He cannot find the right words (*amnestic aphasia*). He is no longer able to name objects, sometimes giving the wrong name (verbal paraphasia), or repeating names monotonously and in no coherent context (paragrammatism, agrammatism) or repeating words that are said to him (echolalia). In so-called *jargon aphasia* the patient speaks formally and mechanically but at times without making any sense. If asked to repeat something he is unable to do so, nor can he read (*alexia*) or write, either spontaneously or to dictation (*agraphia*). He finds it difficult to work with numbers (*acalculia*) and sometimes, if damage is extensive, he finds it difficult to express himself in certain gestures, e.g. winking or threatening, or in mimicry.

Causal associations. Causal factors include cerebral foci of widely varying pathology: disorders of cerebral blood-vessels (arteriosclerosis, apoplexy), cerebral atrophy, Pick's disease, tumour. When cerebral damage is diffuse, it gives rise to a psycho-organic syndrome.

Disorders of speech
Aphonia and dysphonia

These include non-vocalization, hoarseness and aspiration due to paralysis of the 9th cranial nerve or to diseases of the vocal cords (inflammation, tumour). Aphonia may occasionally be psychogenic ('struck dumb with fear').

Dysarthria

Disorders of articulation occur when phonation is affected by respiratory disorder, e.g. in Huntington's chorea, by malformation or diseases of the mechanisms of phonation (cleft palate, paralysis of the tongue, facial paralysis, toothlessness, loose dentures, or also severe general debility and dehydration) and by central motor lesions (bulbar and pseudo-bulbar paralysis).

Stuttering and stammering

Disturbance of the flow of speech, often held to be neurotic.

Logoclonia

Spastic repetition of syllables that occurs in Parkinsonism, when the patient sticks on a word.

Disturbances in talking
Change in the volume of sound

Excited manic patients may talk very loudly, or shout or roar. In severe agitated depression there may also be a kind of tormented bellowing. Schizophrenics may also bellow, when they are in states of catagonic excitement (see *Ego-activity*). Most depressed patients speak softly.

Change in intonation

This may vary between a highly volatile voice, on the one hand, at times with manneristic speech delivered in expressive tones, and a monotonous, uniform way of talking, on the other.

Decelerated talk (bradyphasia)

See *Inhibition of thought, Deceleration of thought.*

Faltering, fragmented talk

Much of the schizophrenic's faltering, fragmented talk is due to thought blocking (q.v.). The patient feels as though his train of thought is suddenly broken (thought withdrawal). This can sometimes be due to the intervention of ideas, delusional experiences or hallucinations. However, in psychogenic disorders, as well as in depression, bewildered patients may sometimes also speak in this halting way.

Accelerated talk (tachyphasia) and pressure of talk (logorrhoea)

The patient talks very quickly and generally too much, there is marked pressure of talk. The content is often connected mostly by the sound of the words (assonance) or by contrast. The patient seems to leap from one word to the next. Sometimes it becomes impossible to follow the flow of his talk, so that a distinction has to be made between coherent and incoherent logorrhoea.

Causal associations. Acceleration of talk and pressure of talk are most frequently found in manic excitement, where they give expression to the excess of ideas; in endogenous mania; sometimes in excited schizophrenics in the form of an autistic rush of talk, with the patient paying no attention to the person with whom he is having a conversation; and sometimes also in aphasias of organic origin (q.v.).

Verbigeration, palilalia, verbal stereotypy

Many aphasics maintain a monotonous repetition of syllables and words, while searching frantically for the right word. Agitated depressives indulge in stereotyped moaning.

EXAMPLE

Protocol 164 (Agitated involutional depression)

The patient kept repeating her miserable complaint 'I would like to die – I can't die'.

Verbigerations of schizophrenics can often be interpreted as self-reassurance, sometimes also as a form of prayer or incantation.

EXAMPLES

Protocol 23 (Schizophrenia)

The patient called out over and over again 'I am a man'.

Protocol 24 (Schizophrenia)

The repeated statement 'I am who I am' can be interpreted as repeated self-reassurance in the face of threatened ego-consciousness (q.v.).

Protocol 20 (Schizophrenia)

The patient kept calling out 'God is omnipotent'. He felt that he and the world with him were perishing; he felt completely abandoned and ran about the street repeating this cry. After his excitement had abated, he said he had felt forsaken and since no one was there he had called on God.

Echolalia

This consists in echo-like repetition of words spoken to the patient and of short sentences. It occurs in great bewilderment following severe disturbance of ego-activity (q.v.) in schizophrenics (see also *Echopraxia*) and at times also in mental retardation and dementia, as well as in aphasia.

Mutism

The patient hardly speaks – or does not speak at all if, as is often the case, he is stuporose (q.v.) – but the speech mechanism is intact. Underlying such mutism there is usually an overpowering feeling of perplexity, anxiety and hopelessness. Mutism occurs in severely depressed patients, when the devitalized patient loses all will to speak and, with no more hope of being understood, is benumbed in mute torment (depressive stupor). The basis of schizophrenic (catatonic) mutism and stupor is likewise usually an overwhelming sense of anxiety and despair, a hopelessness of making oneself understood, a dream-like twilight state, etc. (see *Ego-activity, Ego-vitality*). Less commonly, mutism accompanies experiences of ecstasy and fascination. So-called psychogenic mutism may occur after mental shock and in autistic children. It may be clearly purposive (telephrenic, e.g. in prisoners).

Unintelligible speech

The speech of patients, in spite of correct articulation and reasonable tempo, may be unintelligible for various reasons.

Private symbolism

The patient no longer uses words in the sense in which we use them but gives them a private meaning known only to himself, as in private symbolism, private metaphors, or paralogical thought and speech.

EXAMPLE

Protocol 21 (Schizophrenia)

'I would like to find myself. . . So I must also be extravagant, so that I can experience myself as my own self. Therefore I cannot act like other, ordinary men, therefore I cannot give up the symbols I have worked out for myself.' These are: white stands for notepaper, serviette, handkerchief, car, forget, excuse; green stands for mostly leaves, excuse, forget; crows indicate this – animals obey me; drops means forget.

Parasyntax, paragrammatism, incoherence

Here speech loses its grammatical, logical and emotionally appropriate coherence. It becomes fragmented, disjointed, incoherent and dissociated to the point of complete confusion. In extreme cases all that the patient utters amounts to only nonsense words and syllables (see *Incoherent thinking*). Severe grammatical and logical breakdown of this kind may appear in dementia and in the acute exogenous reaction type. It is also found, though rarely, in very excited manic patients.

Many schizophrenics may be predominantly or at times completely confused (a hotch-potch of words, 'a word-salad', schizophasia). But if the clinician knows the patient well he can sometimes make sense out of the confusion.

The ultimate interpretation of schizophrenic thought and speech disorders as a defence mechanism (in the sense that the patient wants to avoid coming to terms with his fellow men) is certainly *not* true of all such cases. As an interpretation it is plausible if the patient, usually suffering from a chronic illness, speaks in this fragmented way only when confronted with his 'sore points', e.g. delusions or certain earlier experiences. But other patients, especially the acutely ill, enter a confused state because they are overwhelmed by doom, destruction and disintegration, catastrophes, chaos, fear, panic and bewilderment (see *Ego-consciousness*).

Confused speech is found also in other psychoses, e.g. the psychoses of epilepsy.

Many patients in their confused and to a large extent unintelligible talk furnish astonishingly concise accounts of the reality of their existence. If justice is to be done to the patient, even his confused speech should be taken seriously.

EXAMPLE

Protocol 163 (Schizophrenia)

In a torrent of confused words that lasted nearly three-quarters of an hour, this girl made three vital statements: 'That was the biggest crash landing of my life' – a clear and concise indication of her breakdown. 'My clock, it isn't going any more' – the course of her life has been shattered. 'I look to the hills, so that God may help me' – she was aware of her trouble and her need of help from God, whom she located in the mountains.

Talking beside the point (paraphasia)

The patient does not keep to the point, although he has understood the matter correctly. Instead he introduces some quite different topic. Such talking beside the point may occur when the patient cannot or does not want to get into a conversation with the person he is talking to. This may be a form of defence, or it may occur because the patient is so occupied with matters other than those under discussion that he keeps on being diverted from the topics in question.

EXAMPLE

Protocol 15 (Schizophrenia)

This young patient said his thoughts were a 'mixed salad'. A kind of hypnotic influence had been affecting his thoughts, which had therefore become unclear, mixed up. Then after a long silence he finally said: 'Everyone has a sexual complex before they are twenty.' When asked what this meant he first of all said nothing, and later: 'Calderon's great world theatre.'

Neologisms

The formation of new words, frequently by combining heterogenous topics (contaminations), is found almost exclusively in schizophrenics, who thereby express their private symbols, or who are under pressure somehow to express approximately what is incomprehensible in their experience. When the examiner knows the patient well, this kind of talk often becomes intelligible.

EXAMPLE

Protocol 137 (Schizophrenia)

'Blood born...guardianship court sterilization...shooting duty officer's beard...suspensorium shootable duty...womb substitute exchange...'

Cryptolalia and cryptographia

Many schizophrenics make up their own private language, which may be completely incomprehensible (cryptolalia), or even a private written language (cryptographia). This may be considered an extension of private symbolism (q.v.).

EXAMPLE

Protocol 27 (Schizophrenia-like psychosis in epilepsy)

The patient was studying 'gazology' (the doctrine of the Holy Ghost), 'bezalogy' (the doctrine of the angel world). He had been given a diagnosis of hebephrenia, which he termed 'the art of arrogance' (N.B. rising above the poverty of reality). In the brain research laboratory he thought that 'leucopia' should be investigated. 'Pathonia' he regarded as a 'subdivision of hebephrenia'.

10

INTELLIGENCE

10.1 Definition

Intelligence refers to the ability to take correct (i.e. appropriate to the subject and intersubjectively consistent) cognizance of, and to have insight into, the facts of a matter and their interrelationships, as well as to develop planned[1] and directed action on the basis of the data thus assimilated (intelligent behaviour).

10.2 Function

Theoretically there are many separate functions which contribute to this complex operation. Sensory functioning, alert consciousness and orientation, attention and interested application dependent on motivation, drive and affective state, the thought processes of apperception, abstraction, combination, judgement and deduction – all these, influenced by current mood and total life experience (learning), make it possible rationally to review and appraise, to form conclusions, and to plan and execute purposive, goal-directed actions. Insight is conceptualized and communicated by speech, so that it is possible to make intersubjective comparisons and checks.

Intelligence in this sense becomes, in general terms, the ability to live one's life, to cope with and to master the world. This view of intelligence is different from the reductionist, scientific view which sees intelligence as something that is covered by intelligence tests. Intelligence tests can never deal with or measure more than sub-areas of intelligence.

Of the various factors that constitute intelligence (Thurstone, 1935; Jäger, 1967; Pawlik, 1968), the following are of particular practical importance:

(1) The ability to think numerically, counting.
(2) Linguistic understanding, the capacity for self-expression.
(3) Spontaneity, abundance of ideas and ability to make connections, productivity, agility in terms of tempo and flexibility.
(4) Formal logic, judgement, capacity for abstraction, perspicuity.

121

It is not proposed here to deal with psychological aspects of the scientific construct of intelligence or with the question of its factorial structure and development (for the literature see Guilford, 1967; Jäger, 1967; Pawlik, 1968; Thurstone, 1935).

10.3 Foundations

Physical: structure and function of the brain

Intelligence is based on a genetically, presumably a polygenetically, determined development. Genetic influences have been demonstrated particularly in twin and sibling studies as well as in adoptive studies of intellectual concordance (Slater and Cowie, 1971).

Psychological and social influences on the development of the brain and its function

Cerebral function is initiated and fostered by the environment; it is stimulated by upbringing, by parents, by siblings, by competitive games, and by the school. If there is no social stimulation, intelligence may fail to develop fully (see in particular Eysenck on this theme, 1971).

10.4 Examination

In clinical practice a reasonable estimate can be made in the course of a good conversation about different aspects of life and about the patient's development at school and in his work. If more is required, tests can be used to measure particular areas of intelligence (see, for example, Kind, 1973 and Test psychology).

10.5 Pathology (disorders of intelligence)

Possible causes of poor intellectual performance may be:
  Defects of intelligence due to innate or acquired impairment of cerebral structure or function: oligophrenia, dementia.
  Lack of the requisite experience which enables intelligence to develop, e.g. in sensory defects, isolation, deprivation.

Disturbed contact and reality relationships in psychosis.
Affective impairment of perception, attention and motivation
bearing on intellectual achievement, e.g. in depression.

Defects of intelligence

These arise through impairment of the somatic, anatomical and
physiological prerequisites of intelligence.

Oligophrenia

This includes mental deficiency, mental retardation, innate or acquired early in life, i.e. before the brain has reached maturity. The
underlying cerebral damage may be hereditary or may have been
incurred at the intra-uterine, perinatal or postnatal stage. Oligo-
phrenic patients may be grouped as follows, according to degree of
severity (the IQ data giving only an approximate indication of the
range in question):

	IQ (HAWIE, 1955)
Subnormality	80–90
Feeblemindedness	60–79
Imbecility	40–59
Idiocy	Under 40

From the aetiological point of view oligophrenia may be divided
into:

(1) Hereditary oligophrenia:

(a) Genuine mental deficiency with no apparent physical cause.

(b) Deficiency caused by chromosomal abnormalities: auto-
somal (e.g. trisomy 21 or Down's syndrome); sex-chromosomal
(e.g. Klinefelter syndrome XXY).

(c) Hereditary defect – dominant genes (e.g. tuberous sclerosis
(epiloia): mental deficiency, epilepsy, adenoma).

(d) Hereditary defect – recessive genes: errors of protein metabolism (e.g. phenylketonuria: mental deficiency, muscular hypotonia,
hyperkinesis, chloreoathetosis); errors of lipoid metabolism (e.g.
Tay–Sachs's amaurotic idiocy: mental deficiency, muscular weakness, amaurosis (blindness)); errors of sugar metabolism (e.g.

gargoylism: mental deficiency and miscellaneous malformations, particularly in facial structure); errors of water and electrolyte metabolism (e.g. renal diabetes insipitus).

There are many other such syndromes, usually associated with multiple malformations.

(2) Mental deficiency acquired early in life: early exogenous influences:

(*a*) Intra-uterine: accidents to the mother, shock in pregnancy, placental blood supply, etc., due to infectious illness, e.g. rubella, lues, toxoplasmosis. Endocrine disorder, e.g. hypothyroidism in the mother leading to cretinism. Toxic: Poisoning by various drugs, uraemia, e.g. toxicosis of pregnancy in the mother, rhesus incompatibility leading to kernicterus, X-ray damage, etc.

(*b*) Perinatal: birth injury, haemorrhage, hypoxia, etc.

(*c*) Postnatal: nutritional defects, especially lack of proteins and vitamins, infectious illnesses, encephalitis, encephalomeningitis in whooping cough, smallpox and many other traumas and toxicoses.

Since intelligence is an integrative component of personality, the oligophrenias are associated with many disorders of personality, including: defective character differentiation, defective control of desires and instincts, defective motor co-ordination (clumsiness in movement, mimicry, gesture, articulation), disorders of attention and of verbal and non-verbal comprehension, inability to adapt, disorders of thought, poverty of ideas and interests, poor apperception and abstraction, an impaired ability to connect, to judge, to plan and to act accordingly.

Dementia

Dementia is the name given to intellectual defects arising late in life as a consequence of acquired cerebral damage, development having hitherto been normal for the patient's age. Nosologically such syndromes belong to the organic psychosyndrome (q.v.). Causally they involve the whole gamut of cerebral damage:

Degenerative: cerebral atrophy

Example: Alzheimer's disease

Metabolic: (Disorders of metabolism)
   Example: Wilson's disease (errors in copper metabolism)
Inflammatory: Encephalitis
   Example: Progressive paralysis in syphilis
Vascular: Circulatory disorders
   Example: Apoplexy in cerebral arteriosclerosis
Traumatic (Accidental injury)
   Example: Post-contusional dementia
Toxic:
   Example: CO poisoning
Hypoxic:
   Example: Strangulation

Inadequate psychosocial intellectual development

This includes subnormal intelligence due to lack of the basic psychosocial experience that is necessary for intellectual development, and disorders of intellect due to deprivation. Social isolation, isolation due to sensory defects, inadequate care with inadequate stimulation, lack of security, lack of assurance, and fear – all these restrict opportunities for learning and lead to lack of insight and perspective.[2]

Disorders of intelligence associated with disturbances of reality relations

These are found in infantile autism or in severely autistic schizophrenics. In every severe psychosis intelligence is affected, e.g. depressive blocking. In schizophrenics a whole series of transient functional thought disorders has been described (e.g. so-called over-inclusiveness) which can affect intellectual behaviour.

Disorders of intelligence in sensory defects

In severe innate sensory impairment, e.g. of sight or hearing, important prerequisites of intellectual development are lacking.

Disorders of intelligence in reduced vigilance

There is a transient fall in level of performance.

Disorders of intelligence caused by affective disturbance

This is found frequently in severe *depression* with general inhibition of drive and attention and with slowness of thought which may reach the point of complete lack of ideation.

In the increased tempo, volatility and superficiality of *mania*, intellectual capacity may be poorly applied.

11

PERCEPTION

11.1 Definition

To take cognizance of what is presented through the senses.

11.2 Function

Perception and apperception are the artificially separated cognitive stages by which the world is experienced. The distinction between them and sensations, viewed as the building stones of perception, is a relic of the old elemental psychology which has today been superseded by Gestalt and unitary psychology. According to the theories of Gestalt psychology, perception is a process of progressive differentiation and structuralization. The actual genesis of perception resembles a replica of the ontogenesis of perception; it proceeds from a diffuse, unstructured, global whole to structured gestalts, from the protopathic to the epicritic (see Metzger, 1966; Hayos, 1972; for history and development, see Piaget and Inhelder, 1971).

11.3 Foundations, components and determinants

Sensory organs and the brain

These enable us to record and register perceptible data, including those of sight, hearing, smell and taste. The various kinds of bodily sensation are differentiated in various ways, according to different discriminatory functions: touch, pressure, heat and cold, vibration, position and movement, balance. *Epicritic* sensitivity differentiates between quality, quantity and localization; *protopathic* sensitivity is less structured, covering warmth, pain, etc.

The anatomical and physiological prerequisites are the sensory organ (receptor), the nerve (stimulus conductor) and certain cerebral structures (primary projection fields in the cerebrum). Stimulation of the primary projection fields, regardless of whether this stimulation is adequate (i.e. produced via the specific sensory channels) or inadequate (e.g. produced by direct electrical stimulation) can be demonstrated in the electroencephalogram as evoked potential.

General psychological processes
Object character

When an individual grasps what is presented to him, his perception is conscious. What is presented arrives with the character of an object – a physical character of objectivity, an object consciousness in Jaspers' (1959) sense.

Reality judgement

Here there is a conscious reality judgement on what is perceived, whether real or unreal. The process resembles adoption of an attitude (see p. 77). The difference between object consciousness and reality judgement becomes clear through the example of *fata morgana*. Here the observer sees a lake physically, as an object with the character of an object, but then forms a judgement that it is not really a lake (reality judgement).

Gestalt processes

Everything perceived is put into a structured context. In this genetic process we perceive structured Gestalts and wholes. The part is endowed with meaning and sense from its connection with the whole, which is more than the sum of its parts (see *Gestalt psychology*). The organism tend to make incomplete Gestalts whole, to make the unclear clear.

Significance of content

The Gestalt perceived carries a significance that is governed by situation and life history (see *Personal, social and situational influences on perception*, below), as well as by affective resonance for there is an intimate connection between cognition and affect. To have the percept before us more or less clearly with a particular significance attached is to achieve consciousness of meaning.

Personal, social and situational influences on perception
The state of the perceiver

Mood or expectation, affective states like anxiety, and motivation or need all play an essential part in determining what is perceived – 'we see what we expect to see'.

Life experience

Previous experience and learning help to govern perception. Memory makes possible a central organization for the purposes of comparison, evaluation, etc.

Social factors

The group norm and group cohesion also play a part in determining the nature of perception and its relationship to the phenomenon of suggestion. For example, mountain dwellers buried in an avalanche are welded by their common danger into a closely knit group (group cohesion). The group's dominant expectation (group norm) is directed towards rescue. This expectant attitude can make them take any sort of noise for the sound of knocking (illusionary misidentification), or may induce hallucinations of hearing such a noise. If one individual tells the others of such an experience, then this may be shared by the process of suggestion.

Relationship between perception and reality

In operational terms the *real* is what is there to be perceived – something on which normal persons can agree without difficulty. Perception is a compromise between factual (objective) information and a subjective point of view (unique to the individual personality). Pure apperception of reality is not humanly possible.[1] The ultimate extreme is the autistic, de-realistic view of the world encountered at times in delusions and hallucinations.

Relationship between perception and mood

The more sharply circumscribed and structured the object of perception seems to be, and the more neutral the affective state, the more unambiguous will the percept become: it is objective, on target, as close to the object as it can be. The stronger the affective factors, e.g. motivation, the more ambiguous is the Gestalt formation and the more possibilities are there of mood affecting perception.

The relationship between afferent, the coming into being of a sensory percept, and mood seems to be complementary. The significance of an object can largely govern mood: the more overwhelming this becomes, the greater is its influence. Conversely, mood can greatly affect perception. In everyday life, when most percepts are neutral in affect, the relationship is balanced and the control of reality is successful.

Significance and mood

The significance attached to our perception of an object determines our mood, i.e. it puts the perceivers into a certain mood, depending on their predisposition which in turn depends on character and situation. For example, a person of anxious predisposition, seeing a thunderstorm drawing near in the mountains, will tend to experience fear. Exposed and threatened by thunder and landslide, his liability to anxiety is greater than when he is in the safety of a mountain shelter.

Mood governing perception

On the other hand, mood determines to a large extent what is perceived. Predisposition governs the way in which the world is viewed. The stronger the effect of mood, the less easy is it to achieve reality control. To give an example from normal psychology: a child may have to go alone through a wood at night. He is anxious and keeps a tense watch on the bushes. At first these seem familiar. As his anxiety increases, he still sees the bushes, but thinks they are threatening figures (*delusional perception*). As fear gets the better of him, he no longer sees the bushes but 'recognizes' a lurking figure, i.e. fear makes him perceive another Gestalt with another meaning (*illusionary misidentification*). If the child is now paralysed with fear, or runs away, he can see his pursuer running after him, can hear his footsteps, feel arms catching hold of him: he is hallucinating (visual, acoustic, tactile – cf. Goethe's *Erlkönig*). Similar examples are to be found in clinical psychiatry. In *depression*, to a severely downcast and melancholy man his surroundings seem less lively, colourful, clear and distinct. Sometimes it is as though he were experiencing them at a distance. A depressed patient may experience himself as falling to pieces; feeling putrefied, he may even smell the decayed odour that emanates from him (see olefactory hallucinations). A man with delusions of sin and damnation may see a skeleton of death, or the fires of hell, or the devil's face with its scornful sneer. His mood determines his experience of himself and of the world in the various modalities available to him, in his brooding, his fantasies, his ideas and his perceptions. In *schizophrenia*, a young schizophrenic felt the physical pain of being torn between opposing powers.

These are all sensory experiences that have the character of perception. Ideas, on the other hand, even when they are vivid and pictorial, do not have this character of a sensory experience. They belong to another modality of experience.

11.4   Examination

In clinical psychiatry disorders of perception can be elicited by questioning or can be inferred from behaviour.

For experimental research in perception consult the literature in neuropsychology and experimental psychology. For experimental research on the perception of schizophrenics, see the work of Schooler and Feldman (1967).

11.5   Pathology

Summary:

Perceptual impairment
  Organic
  Psychogenic

Perceptual abnormality
  In intensity
  Changes in perception of size and form (Gestalt)
  Qualitative (abnormal change in the character of perception)
Hallucinations
  Definition
  Classification
  Quasi-hallucinatory experiences
  Hallucinations and delusion

Perceptual impairment
Organic

When a sensory organ is damaged or absent, or when there is circumscribed cerebral damage, the perception function in question will be defective and result in:
  Blindness (amaurosis)
  Deafness (anacusis, hypacusis, surditas)
  Loss of smell (anosmia)
  Loss of taste (ageusia)
  Loss of sensation (disorders of sensibility, loss of sensibility, hypaesthesia, anaesthesia) in various modalities
Although the sensory organs and the afferent nerves may be functioning normally, recognition (visual, acoustic, tactile, etc.) may not take place if the actual sensory impressions are not co-ordinated with previous memories: every cognition is a re-cognition. When recognition is disturbed in this way, with no impairment of consciousness and no defect in intelligence to account for it, the disorders are called agnosias. They come within the province of neuropsychology and are only briefly mentioned here because of the part they play in differential diagnosis.

There are various forms of *visual agnosia*:

(*a*) Disturbances of video-spatial (geometric) orientation in a concrete situation and of video-spatial ideational ability occur in parieto-occipital lesions, usually of the dominant hemisphere. Patients whose consciousness and intellect are unimpaired are no longer at home in familiar surroundings, e.g. house, room, streetcar. They cannot dress themselves because they no longer know the spatial structure of their clothes. They can no longer describe how the street runs, or the spatial arrangement of their room. At the same time they may still be able to recognize the physiognomy of individual objects.

(*b*) Agnosia for objects and persons: Distinctive visual character-istics of objects and persons are no longer recognized. In most cases there is bilateral basal occipital lobe damage. Patients can no longer recognize objects or persons, though they apprehend their size, shape, category (e.g. man, animal, house) and spatial disposition.

(*c*) Colour agnosia: Patients no longer recognize the semantic content of colours. They no longer recognize, for example, the significance of traffic lights, cannot copy colours on to an outline drawing, cannot sort similar colours according to their shades.

(*d*) Letter agnosia (sensory alexia, inability to read) or number agnosia (acalculia).

In *auditory agnosia* the meaning of words is no longer recognized: there is disorder of speech and of the understanding of speech, sensory aphasia. Patients cannot appreciate the meaning of other sounds, e.g. rattling of a bunch of keys. Tunes are no longer recognized (sensory amusia). These phenomena are encountered in temporal lobe damage.

Somatagnosia is agnosia in regard to body orientation, occurs in parietal lobe damage.

(*a*) Autotopagnosia: Inability to recognize, point to or name parts of one's own body, of the bodies of others, of body drawings. (This should not be confused with aphasia.)

(*b*) Finger agnosia: The patient cannot tell his own fingers apart.

(*c*) Right–left agnosia: Impairment of ability to distinguish right from left, even in regard to one's own body. This should not be confused with anosognosia in which there is an inability to recognize, an unwillingness to admit to a functional deficit in one's own body, e.g. paralysis, amounting to a denial of such deficit. This is not a gnostic disorder which might be attributed to a circumscribed cerebral lesion, but occurs in diffuse cerebral damage, often with dementia, or may be psychogenic, e.g. a form of defence. For example: a patient who was paralysed on one side after a stroke had no knowledge of his disability, did not notice it, did not want to admit that he could not move one side of his body.

Tactile agnosia (*stereoagnosia, astereognosis*) is an inability to recognize objects by touch. It is a complex disorder, involving impairment of various peripheral sensations and of fine motor functioning, which cannot therefore be attributed exclusively to a central disorder of recognition.

Psychogenic perceptual defects

These may follow traumatic experiences, e.g. psychogenic blindness, deafness, loss of smell or taste, disorders of touch. The motivation for such psychogenic disorders varies: at times they are symbolic (not wanting to see or hear), at times they occur in a framework of envy, fear or compensation neuroses. In such cases it may be difficult to distinguish between simulation and aggravation. The psychogenic anaesthesia in accident neurosis may be cited as an example.

Perceptual abnormalities
Changes in intensity

Decreased intensity of perception means that the character of perception is less lively and fresh than usual; for example, everything seems flat and grey, bleak and colourless, as if shrouded in mist. This decrease in the intensity of perception is found in severe depressive states of various kinds and also in severe general exhaustion, in psychaesthenia, and following high dosages of neuroleptic drugs.

Increased intensity of perception means that the experience of perceiving is richer, more lively, more colourful than usual. It occurs at times in mania, under the influence of hallucinogens (LSD, mescaline, hashish) and in the rare states of hysterical ecstasy.

Changes in perception of size and shape (Gestalt)

This is called metamorphopsy and may refer to external objects or to the patient himself.

With *external objects* changes in the perception of space, of proportion and size, and of Gestalt are mostly of short duration (seconds or minutes). When there is alteration in size (dysmegalopsy), everything may be seen as smaller (micropsy) or as larger (macropsy).

Alteration of shape (dysmorphopsy) is also reported. For example, in an epileptic aura a patient reported that a picture on the wall seemed to recede into the distance, becoming smaller and smaller. The most common change is change in perception of the Gestalt. Metamorphopsy can occur in normal persons, in childhood, in states of fatigue and when falling asleep, as well as in temporal lobe epilepsy, in schizophrenia (especially in the initial stages) and in acute organic psychoses, e.g. following the use of hallucinogens. In neurotic dysmegalopsy a symbolic content may be evidenced, e.g. a mother whose attitude to her newborn child is ambivalent may see its head smaller.

Heautometamorphopsy refers to the *patient's own body* or to separate limbs. For example, the feet may seem to be miles away and yet gigantic. This may happen when falling asleep in a state of fatigue and is frequently reported in states of drug intoxication with such substances as LSD and mescaline. Closely related to heautometa-morphopsy is heautoscopy, in which there is a hallucinatory vision of one's own figure, similar to a *doppelgänger*. This may occur in normal people when overtired or when falling asleep, but is more frequently reported in epileptic aura and by many patients with cerebral tumour.

Qualitative anomalies of perception (abnormal character of perception in the broad sense)

With *derealization* everything in the environment seems unreal, veiled, strange and unfamiliar, objects appearing partially to lose objective character. The symptom is found sometimes in normal persons. It is frequently seen in organic psychoses and in schizo-phrenia, as well as at times in depressive illnesses, particularly neurotic depression. It is generally associated with depersonalization (see p. 50).

A feeling of *abnormal distance or proximity*, the less common 'split perception' (Jaspers, 1959), is akin to derealization. There is an extraordinary lack of connection between the object perceived and the person perceiving it. There are similarities, too, between this state and depersonalization: not only do the surroundings seem strange and far away, but the patient feels that he himself is at a distance and not in touch with things. This occurs in hallucinogenic psychosis due to LSD or mescaline, and in schizophrenia. Alternatively, there may be a feeling of greater proximity – an experience which is akin to that of increased intensity.

Changes in the character of perception may include, for example, changes in the affective responses to colour, music, space perception. Such changes are akin to depersonalization and occur particularly in toxic psychoses associated with LSD and mescaline.

Synaesthesia, which resembles perception, is usually associated with the hearing of music, though sometimes also with touch and other bodily sensations, when the individual sees colours (auditory-visual synaesthesia, *audition colorée*). Synaesthetic states come within the sphere of normal psychology and occur as individual experiences in predisposed persons. They are frequent and marked in the 'psychedelic' psychoses caused by LSD and mescaline. Hallucinations in various modalities may be synaesthetically linked.

In *spurious recognition* a new perceptual experience is felt to be familiar (*déjà vu, déjà vécu*, etc.). Such experiences, sometimes spoken of as falsifications of memory and identification, are often associated with depersonalization and derealization. They are not specific to any particular illness, though they occur mainly in psychomotor epilepsy. They are also reported in healthy persons.

EXAMPLE

A female patient (*Protocol 167*) in an epileptic confusional state, with partial disorientation and incoherence of thought, said of the voices of the nurses and of her fellow-patients: 'The voices remind me so much of home. I know them.' To the doctor she stated 'I have seen your face before. I know you. You are my teacher, Miss B., you are certainly Miss B.'

Hallucinations
Definition

Hallucinations, or false perceptions, are diagnosed when someone hears, sees, smells or tastes something, or feels something on or in his body, for which other people can find no objective basis. They may occur in any sensory modality, or simultaneously in more than one (combined hallucinations).

Hallucinations represent a modality of experience that is closely related to sensory perception: their character fluctuates in the following respects.

Character of the perception. This ranges from an unambiguous sensory experience to one that is closer to imagery. This is seen particularly in auditory hallucinations, which may consist in straightforward hearing, or in 'hearing but not with the ears'; in a feeling of voices in one's body 'like waves', i.e. contaminated with bodily sensations; or in 'knowing' the voices in an extrasensory manner, a transitional phenomenon to thought echo (see *Auditory hallucinations* below).

Intensity. This ranges from the almost real, with its intensely physical obtrusiveness that is close to sensory perception, to the faintest of manifestations.

Clarity. The character and intensity of hallucinations may also show fluctuations in clarity, ranging from clearly outlined and structures Gestalts to shadowy, shifting scenes.

Object consciousness. This may vary with the intensity of the experience, ranging from what is judged to be physical to experiences in which object consciousness has almost disappeared. In the latter case the hallucinations are less vividly perceived, though they may still have a specific spatial location.

Reality judgement. This may vary between assessments of objects being 'really there', via 'doubtful' to the 'not real' of pseudo-hallucinations (q.v.).

Spatial location. Visual and tactile hallucinations are usually experienced as originating outside the body. But hallucinations are by no means necessarily confined to the sensory field. Thus something may be seen in a place that is outside the field of vision, so-called extra-campine hallucinations. Auditory hallucinations are located in a much more changeable way, for it is more difficult to place sounds; the character of the perception is correspondingly variable.

Classification of hallucinations

Subdivision according to *complexity* is into simple, elementary hallucinations (e.g. amorphous noises, flashes, lights) and complex or scenic hallucinations (e.g. pictures, dramatic scenes, pieces of music).

Subdivision according to *sensory modality* is set out below.

(1) *Auditory hallucinations.* The patient experiences noise or sounds, amorphous or unstructured auditory percepts (achoasms) or he hears speech, words, sentences, whispers, voices (phonemes). These may be heard distinctly or they may be just a distant murmur, indistinct and barely perceived. Sometimes the source of the sound is outside the body; sometimes it is located in the body – 'as if I had swallowed a little man'.

The hallucinated material may be wholly or partly intelligible, or quite unintelligible. At times the patient can recognize who is speaking. He may hear one or several voices which speak directly to him and comment on his actions or thoughts or feelings, or tell him to do things, give him orders and put thoughts into his head. Voices heard in this way are characteristic of schizophrenia and the symptom may gradually progress into that of having thoughts put into one's mind. At the same time the schizophrenic may feel that he is hearing words not through his ear but 'in his brain', 'in his head', or he feels them coming through his body. Often it is his own thoughts which are spoken aloud, or it may be those of other people (cf. consciousness or experience). Depressed patients may 'hear' reproaches, threats or scoldings.

Other patients hear several people talking about them, e.g. mockingly or threateningly. In classic alcoholic hallucinosis the voices may be concocting a plot against the patient; in a wide variety of other psychoses the patient may conduct a conversation with someone existing only in his state of auditory hallucinosis, e.g. in delirious states caused by alcohol or other intoxicants. Sometimes surrounding noises are heard as a 'summons' to the patient.

These phenomena must be distinguished from noises in the ear, or tinnitus, occurring in diseases of the ear and taking the form of murmuring, buzzing, or ringing. The case history and otological examination should establish the diagnosis.

(2) *Visual hallucinations* may be elementary, amorphous visual experiences (photomes) in the form of lights, colours or flashes, occurring primarily in diseases of the eye, the visual pathways and the posterior cerebral lobes. They may also take the form of more or less distinct Gestalts, figures and scenes, either static or moving, coloured or uncoloured. Small moving objects and small or miniature animals appear to patients with alcoholic delirium and at times also in hallucinatory confused states in other organic psychoses, e.g. cerebral arteriosclerosis. Dwarf-like figures may also appear, the so-called Lilliputian hallucinations.

Melancholics oppressed by feelings of sin and damnation may briefly see devils' faces or shadowy figures of death. In schizophrenia intense and clearly formed visual hallucinations are rare; they occur mainly in states of religious ecstasy in schizophrenia and particularly in epilepsy, in some circumstances as elaborate visionary scenes.

(3) *Olfactory and gustatory hallucinations* (hallucinations of smell and taste) are usually intermingled. Distinct hallucinations of smell and changes in taste may occur with tumours of the olfactory area of the brain and at times also in the part of the aura that precedes epileptic fits. Deluded patients with fears of persecution and poisoning may think that they smell or taste poison. Many schizophrenic patients think that they are being hypnotized by unpleasant smells. When closely questioned, deeply depressed patients with reduced vitality and fears of putrefaction not infrequently admit to smelling a foul corpse-like odour, often associated with the delusional idea that their own odour is harmful to other people or at least that other people have noticed it and are avoiding them.

(4) *Tactile hallucinations* (haptic hallucinations, hallucinations of touch) refer to cutaneous sensations, and as such are often indistinguishable from general bodily hallucinations. The patients think that they are being seized, held firmly, blown upon, burned, stung, pierced, scratched, scorched, strangled, or even sawn through.

The experience may or may not be accompanied by pain. There may be an additional feeling of being touched by something hot or cold (thermic hallucinations) or by damp (hygric hallucinations). The hallucinations occur particularly in organic psychoses (toxic delirium, cocaine delirium).

In *chronic tactile hallucinosis* small animals, e.g. worms, beetles or vermin are felt crawling on the skin (*dermatozoic delusion*) or burrowing under the skin, inside the body, in the bowels and in the sexual organs (*enterozoic delusion*). This clinical picture is found mostly in diffuse cerebral disorders, i.e. as part of an organic psychosyndrome.

(5) *Bodily hallucinations* (coenaesthetic hallucinations):[2] Although these may at times merge into tactile hallucinations, they can be extraordinarily varied: for example, the patient may feel that he has been turned to stone, dried up, shrivelled, that he is empty, or crammed full, that his insides have been turned to gold, or to stone. The body is felt to be penetrated by currents or rays; many words are used to describe this experience – flowing, pulling, moving – and at times new words have to be invented. The experiences may be felt all over the body, or they may be localized. They often appear to affect the sexual organs, e.g. drawing off semen, electrical stimulation, delusions of coitus in erotic delusions.

Occasionally the patient may think that he is being lifted up, elevated or suspended (vestibular hallucinations), or that he is being moved (kinaesthetic hallucinations).

Experience of bodily distortion: Here the body appears to increase in size, to become distorted, or fatter, or heavier, or lighter; separate parts of the body may seem to change in size and shape.

In schizophrenia many such hallucinations are experienced passively – they are 'done' to the patients, inflicted on them: the patients may complain that they are electrified, that rays are passed through them, that they are hypnotically tortured or sexually abused. The agents accused vary according to cultural background and may include ghosts, witches, hypnotic forces or technical media. In melancholia and in delusional hypochondriasis the feeling of lowered vitality provides a basis for experiences of decay or putrefaction, the hallucinations then being seen as a confirmation of the mental state. Delirium tremens is occasionally accompanied by massive vestibular and kinaesthetic hallucinations.

Classification may also be according to the *circumstances in which the hallucinations occur.*

(1) In *local physical diseases* they are practically always elementary hallucinations. Visual hallucinations are associated with injuries or other diseases of the eye and the visual pathways. Auditory hallucinations may at times occur in diseases of the ear, though it is more usual to find a kind of inner hearing in patients suffering from noises in the ear. Hallucinations of smell may accompany tumours of the olfactory area or of the basal temporal lobes.

(2) ' *Physiological'* hallucinations include hypnagogic hallucinations which occur on the point of falling asleep and hypnopompic hallucinations which precede the process of waking. Sensory illusions of varied kinds, mostly visual and auditory, also occur when falling asleep or waking up. There is no conscious activity or clarity of consciousness. The content of such hallucinations is mostly governed by the affective state; it may, for example, be personal, e.g. a son sees his dead mother, or religious, e.g. a vision of the Madonna. Such hallucinations are not morbid. They often resemble pseudo-hallucinations (q.v.). Individuals vary greatly in their capacity for such experiences which at times depends also on the cultural background.

(3) In certain *sensory situations* visual and auditory hallucinations may accompany sensory deprivation, either natural or experimental, and may also occur in sensory overloading.

(4) Certain *life situations*, e.g. solitary confinement, with sensory deprivation as a contributory factor, may lead to hallucinosis. Such hallucinations occurring in isolation are largely governed by mood. For example, anxiety can govern delusional feelings of persecution and the hallucinations occur as if in confirmation of the delusions, underpinning them and providing them with a foundation. Patients may hear people whispering about them, plotting against them, arranging their execution: they also hear the executioner's steps, smell gas that is being brought in to poison them, or believe, because of the taste, that their food has been poisoned. Alternatively, a longing for freedom and mercy may become a delusion of reprieve. Voices may then be heard speaking about this autistic wish fulfilment.

This group of hallucinations also includes the visionary experiences of deeply religious people, especially if they have prepared themselves for such experiences by fasting, by withdrawal from the world (sensory deprivation) and by meditation.

(5) In *acute psychoses of organic origin* (acute exogenous reaction type, especially delirium) hallucinations often occur in several sensory modalities. If the hallucinations are very prominent and consciousness is not clearly affected, we may speak of hallucinosis. This group of hallucinations occurring in acute organic psychoses also includes the toxic hallucinations which may appear under the influence of drugs, hallucinogens, etc. In these various hallucinated and delirious states, including alcoholic and arteriosclerotic delirium, the hallu-cinations are mostly visual, though vestibular and kinaesthetic hallucinations are not infrequent. They occur mainly in association

with other perceptual changes, e.g. changes in spatial perception, in colour intensity, synaesthesias.

(6) *Chronic organic psychoses* may be accompanied by hallucinations, e.g. dermal and enterozoic delusions in senile dementia. Visual hallucinations occur in arteriosclerotic and other chronic cerebral impairment.

Hallucinatory experiences are also associated with *epilepsy*, e.g. visionary ecstasy, bodily and olfactory hallucinations, both within the framework of acute psychotic episodes (psychomotor attacks, twilight states) and in the more persistent paranoid-hallucinatory psychoses of epilepsy (often schizophrenia-like, so-called productive psychoses).

(7) In *schizophrenia* the most common hallucinations are auditory (q.v.) and various bodily hallucinations. Other hallucinatory experiences are less frequent, those in the visual modality being atypical, though they may occur in acute dramatic schizophrenic episodes with dream-like confusion (oneiroid, schizophrenic delirium). Hallucinations in schizophrenia are almost always associated with delusions but this is not generally the case in the organic psychoses.

(8) In *endogenous depression* hallucinations are not on the whole frequent, though close questioning of a group of severely depressed inpatients with greatly reduced feelings of vitality revealed that olfactory hallucinations were fairly common: smelling like a corpse, smells of putrefaction and decay, at times smelling a mortuary, even in the open fields, or a cemetery. Many melancholic patients see fleeting shadowy figures, skeletons, figures of death or of the devil on the wall. Like the delusions of melancholia, the hallucinations are here completely appropriate to the patient's mood – so-called synthymic hallucinations.

(9) In *obsessional* syndromes of various nosological types, obsessional neurosis, endogenous depressions, schizophrenia, organic psychosis, the patient may experience hallucinations: for example, an obsessional patient saw the knife which he was afraid he was going to run through someone's body.

Modes of experience that are closely related to hallucinations

These are set out below and in Table 2.

Pseudo-hallucinations, unlike true hallucinations, which to the patient are very similar to sensory perception, are experienced more as a kind of plastic image or inner picture, not as phenomena evoked by an external object: unlike hallucinations, they do not have the character of objects and are not located in space. Their illusionary nature is recognized and they are judged to be not real. Between hallucinations and pseudo-hallucinations there are shifting transitional stages. Sometimes when a conversation with a patient is going well, one can see his hallucinations 'breaking down' into pseudo-hallucinations, only to flare up again at times as true hallucinations when the patient is left alone and withdraws once more into his own world. Such fluctuations occur in all modalities of experience, as can be observed particularly well when one is on the point of falling asleep.

Illusions. In illusionary misidentifications there is always something regarded as really there, something objective which is transformed and taken for something other than it really is, i.e. it is misidentified. Illusions are thus false percepts, errors in perception, false forms of recognition. For example, a bush is taken for lurking man. A patient waking from an anaesthetic thinks the nurse is a member of his family. Over-tired soldiers mistake trees for enemies.

Illusionary misidentifications are more liable to occur when conditions of perception are difficult so far as the object perceived is concerned, e.g. half-light, confusion of voices, or so far as the person perceiving is concerned, e.g. clouded consciousness, over-tiredness, a state of expectation or emotional tension. For example, a patient in a delirium takes rays of light to be spiders' webs, spots on the wall to be animals.

There are transitional stages between illusions and hallucinations, pseudo-hallucinations and delusional perception.

Pareidolia is seeing images in a poorly structured visual field, e.g. in old walls, clouds, wallpaper, carpets. The hearing of words in amorphous noises also comes into this category. The object and the fantasy exist side by side, and the object itself is not misidentified. Pareidolia may be deliberately created and controlled by those with

Table 2. Modalities of experience: summary

Concept	Object of perception present at time of perception	Perception-like character	Spatial location	Object consciousness	Reality testing	Correct object recognition	False interpretation
Perception	+	+	+	+	+	+	–
Illusion	+	+	+	+	+	–	+
Hallucination	–	+	+	+	+	–	–
Pseudo-hallucination	–	+	+	+	–	–	–
Pareidolia	+	+	+	–	–	+	–
Eidetic imagery	–	+	–	–	–	+	–
Delusional perception	+		+	+	+	+	+
Bodily experiences	–	±	+	±	±	–	+
Fantasy	–	–	–	–	–	–	–
Dream	–	+	±	+	–	–	–

a predisposition in this direction. In feverish delirium pareidolia may become so insistent that the real object disappears, i.e. the pareidolia becomes an illusion.

In some circumstances this process may develop into hallucinations. For example, a child looks at the curtain, where he sees a figure (pareidolia). At night he is anxious and thinks he recognises the figure (illusion). In panic he thinks he sees the figure moving and reaching out towards him.

Eidetic imagery covers quasi-perceptual sensory impressions, usually visual or auditory, that have the clarity of real perception. They are closely related to perceptual experiences and, like them, are located in space; unlike them, however, they have not the characteristics of objectivity and are not subject to reality testing. They are, nevertheless, based on a genuine perceptual experience which is vividly and concretely recalled. Eidetic personalities (people with eidetic ability) are able to reproduce details from eidetic images, which can be recalled voluntarily or may come to mind involuntarily.

Eidetic ability is more widespread among children than adults. There are transitional stages between eidetic images and images of varying sensory intensity. There is nothing pathological about eidetic experiences.

Delusional perception. Correct sensory perception may, because of a delusion, be endowed with an abnormal meaning, mostly self-referring, which does not objectively belong to it. Delusional perception (Schneider, 1967) is thus a delusional misinterpretation of real perception. For example, a patient may see two men talking in a cafe and perhaps hear their voices without understanding what they are saying. This perception he refers delusionally to himself, believing that he is the subject of the conversation.

False physical awareness (*leibhaftige Bewußtheiten*) (Jaspers, 1959) is a bodily experience which resembles perception and which carries great conviction, for example in schizophrenia or under the influence of drugs (LSD, mescaline). The patient may say: 'Someone is behind me, is trying to touch me, is touching me, speaking to me, putting thoughts into my head'. Such convictions have little or no sensory vividness but are given a spatial setting and thus seem like sensations. They partly resemble extra-campine hallucinations. The patient may judge them to be real or unreal. Sometimes a bodily experience of this kind may be so concrete that the patient turns round to see who is behind him. The 'experienced' patient, however, often says something like 'I feel sure that someone is behind me, but I know that no one is there' (negative reality judgement).

This purely delusional experience has no sensory or spatial accompaniment and always has a special meaning for the patient within the context of his delusion.

Hallucination and delusion

Delusions may exist without hallucinations, e.g. delusions of guilt, of illness, of sin and perdition, many chronic paranoid delusions of schizophrenics. There are also hallucinatory experiences of the most varied nosological types in which there is no question of delusion. Frequently, however, hallucinations and delusions are found together. To an unbiased observer it sometimes seems as though in cases of marked delusional mood and strong delusional dynamics the hallucinatory experience serves to confirm, underpin, strengthen and 'prove' the delusional experience.

In other words, mood determines total experience, regardless of commonly accepted reality, and this extends even into the area of perception: affective predisposition shapes the world (the autistic experience of the world pays no regard to any common consensus about facts). In his hallucinations the world which appears to the patient, as if by the process of perception, is his own fantasy world, the world in which he is engrossed. Thus to the depressed patient with a delusion of putrefaction, his rotting existence manifests itself in the smell which emanates from him. To the schizophrenic with disturbances of ego-consistency and ego-boundary (q.v.) his thoughts, whether his own or allegedly alien to him, appear to him as voices. Such a disturbance of boundary is, of course, not specific to schizophrenia, as may be seen by reference to psychedelic toxic psychoses.

APPERCEPTION
(*Auffassung*)

12.1 Definition

Apperception is the ability to understand perceptions in their interpretative context, to connect them one with another and to incorporate them into one's store of experience.

12.2 Function

Apperception, by integrating sensations, continues the structural synthesis which begins in the process of perception. This process starts with sensation and proceeds, by way of perception, interpretation and organization of complex perceptual experiences, to knowledge and recognition, including the development of mental and verbal concepts and the apprehension of meanings, ultimately to form one contextual whole. These advanced stages of apperception are intellectual processes. Apperception is a prerequisite of practical living.

12.3 Necessary conditions and determinants

The prerequisites of successful apperception are vigilance and clear consciousness, ego-consciousness, intact perception, orientation, attention and concentration (registering and connecting), intelligence (ability to combine and judge, to organize one's store of experience) and memory (to have this experience at one's disposal).

The determinants of apperception are total life experience, age, situation, personal and cultural characteristics, mood and motivation.

12.4 Examination

Apperception can be judged in conversation and by observing whether the patient's behaviour is in keeping with his situation.

Alternatively, the patient can be asked to explain the meaning of pictures, proverbs or stories told to him. One can test object recognition, with the proviso that amnestic aphasia, the inability to find the right word, may lead to difficulty in naming objects. The Thematic Apperception Test (TAT, Murray, 1943) seeks to reveal unconscious attitudes and complexes, by studying apperception.

12.5 Pathology

Apperception (see 12.3), being a highly complex, multiconditioned operation, may be disturbed in any number of ways. Disorders in apperception have therefore no particular nosological significance of psychopathology, though they are of considerable importance when it comes to judging a patient's capacity for practical living.

Apperception may be lacking, e.g. in disorders of consciousness, mental defect, disorders of understanding and judgement in dementia, or may be false, e.g. false interpretation in delusion.

Apperception may be slowed down in states of fatigue and depression; it can be volatile in mania or toxic psychosis, e.g. due to alcohol. It can be widely scattered, as in mania; fluctuating, as with fluctuations in consciousness, changes in drive and mood; or narrowly concentrated, as with the fixation of delusions and hallucinations, and twilight state.

12.6 Causal associations of disorders of apperception

These occur in global acute and chronic cerebral damage, i.e. in acute exogenous reaction type, in the psycho-organic syndrome, and in all disturbed states of consciousness of whatever genesis, in mental deficiency and in dementia.

Psychogenic disorders of apperception occur under strong affective pressure, in panic states, e.g. following catastrophes, in hysterical reactions and twilight states. Neurotic disorders of apperception, e.g. blind spots and scotoma, are often determined by complex factors.

Disorders of apperception are also associated with the functional psychoses. In schizophrenia apperception is sometimes blocked. The autistic, de-realized delusional existence of schizophrenics may lead to strange, paralogical apperception which it is not easy for others to understand. In depression apperception becomes more difficult and narrowed, in mania it is volatile and diffuse.

Disorders of apperception and recognition in localized cerebral damage are called agnosias and have been described in Chapter 11 under *Perception*.

13

DELUSION

'My life, my freedom, my goal' (*Protocol 29*)
'It always refers to me' (*Protocol 38*)

13.1 Definition

A delusion is a man's private, overriding, isolating conviction about himself and his world. As a mode of private reality, a delusion becomes morbid only when it hampers the conduct of life. Its assessment therefore calls for an awareness of cultural and social relativity.

(*a*) A delusion is a completely *personal and rigid conviction* about one's own life and reality. For the patient it is a self-evident reality. It is experienced as certain, requiring no proof, no evidence. It is a matter of knowing, not of faith and belief.[1] Neither previous experience nor compelling counter-arguments can shake the certainty of a delusion. Doubt is not admitted. No change in standpoint or shift in conviction is possible.

When a delusion is building up or breaking down, or in some transient unsystematized forms of delusion, it may be more a question of supposing, opining, suspecting, in which case there is still some doubt.

(*b*) A delusion is an *overriding* reality that governs the patient's life. It is legitimate to speak of delusion only when it controls a person's experience and action, when his life and behaviour are governed by his delusional existence.

(*c*) A delusion is a *private* conviction of reality. Delusional reality is not the reality which normal people of a given socio-cultural and situational background agree upon in their common world. The special private delusional conviction is firmly adhered to, even when it runs counter to the general communicable reality of mankind and contradicts the patient's own previous experience of this reality and the experience of normal fellow-men, as well as their collective beliefs and opinions.

It is not the content of a delusion, its rightness or wrongness, that

150

constitutes a general criterion of delusion. From the normal point of view the content may be inappropriate, false or quite impossible, but in all supersensory forms of delusion, this content is basically incapable of proof.

It is not the content which is the morbid factor in delusion, but the relationship to the world and to fellow-men which has lost all generality, become deranged. Delusion is a disturbance of the common experience which a person shares with his fellow beings.

(*d*) A delusion is an *isolating* conviction. The private reality of the delusion separates the patient from the community. He is alone with his delusion in a state of isolation, removed from the common world of his fellow men by virtue of his alienation.

In general delusions are not communicable, with the exception of symbiontic delusions (see p. 191).

(*e*) Delusional reality is the *reality of an individual*, referring to himself and through him to his world – 'It always has to do with me' (*Protocol 38*).

The reference is always to the individual's own self, even if in the foreground the so-called external world seems changed.

(*f*) *Man is basically liable to delusions.* This is part and parcel of the way in which the world exists for him. The world is only what it seems to be in the receptivity of his existence ('openness' in Heidegger's sense (1927) – *Offenheit des Daseins*).

Human existence and the human world thus belong together. Normal people can have a common area of receptivity and agree about a common world in a way which is not possible for many mentally ill patients. Experience of the self and of a world that is destructive, split, dissolved, confined, oppressed, persecuted or poisoned correspond to modes of existence that are warped, imprisoned, confined, divided or disintegrated.

Delusional mood, sudden delusional ideas, delusional thought, delusional perception, delusional elaboration, delusional system

A delusional conviction may appear suddenly (sudden delusional idea) or may develop gradually. Delusions generally develop from a *delusional mood*. The patient feels a sense of alarm, that 'something is wrong' or something strange is happening to him, that he himself or his surroundings are changing (depersonalization, derealization); there is a feeling of shock, fear, menace, of anxious anticipation, of suspicion, uncertainty, bewilderment or oppression. More rarely the mood is elevated to one of rapture and conviction. The delusional mood will then be without any systematic content.

The delusional patient is characteristically engrossed in his delusion, his experience is governed by it, he broods and meditates over it (*delusional thoughts*). The delusion may be shaped by further sudden ideas, by 'confirmatory' hallucinations and observations which are interpreted in the context of the delusion (*delusional perception*), by 'reasons', 'proofs', inferences and connections (*delusional elaboration*). When a coherent, self-contained structure has been clearly evolved, we speak of a *delusional system*.

The concept of *delusional dynamics* has been inferred from the way in which the patient's affective state accords with his experience and governs his actions. These dynamics vary from stormy productivity with marked concomitant mood swings to the seemingly affectless, grinding (*eingeschliffen*) repetition of old delusional ideas (residual delusion).

13.2   The nature of delusion

Delusional reality and reality
The relationship between delusional reality and reality may be described as follows:
    Delusional reality as the only reality
    Delusional reality as the dominant, but not the only, reality
    Delusional reality and reality existing side by side in parallel (Bleuler's 'double registration', 1911)
    Delusional reality and reality inextricably intermingled

Delusional reality as the only reality

The delusion may take the place of general human reality, which thus loses its validity. The patient is then trapped in his delusional world, removed from the common world into Bleuler's (1911) autistic, derealized experience of the world. This state is found particularly in acute, overpowering delusional existence.

EXAMPLES

Protocol 162 (Schizophrenia)

This girl believed at times that she was a saint, at times a whore. She was afraid that she would be murdered. This mood governed the way in which she experienced the world. For her there was only this hostile world; the ordinary human world no longer existed. From the standpoint of normal people, her misinterpretation of the world was complete.

Protocol 151 (Pick's Disease)

The patient thought he was President of the Federation and that he was driving up to the entrance of his office in the Federal capital. Impoverished, alone, severely affected by his psycho-organic illness, the reality of his situation was completely abandoned in favour of his delusion. His life and his actions were entirely governed by his new delusional interpretation which brought him higher status.

Delusional reality as the dominant, but not the only reality

Here delusional reality may be the more important reality for the patient, because it is more pressing, but general human reality does not completely lose its validity.

EXAMPLE

Protocol 19

A chronic paranoid schizophrenic thought she was the child of a royal family (delusion of origin) and felt she was being influenced and persecuted (delusion of persecution) and devoured by snakes which had eaten her brain.

Her delusional experience was undoubtedly real to her. But there was also another reality. She said: 'It is not as strong as reality. It is like dreaming while you are awake, it is like a fairy tale. It is not really real. But yet it is real, it is like another world. There is no connection.'

Delusional reality and reality existing side by side

The delusion may exist alongside a complete apprehension of reality, the one in no way disturbing the other. They bear no relationship to one another. The two worlds exist in parallel, in 'double registration' (Bleuler, 1911).

Protocol 133

A chronic schizophrenic thought his bowels had carbonized and that his lungs had withered, but for years he was able to support himself and follow his profession of building overseer.

Protocol 27 (Chronic paranoid psychosis in epilepsy)

The patient thought himself to be Director of the Institution but was still able to concern himself diligently with the work of his department.

Protocol 64 (Schizophrenia)

Mr B. insisted that he was not the son of Emil and Ida B., but the son of Edward VIII of England, and that his mother came from France. The world of the Bs remained his real world, but he still had no doubts about the other. He had been working for years as a bookkeeper.

Delusional reality and reality intermingled

Sometimes general human reality and delusional reality can barely be kept apart. The patient struggles to retain his consciousness of reality (q.v.), often at the cost of much anguish.

Many patients become severely anxious and bewildered. 'Everything is mixed up, a "salad lettuce".' Their thinking is confused. They may be benumbed and stuporose. Others try to test reality, which only renders their behaviour more conspicuously odd.

EXAMPLES

Protocol 20

This young schizophrenic said of the voices he heard and of his threatened feeling, which had not yet been systematized:
'I ask myself whether they have been put into my head or whether perhaps it really happened...I started asking myself in despair: what is real? I couldn't make out any more what was coming from outside, what was right – and what only seemed to me to be so, what I imagined...I couldn't tell the difference between what was real and what I invented. That was terrible, it was as if my world was ending.'

Protocol 129 (Schizophrenia)

The patient was not sure whether his feeling of being in telepathic communication with a deaf and dumb mute was real or not. So he decided to test it by walking naked across the street to her – if the telepathy were real, he argued, she would be expecting him to come naked.

Delusional interpretation

In a delusional state the ordinary world of one's fellow men acquires a new interpretation. The existence of the deluded patient, his receptivity (*Offenständigkeit*), and his ability to share with his fellows a common understanding of the world he encounters, all these are changed: he is a changed man living in a changed world. The change within him is often not as clear as the effect upon him of his changed interpretation of the world around him, especially in the frequently encountered delusions of reference and of persecution. In psychotic withdrawal from the world, on the other hand, the ego-change may appear to be the only obvious one; there is no apparent change in the world, because the world no longer exists for the patient.

Delusional interpretation may affect exclusively or predominantly the patient himself (his self-existence); or the world around him; or both the ego and the world.

Change in self-existence

This may be systematized in the following areas: conscience; health; vitality; economic status; origin; role; identity, shape, physiognomy, age; ego-consistency; ego-demarcation; ego-activity.

Conscience (*conscientia*) – delusion of guilt:

EXAMPLES

Protocol 90 (Schizophrenic depression)

This young man showed poverty of movement; he was sunk in himself, spoke in a soft voice and displayed little mimicry. During the day, while fully awake, he distinctly saw black eyes in front of him, which he took to be the eyes of the devil. The devil, he said, had come to him because he had once, years ago, invited a girl to go skiing with him but had never visited her again. He felt guilty about this event and worried lest perhaps he had also 'harmed other people mentally'.

He felt anxious, oppressed, unsure, at times completely changed, as if he were no longer quite master of himself.

(The diagnosis of schizophrenia was based on an earlier psychotic experience and on other symptoms not detailed here.)

Protocol 8 (*Depressive schizophrenia*)

The patient was plagued by devilish voices which reproached him for earlier, trifling sins. The voices threatened him with damnation, with no possiblity of redemption. Subjectively the worst feature of the mental state was the feeling of being completely given over to guilt.

(The diagnosis of schizophrenia was based on further symptoms not detailed here.)

Health – hypochondriacal delusions:

EXAMPLES

Protocol 56 (*Depression*)

The patient, a despairing old man, felt that he was lost and had to die. He said that his bowels no longer functioned, his stools were accumulating, and that he could no longer eat anything. He knew that he was decaying and had already smelt the smell of decay.

Protocol 110 (*Depression*)

The patient thought he had cancer of the stomach and that his bowels were closed because of cancer. He could not defecate and had lost 7 kg in three weeks, this furnishing proof of his conviction.

Protocol 113 (*Depression in a schizophrenic*)

The patient felt that she was changed, that her body was ill. She felt that her insides were cancerous, rotten, dead, and that a bad smell was emanating from her.

Vitality – delusion of physical disaster, putrefaction, death:

EXAMPLE

Protocol 16 (*Schizophrenia*)

The patient became more and more aware that she had no strength. Eventually she complained of uncanny happenings. 'One doesn't know any more that one is oneself.' Her body felt 'as if deformed' and a ripple passed through her like an electric current. She was no longer in control of her own thoughts and actions, but felt as if spellbound or enchained. At the same time there was a growing fear of being overwhelmed by external influences and she felt that she was being manipulated and persecuted.

In her anxiety the patient became mute ('so hopeless and desperate that one can't speak with anyone any more') and paralysed (catatonic stupor). One night she cried out in fear. She exhibited feelings of devitalization and delusions of disaster and persecution. There was disturbed ego-activity and feelings of external influence, which led to mutism and stupor.

Economic status: delusion of financial ruin, delusion of poverty:

EXAMPLE

Protocol 57 (Involutional depression)

This 60-year-old man was constantly tormented by thoughts of financial ruin. In his feeling of inadequacy he was convinced that he was no longer capable of following his profession, that he would achieve nothing more, and that his memory and powers of thought were failing. He tormented himself with feelings of guilt towards his wife, since his incompetence had reduced her, too, to misery and want.

Change in self-existence: delusion of change (delusional metamorphosis) (see also *Ego-identity*):

Change in origin – delusion of descent:

EXAMPLES

Protocol 29 (Chronic paranoid psychosis in genuine epilepsy)

The patient lived in a world of exaggerated status and high connections, e.g. great wealth, mother of many children and influential husband. She had traced her descent from the House of Windsor.

Protocol 64

See p. 154.

Changes in role, status, ability: Here there may be an exaggeration of role, or the assumption of a different and important mission in life. In worldly or religious terms, the patient may campaign for a better world, for better conditions for mankind, against a world cataclysm, for a new fellowship of man, a new religion. The delusions may include being a prophet or a Messiah. Cosmological delusion (the ability to create a new world) and delusions of omnipotence also occur.

EXAMPLE

Protocol 4 (Schizophrenia)

The patient suspected that something great and significant was happening, which made him happy but at the same time anxious. He sensed the dawning of a new world in the coming of which he himself was of special religious significance. He rejoiced in the great task before him and in his guidance by God. But he was also uneasy about his task, worried that the new world would not come so quickly and that he was perhaps not well enough equipped for it.

Change in person (delusional change into another person):

EXAMPLE

Protocol 17 (Schizophrenia)

This young patient suddenly felt that she was an old woman, that she had changed into her mother.

Change in physiognomy: sometimes a feeling of changed identity may crystallize only as a change in facial features, perhaps only in the nose. It is possible that the hands, too, have a special significance: many catatonics stare wonderingly at their hands – see *Ego-consciousness.*

EXAMPLE

Protocol 130 (Schizophrenia)

'My head is not my own head...I am the only one that has a nose...a new nose.'

Change in shape:

EXAMPLES

Protocol 53 (Schizophrenia)

This 63-year-old patient believed that for 40 years she had been followed by a man who was 'trimming' her, so that in the last few months she had lost

17 cm in height and had acquired a beard. She also maintained that the man was 'infiltrating' her thoughts. Physically she was of pyknic build and displayed oxycephaly and hirsuitism.

Protocol 68 (Schizophrenia)

This 24-year-old patient felt changed in her figure, her hands and her feet. Her blood, she believed, had become thinner, perhaps because of something she had eaten.

Protocol 35 (Schizophrenia)

'My skeleton has changed, I have a crooked hand – that is how I know my body.'

Change into an animal:

EXAMPLE

Protocol 34 (Schizophrenia)

'I am an animal...I am in the family way and will give birth to an animal...'

Change into a monster:

EXAMPLE

Protocol 34 (Schizophrenia)

'I have four heads to carry around.'

Ego-consistency (q.v.) – splitting

Ego-demarcation (q.v.), alien influence, loss of ego-boundaries, expansion

Ego-activity (q.v.) – alien influence

Change in the external world

It should be emphasized again that *changes in the external world are never isolated (because ego and world are always one) and that if the external world at times seems alone to change this is only superficially so – the patient is no longer capable of realizing that he too has changed.* There may be different reasons for this phenomenon. In oligophrenia and dementia, self-perception is lacking or is defective because of impaired apperception and judgement. In states of clouded consciousness, in all experiences of fascination, in exogenous or endogenous psychoses of acute onset, self-perception is impossible. In depersonalization, especially when the patient is unsure of his own identity, he detects changes in the self chiefly from outward signs, e.g. facial expressions, what other people say about him.

Derealization and delusional mood. Initially these changes may be hard to define; they often begin with a vague feeling that the external world has changed, that it is unfamiliar (derealization), peculiar, full of signs which cannot yet be interpreted and of meanings which are still unknown (delusional mood, not yet thematized). Derealization, like depersonalization, and delusional mood belong together.

EXAMPLE

Protocol 37 (Schizophrenia)

'You know, everything has a terrible significance for me.'

The delusional patient's experience of the external world. As long as the patient can remain receptive to the world, which still exists for and is accessible to him, so the world seems different from what it used to be. The meaning he attaches to what appears before him, is determined by his mood; and this mood is usually one of anxiety.

To the anxious person the world seems frightening, hostile, threatening, restrictive, destructive or poisonous; it may exert a negative influence, or it may exhibit signs. To the dejected person, everything is too much; he carries an oppressive, unmanageable burden.

Even the healthy man with a bad or disturbed conscience can be tormented by mistrust and by anxious suspicion, so that events which would otherwise seem harmless are taken as signs that he is under suspicion. However, the normal but mistrustful man can still take account of ordinary common realities, even though his bad conscience may make them appear in some circumstances to be not quite the same, and he organizes his behaviour accordingly. By contrast, the delusional patient can no longer change the point of view to which he is mistakenly committed.

It is not only in the fairly common delusion of persecution that the world seems full of negative signs: hypochondriacs too, and even manic patients, may find their world full of such negative portents (see p. 186). In both conditions the patients themselves have changes in their own way; their mood is not what it used to be, and so they experience a different world.

EXAMPLES

Protocol 157 (Alcoholic hallucinosis)

The patient heard men plotting to kill him; he saw in the forest figures which were watching him, he heard the steps of his persecutors, and ran away in terror.

Protocol 95 (Schizophrenia)

The patient experienced acute delusions of persecution on a journey to Prague. There were many signs that made him certain that he was being threatened and watched. Thus, the curtain in his room had moved in a curious way, and the mirror had been placed so that he could be observed. There was a listening device in the radio. The waitress would not speak to him at first, and then spoke in German. The waiter went to the desk in a peculiar way, presumably to photocopy his notes secretly. It appeared very strange that the waiter brought ice to his room, though he had not ordered any. An acquaintance arrived a few days after the date on which they had agreed to meet. A colleague said things which all referred to the patient. Pains in his hips were caused while he was drugged, by something being implanted which was intended to turn him into a criminal.

More rarely the delusional world is more beautiful than the ordinary world which in some circumstances may be rejected. The deluded patient is sometimes successful, or partly successful, in creating for himself a happier world, at the cost, of course, of psychotic isolation: there may be boosting of the ego in delusions of descent, of greater power, or of more possessions (see p. 157).

Such reshaping of the world for the better is found in schizophrenia and also in other chronic delusional psychoses, e.g. in epileptics. Ecstatic bliss is experienced in twilight states, e.g. in epilepsy and in the oneiroid states of acute schizophrenia, e.g. religious inspirations, talking to God, erotic happiness.

EXAMPLES

Protocol 35 (Schizophrenia)

'All the rulers of the earth live in Paradise to make themselves smaller, to become boys and girls...I am the gardener in Paradise.'

Protocol 75 (Schizophrenia)

The patient went through an oneroid phase. 'These pictures there are of my bridegroom's brothers and sisters...He is speaking to me, the Lord Jesus...I am pregnant with twins, look, the little dolls, there they are.'

Protocol 135 (Schizophrenia)

This young patient felt himself to be led by God, first through Hell and then into Heaven, cf. Dante. 'Heaven is empty, there are no angels, no people. It is like a gentle land in early spring, with green meadows, gentle valleys, a couple of cherry trees in blossom.'

Changes in the ego and in the world

On closer examination it is nearly always possible to see that the ego and the world are inseparable. This is often self-evident to the patient, and is expressed in the delusion in which the patient himself feels changed and at the same time the everyday world acquires a new significance.

EXAMPLES

Protocol 56 (Depression)

The patient experienced his own physical decay, smelt his own putrefaction. From the behaviour of those around him he knew that other people were aware of his rotting state and were avoiding him. Even a blackbird, he said, flew away from him. Here there were hypochondriacal delusions and delusions of reference.

Protocol 11 (Schizophrenia)

'I know that I have cancer...I can feel the lumps, I see little animals in my throat...The doctor has examined me and says he can find nothing. When he said goodbye and shook hands with me, he nodded his head and I knew it meant that I really had got cancer.' Here too there were hypochondriacal delusions and delusions of reference.

Certainty of interpretation that takes no account of experience

In this state delusions appear on the scene as *a priori* evidence. The patient needs no proof in order to be convinced that his interpretation is correct.

EXAMPLE

Protocol 38 (Schizophrenia)

'It is an inner proof, an intuitive proof, it is simply certain.'

From the standpoint of other members of the patient's group, the delusional interpretation is not well founded and there are no compelling grounds for it: in other words, a normal person would not find the same conclusion inevitable.

N.B. This is not to say, however, that the delusion is basically beyond comprehension. If we know the life history of the patient and his mood, the delusion, i.e. the theme of the delusion (its 'being just so' (*Sosein*) in Kurt Schneider's sense, 1967), often becomes understandable. Not every delusion can be comprehended, however, nor can the how and why of delusions always be explained.

Dissent from and resistance to the general experience and the group conviction

Delusional reality is a valid reality for the patient, no matter how improbable and incredible the content of the delusion and how much it is at variance with the categories of apperception to which the patient formerly adhered and with those of his group.

The delusion is therefore resistant to logical argument. It is only when the delusion is breaking down (q.v.) that the patient may be induced to doubt it. However, such a breakdown of belief cannot be accomplished by counter-argument.

The patient is likewise not bothered by the difference, or even the contradiction, between his belief and the collective beliefs, opinions and attitudes of the society to which he used to belong. In his illness he is removed from society in a state of isolation or alienation.

Inability to change one's point of view

The normal person, and the neurotic, lives in a world which can be shared with the members of his socio-cultural environment. He is able to compare his experiences with those of others and to modify them. He can change his attitude, his point of view and his perspective, either as a result of his own reflection or by coming to an understanding with others, which reaches agreement in objectivity or so-called reality – by all such means he can adapt to new facts in an elastic and flexible manner.

None of these possibilities is open to the delusional patient. He has no insight into his own standpoint and cannot place it in perspective; he is caught, overpowered by the certainty of his new interpretation and he is frozen by the new evidence (Conrad, 1958) which he no longer shares with his fellow men. His mood, his affect, governs his experience of the world – and separates him from other men. In his delusion he is removed from the world of other people; he is deranged in a private world whose validity exists for him alone.

This inability to change one's point of view is not by itself a criterion of delusion. The depressed patient who sees the whole world as dark, burdensome and oppressive, is also unable to accept other points of view. He too can no longer see things in perspective.

Isolation and alienation

Delusion means isolation, removal from the common world of fellow men. The delusional patient is alone.

EXAMPLE

Protocol 20 (Schizophrenia)

This young man faced the 'despairing question, what is then real?...it was as if my world was ending...'

He repeatedly called out in anxious agitation: 'God is all-powerful'. He pinned his hopes on this imploring cry for help: 'God give me help...I did not think he would abandon me.' In his state of anxious agitation he ran naked on to the street. 'I was so abandoned and thought there was no one left any more. I thought it was the end of the world, that chaos had come. So I ran out on to the street.'

It is in the delusional state that we see most clearly the isolation and alienation of the psychotic. His relationship to the people and the objects of his world is disturbed (cf. disturbance of sympathetic feelings in the sense of Scheler, 1913; Mayer-Gross, 1932; disturbance of the intersubjective constitution of man, Blankenburg, 1971). It is not that he does not perceive them, for even the autistic patient is very attentive to his surroundings. It is rather that his apperception of what he perceives is special, peculiar, different from the usual, i.e. from his own previous apperception and from that of his group. Thus even his closest associates are unable to share his experience and in general his delusions cannot be communicated in that no genuinely mutual understanding can be reached. Only in symbiontic psychoses (Scharfetter, 1970) are shared delusions encountered.

From the standpoint of the normal man the deluded patient is set apart by the fact that normal people cannot accept a delusion, since it goes against both their reasoning and their capacity for empathy, which is not to say that the delusional state and the content of the delusion are incomprehensible. The patient's delusional conviction, which is not based on experience but to which he desperately adheres (the evidence of 'I know'), gives him an autistic, private, restricted and hence privative view of the world and makes it impossible for him to reach a common understanding with others. In consequence he is set apart from the community of his fellow men.

13.3   Conditions which promote the development of delusions

Basically a delusion is a special form of apperception of the self and of the world, and as such it is separative (privative). It sets the patient apart from his fellow men. Everyone is always in some frame of mind, or mood, which determines his experience of himself and of his world: mood disposition (*Gestimmtheit*) is, in other words, the way in which an individual exists in the world and the way in which the world exists for him.

Even in normal people a change in mood can modify their view of the world, making it different from their own previous view and from the views of their fellow men. To a man who is sad the whole world is grey and difficult, dreary and empty, and he cannot elect to have another point of view. To a man in high spirits everything seems easy and rapid. The suspicious man reads signs into harmless events, words, mimicry and gestures, that tell him people know the reason for his suspicion (cf. delusional suspicion), that they know about his bad conscience, his weakness, his defencelessness or his isolation.

To the person in love the world is a changed place and is full of signs and portents which announce the presence of his beloved. To the anxious man things that are otherwise harmless become threatening. The more mood governs experience, the more difficult it is even for the normal person to adopt another point of view, to change his standpoint. But he does manage to do this, so long as he still can come to an understanding with other people, so long as he still recognizes his own experience as special and in some circumstances controlled by identifiable events, so long as his own experience can be seen in perspective.

Delusion and age. Age plays a part in determining the choice of theme (see Berner, 1965). In our own material, hypochondriacal delusions were found to be independent of age, though other authors have shown them to be related to puberty and to old age. Delusional change of identity, including delusions of origin, did not usually develop after the age of 30. Over the age of 50, the predominant themes were persecution, hypochondriasis and religion.

Delusion and sex. Erotic delusions are more frequent in women than in men. Delusions of grandeur are almost entirely confined to men. The other delusional themes show no significant correlations with sex.

Delusion and intelligence. The development of delusions has no direct connection with impairment of intelligence. People of high intelligence are just as liable to delusion as the less gifted. Intelligence does, however, play a part in the elaboration and verbalization of delusions. Chronic patients of good intelligence are able to develop complicated and elaborate delusional pictures. The delusions of the mentally deficient and of dements may be very blunt and crude.

EXAMPLE

Protocol 180 (Schizophrenia in a mentally defective patient)

This peasant boy dreamed of a new farm on a sunny slope and of new cattle. He heard voices which advised him to set fire to the existing farm so that a new one would be built. He saw beautiful cows coming through the air from a mountain pasture. Then he started the fire and went off to an inn. When arrested, he asked whether the new farm was now being built where he wanted it.

Mood disposition always governs experience of oneself and of one's own world: this applies equally to delusion. Depending on the mood of the patient and the way in which this is governed by his life history and situation, we may say that there are four groups of conditions which favour the development of delusions:

Delusion as a hardening of affective disposition

Delusion 'determined' by life history and situation

Delusion as a transient reaction to certain sensory situations and to hallucinogens

Delusion as an expression of, and an attempt to overcome, changes in self-experience

This classification has been drawn up purely for didactic purposes and is based on associations which are often, but no no means always, in evidence.

Delusion as a hardening of affective disposition (Table 3)

Sometimes the mood governing the delusion is uniform and unambiguous; the delusion is then *synthymic*, i.e. content and mood are concordant, and *holothymic*, i.e. the mood takes the patient over entirely and uniformly without any great inner conflicts. This is seen in the delusions of depressed and at times also of manic patients.

Depression

The delusions of depressed patients are governed by lowered vitality, fears of perishing, and feelings of guilt.

Delusion of personal disaster	Delusion of perishing
	Delusion of decay
	Delusion of death
Delusion of personal disaster through illness	Hypochondriacal delusion
Delusion of personal disaster through poverty through starvation, etc.	Delusion of poverty

Delusion of personal disaster
  through guilt and sin
  through punishment

Delusion of complete personal
  and general catastrope
  (cataclysmic, with the end
  of the world)

Delusion of sin
Delusion of damnation
Delusion of punishment
Depressive delusion of
  persecution
Nihilistic delusion

Mania

The heightened feeling of vitality found in manic patients may increase their sense of their own strength and power, their belief in their own abilities and their own possessions. At times this amounts to *delusions of grandeur*. These may be followed by a (secondary) fear of being robbed of greatness and possessions, leading to *delusions of harm*.

So far it is possible to infer how a patient with such a definite melancholic or manic disposition comes to have delusions. However, this does not explain why one such person becomes deluded, and in a particular way, e.g. with delusions of guilt or illness, while another does not. The reaction is governed by the degree of affective upset and by the personal life history and the social and cultural experience.

Where religious creeds offer concrete threats of Hell, delusions of damnation will flourish, as indeed they do in Catholic areas, though very little in Protestant neighbourhoods. Where religious feelings of guilt are indoctrinated, these will be incorporated in the illness. Where medical enlightenment and rudimentary anatomical knowledge make minds uneasy, as, for example, when a prominent person or a relative or close acquaintance has suffered or died from heart failure or cancer, then this theme will be adopted.

Where sexual potency is decisive in determining self-esteem, the patient will experience devitalization in his own sexual organs, e.g. withering of the genitalia in India.

These considerations do not, of course, cover the ultimate why of delusion (its 'being there' as opposed to its 'being so' (*Dasein* as opposed to *Sosein*, Schneider, 1949, 1952): the ultimate cause of the

Table 3. *Delusion as a hardening of affective disposition:*
mood entirely governs experience

Motive/affect	Form of delusion	Occurs in
Lowered feeling of vitality	Delusion of illness Delusion of disaster	Depression
Depressed mood	Nihilistic delusion	Schizo-affective psychosis
Feeling of guilt	Delusion of poverty Delusion of guilt/damnation	
Heightened feeling of vitality	Delusion of grandeur	Mania

change from the real experience of the world, in the sense of a common, shared reality, to the de-real, autistic experience (Bleuler, 1911), the reasons why the patient deviates and becomes deranged, remain unknown.

Delusion 'determined' by life history and situation[3] (Tables 4, 5, 6)

The patient's life situation, combined with additional personality factors, either innate or acquired, can often lead to delusion. The constellation of life events provides the framework for an 'affective need of delusion' (Bleuler, 1911).[4]

The affective states in question take many forms but may be grouped roughly as follows:
Insecurity
Restriction of freedom
Isolation
Intolerable injury to self-esteem
These factors are often found in association, especially insecurity and isolation.

Delusion as a thematization of insecurity and isolation

When a person in *old age* feels that his strength and intellectual abilities are declining, he may become insecure. If, in addition, he is

Table 4. *Delusion determined by life history and situation –*
delusion as thematization of insecurity and isolation

Situation providing motivation for the delusion	Motive affect	Form of delusion	Nosological classification
Weakness of old age	Insecurity Isolation	Delusion of harm, of persecution, of robbery	Paranoid development
Sensory defect (e.g. hearing difficulties)	Insecurity Isolation Mistrust	Delusion of reference, of harm	Paranoid development
Exile in country where he cannot understand the language	Linguistic isolation	Delusion of harm, of persecution	Paranoid development
Political persecution Concentration camp	Insecurity Apartness Isolation	Delusion of persecution	Paranoid development

alone, he may well feel abandoned and defenceless and in his anxiety,
combined with advancing psycho-organic decline, he may lose
control of reality. Anxiety is then the governing mood that makes
him feel persecuted, spied upon, robbed or harmed. In his isolated
state he can no longer discuss this experience with his partner and
perhaps rectify it. A similar experience may befall those who suffer
sensory impairments and who also are often isolated. Impaired
hearing and deafness are conducive to suspicion, which can lead to
delusional convictions, e.g. delusions of reference, of harm. Delusions
occur more rarely in cases of impaired sight.

Exiles who cannot understand the language of their new country
often feel exposed and abandoned. They cannot make themselves
understood and, becoming increasingly mistrustful, may develop
delusions of harm or persecution. The same reaction may occur over
years with the politically persecuted.

Table 5. *Delusion determined by life history and situation –
delusion resulting from intolerable insult, impotence*

Situation providing motivation for the delusion	Intolerable injury to self-esteem	Forms of delusion	Nosological classification
Bad conscience	Feeling of moral inferiority Mistrust	Delusion of reference	Sensitive delusion of reference Paranoia
Unfair legal decision	'Juridical' feeling of inferiority	Querulant delusion	Fighting paranoia
Sexual impotence	Sexual feeling of inferiority	Delusional jealousy	Delusional development, e.g. in alcoholism

Delusion in intolerable injury to self esteem

A bad conscience can lead even normal people to watch their
surroundings tensely and to read meanings into objects, gestures or
words that would otherwise be regarded as harmless.

A feeling of *moral inferiority* arouses mistrust and the suspicion
that everything around is in code. It may lead to the delusion that
other people know of one's lapse, that they are spreading rumours
about the 'conscience-stricken man' which expand into ever widening
circles – *sensitive delusion of reference* (Kretschmer, 1966).

Sometimes the sensitive patient may battle with the rumour-
mongers and take violent revenge: *fighting paranoia* (see the case of
Wagner, Gaupp, 1920, 1938; and Kretschmer, 1966).

Many sensitive people may greatly exaggerate a slight injustice.
The feeling of being wronged by the law, 'juridical feeling of
inferiority' when defeated in law, may become unbearable and
develop into a permanent goad that makes the patient fight, protest
against alleged injustices, or submit endless petitions to the courts
– *querulant delusion* (cf. Kleist's *Michael Kohlhaas*).

Feelings of *sexual inferiority* when potency decreases or is lost, e.g.

as a result of diseases of the sexual organs or spinal cord, or in alcoholism, may develop into a persistent ego-sickness leading to a delusional conviction that one's partner is being unfaithful – *delusional jealousy* – though this is not to say that every case of morbid jealousy is so caused.

Homosexuality, if unacceptable because of social pressures, may also perhaps lead to delusional hostility (see the case of Schreber, Freud, 1911).

Delusion as a substitute reality when reality is inadequate

Poverty, low birth, unfulfilled erotic desires or desire for pregnancy may in some circumstances induce a permanent ego-sickness.

A normal person is aware of his unfulfilled desires, looks for means of fulfilling them, and suffers if he does not succeed in doing so. Some people, however, not only suffer but have to and are able to convert this pressure into a *delusional compensation*; this is, of course, an hypothetical explanatory interpretation. The patient, at the cost of psychotic derangement, finds his desire fulfilled in his delusion: the delusion becomes a substitute reality, the so-called 'desiderative' delusion.

EXAMPLES

Protocol 116 (Schizophrenia)

This 24-year-old unemployed girl thought she had been wooed in Spain by a diplomat. She had never seen him, he made contact with her only through intermediaries and signs: the conduct of strangers or the presence of road-blocks, for example, were seen as signs from him to her. She heard his voice and could speak to him by radio. By opening the boot of his car he had spoken to her of marriage, saying that they were 'spiritually married'. He spoke to her about their two children, she being one of them and he the other.

Protocol 83 (Schizophrenia)

This 35-year-old chronic patient had a delusional relationship with a nurse, which she controlled by her choice of certain foods. When she saw the nurse or was in delusional contact with her, she experienced bodily sensations as if in sexual intercourse with her (homoerotic delusional love).

Erotic lack of fulfilment and loneliness may thus be regarded as the motivation for delusional love, for the delusional conviction that one is loved and is the object of erotic desires or, in a more negative way, the object of erotic attack or even rape. Delusional love can then lead to erotic delusions of persecution.

EXAMPLE

Protocol 33 (Schizophrenia)

An older women, living alone, wanted to break out of her state of lonely isolation and was looking for an admirer. At the same time she was anxious about the situation and rejected suitors who were available. She then developed an erotic delusion of persecution, believing that she had been captured and carried off by white slavers.

In psychoses an unfulfilled desire for children may be elevated into a delusion of being pregnant or of having borne many children. This does not mean that such an interpretation can be applied to every delusion of pregnancy, especially the rare delusion exhibited by schizophrenic men who believe that they will bear children.

EXAMPLES

Protocol 156 (Epilepsy and mental deficiency)

This young patient thought that she was pregnant and that a rotating sphere in her stomach was her child. She had, in fact, been sterilized.

Protocol 34 (Schizophrenia)

'I am an animal...I am in the family way and will bring an animal into the world.'

Poverty, low intelligence and insignificant group role, plus the feelings of unimportance and inferiority that accompany them, may sometimes be elevated into a *delusion of wealth*, often associated with a *delusion of origin*.

EXAMPLE

Protocol 29, see p. 157.

Table 6. *Delusion determined by life history and situation –*
delusion as a substitute reality when reality is inadequate

Situation providing motivation for the delusion	Intolerable injury to self-esteem	Form of delusion	Nosological classification
Erotic lack of fulfilment, and loneliness	Erotic need, isolation	Delusion of love	Sensitive delusion of reference, schizophrenia
Unfulfilled desire for children	Unfulfilled motherhood	Delusion of pregnancy Delusion of motherhood	Schizophrenia, organic, including epileptic, psychoses
Poverty, insignificant role	Feeling of inferiority	Delusion of wealth Delusional rise in status	Organic psychoses (GP)
Lowly origin	Feeling of inferiority	Delusion of origin	Schizophrenia, organic psychoses
Imprisonment, especially life imprisonment	Loss of liberty, especially isolation, no future	Delusion of mercy Delusion of innocence	Paranoid reaction

Insignificant lowly origins may likewise produce a persistent, driving feeling of inferiority which can form the basis of a *delusion of origin*. Again, however, this is not to say that all forms of delusional origin can be interpreted in the same way.

Imprisonment, especially solitary confinement for life, is one of man's intolerable situations. Loneliness and lack of liberty hem him in, not only in the external sense of restricting his movements, but also in the sense of his lack of a settled future. He sees there is no more hope. In such a situation he may develop a *delusion of mercy* or a *delusion of innocence*.

It is conceivable, though it has not been proved, that some *delusions of salvation* (such as occur at times in schizophrenics) may have their roots in anxiety about feeling ill and may represent a delusional attempt to overcome this intolerable situation.

Delusions as a reaction to certain sensory situations (*deprivation, flooding*) and to hallucinogens (*Table 7*)

Sensory deprivation may occur extraneously, e.g. in shipwreck, on Arctic expeditions, in desert expeditions, or in sailing single-handed across the Atlantic (Lindemann, 1957). Reports of such experiences speak of depersonalization, derealization, delusional misinterpretation of the situation, delusional and hallucinatory wish fulfilment: the seeing of land, coming to an oasis, hearing encouraging voices, feeling oneself raised up and guided.

In experimental sensory deprivation, too, in which the lack of sensory afference is usually more complete than in accidental isolation, delusional misinterpretations are frequent: for example, the subject may state that the cell is not soundproof, that noises are coming in, that something is being introduced into the experimental cell, that gas is entering. In thus misidentifying the situation, the subject may be attacked by panic and he may become deluded.

Table 7. *Delusion as a reaction to a given situation – delusion in sensory deprivation and under the influence of hallucinogens*

Situation providing motivation for the delusion	Motive/affect	Form of delusion	Nosological classification
Sensory deprivation Hallucinogens	Depersonalization Derealization Hallucination Illusion Anxiety	Delusion of threats Delusional interpretation of situation	Paranoid reaction Hallucinogenic psychosis, experimental, accidental

How far the same effects may be produced by *sensory flooding* is not known.

Under the influence of *hallucinogens*, accidental or experimental, there may be similar anxious experiences of depersonalization, derealization, hallucinations or illusionary misidentification. In some circumstances the affected subject then no longer knows that he is in an experimental situation; he delusionally misinterprets the situation, e.g. he thinks the dose was too high, or that he is mentally ill, and he may feel delusionally threatened.

Normal people, too, may experience delusion-like misidentification of a situation, particularly if they are overtired, or in a state of anxious anticipation or find themselves in surroundings that favour misidentification, e.g. at night or in fog.

EXAMPLE

Protocol 159

After a party a young women frantically kept herself awake with coffee and nicotine. She then felt 'funny' and uncertain and suddenly had the idea that she had been given a drug (hashish) in her coffee. She spoke freely about her fears and became calmer. She then drove off alone in her car and at night in the avenues of trees she seemed to see ghostly faces, though she knew these were hallucinations. She became worried that she might be becoming mentally ill. The next day she went to see a friend, still anxiously anticipating new hallucinations, and in her friend's heavily made-up face she saw a death's head.

Delusion in altered self-experience (*Table 8*)

In our discussion of ego-experience we mentioned the possibility of delusional interpretation of disturbances in the various ego-dimensions.

It cannot be said that the patient is mistaken when he constructs a threat to his ego-vitality. Through his delusion the patient is telling us of the threat to his existence, the disintegration of his existence, the destruction of his self-being and of his world; he is telling us how he has been overwhelmed by people and things which are persecuting and poisoning his threatened, vulnerable, restricted existence. He is describing to us the reality of his life. We can do the patient justice only by recognizing that this is his life's reality, only by taking it seriously, never if we treat it as delusion or fantasy. To do this is to brush the patient aside, to push him further into his isolation.

Disturbance of ego-vitality may be divided into: hypochondriacal delusion; delusion of personal disaster; delusion of the end of the world; delusion of persecution, delusion of poisoning.

It would seem that the delusional development does not necessarily stop at this declaration, as it were, of the patient's suffering (expressed at times symbolically in an abnormal modality) but that in special conditions, which still have to be investigated and which may conceivably correspond to the psycho-dynamic construct of 'defence', the development of a delusion brings relief. It is possible that the *delusion of healing* is a compensatory or over-compensatory means of mastering the fear of one's own illness, and that fear of the end of the world, by compensation or over-compensation might become a *delusion of a new world, a new creation, a reformed world*, or in religious guise a *prophetic, redemptive or messianic delusion*.

If the patient loses reality control, such an imagined, or imaginable, triumph over his suffering becomes a life-reality in delusion.

Sometimes feelings of guilt may be extended beyond the patient's own conscience and he becomes convinced of the wickedness of the whole world. This can provide a reason for him to overpower the evil world.

EXAMPLE

Protocol 31 (Schizophrenia)

After being the victim of attempted rape, this patient became depressed, with feelings of guilt and fears of pregnancy. The feeling of guilt led to the delusion that she should conquer the wicked world and found a new one.

Disturbances of ego-consistency may also, if the feeling of splitting spreads, become a delusion that the world, or the whole universe, is splitting or exploding. The patient's remedy lies in a delusion of a new world, a delusion of salvation.

EXAMPLE

Protocol 129 (Schizophrenia)

In 1971 this young man experienced a series of ego-disturbances. He stated, 'I am not like other men' – alienation, identity as man, feeling of his own difference. 'Probably I don't belong to this world... how should I have a name?... I am engaged in a cosmic battle between two galaxies, in which this world is involved too. The battle is being waged in the mind... I am complete chaos' – ego-splitting, cosmic struggle. He was afraid the world would be destroyed by an atomic explosion.

He remained in this state till 1974, when the pressure of his torment was successfully liberated in an upsurge of energy. Formerly depressed, the patient became manic and filled with a feeling of power. The cosmic struggle was reduced to a more contemporary and appropriate sense of the atomic destruction of the world: this could then be handled prophylactically – the patient developed proposals for preventing atomic war by founding a harmonious community of nations and was actively engaged in averting the danger. He was no longer disorganized, and felt at one with himself.

Sometimes the process of splitting results in double or plural identity – *delusions of plurality*:

EXAMPLE

Protocol 38 (Schizophrenia)

'I am we.'

Disturbances of ego-activity and ego-demarcation are associated with *delusions of alien influence* and *delusions of persecution*. If the patient's own activity is lost, then all power is in the hands of other people. It might be speculated that the loss of ego-boundary and the cessation of activity become, by overcompensation, a delusional feeling of *omnipotence*, of magic powers and creativity:

EXAMPLE

Protocol 40 (Schizophrenia)

'Since Christmas the tide has spiritually turned for me. Now I have absolute power and insight.'

The patient felt that he could read people's thoughts, influence their thoughts, communicate by telepathy or hypnosis.

'I can be God – and I will be God.'

'My spirit can enter into another body and do with it what it will.'

Table 8. *Delusion as an attempt to overcome changes in ego-experience (interpretation, explanation, supplementation, compensation, over-compensation)*

Dimension of ego-experience affected	Interpretation	Compensation and over-compensation	Occurrence
Ego-vitality	Hypochondriacal delusion Nihilistic delusion	Delusion of healing	
	Delusion of personal disaster	Delusion of healing Messianic delusion Delusion of reforming the world	Schizophrenia
	Delusion of the end of the world Delusion of persecution	Delusion of creating a new world	
Ego-activity	Delusion of alien influence Delusion of persecution	Delusion of omnipotence	
Ego-identity	Delusion of change of identity	Delusion of origin	
Ego-consistency	Splitting, disintegration, personal disaster, end of the world, ego-plurality	Messianic delusion	
Ego-demarcation	Delusion of alien influence Delusion of persecution	Magical extension to cover the whole world Experience of coalescence	

Omnipotence may also manifest itself as involvement in cosmic events: the *cosmic-astronomical delusion, or cosmogenic delusion* of world creation.

EXAMPLE

Protocol 30 (Schizophrenia)

'The sun and the moon have become one... The sun is eating up the stars; when it has eaten a lot of stars it will be stronger. According to whether it eats blue or red stars, there are sunspots or no sunspots.' The patient claimed to have power over the sun, to be able to pull it out from behind the clouds, to make the weather. When the moon is waxing, he said, it speaks to him and calls to him 'Come', meaning that he must die. This extension of the boundlessness of existence and of its power is clearly associated with the threat of the dissolution of existence and his own death.

13.4 Etymology of delusional thinking and delusion

What does language tell us of the essence of delusion? According to the etymologists, the words *Wahnsinn* (delusional thinking), *Wahn* (delusion) and *Wahnwitz* (delusional wit – cf. 'de-mentia') have various derivations (see Duden, 1963; Hofer, 1953; Wasserzieher, 1963).

Wahn (delusion) in Old and Middle High German is *wan* (empty) and is closely related to the Gothic *vans* (deficient, empty), the Latin *vanus, vastus* (empty). The word *Wüste* (waste or desert) comes from the same Indogermanic stem. Sinn (sense, mind) is originally direction or way of thinking. *Wahn-sinnig* (deluded) therefore means empty of sense or mind, defective in reason (wit).

Wahn (delusion) comes from the Indogermanic root *wen* which is still encountered in the New High German *gewinnen* (to win), meaning to look for something, to aspire to something, to wish, desire hope, long for, or assume in the sense of suppose. This is related to the Old and Middle German *wan* expectation, supposition, opinion, suspicion (cf. *Arg-wohn* = bad-expectation, suspicion). From the same Indogermanic root we obtain the English 'to win', the German *Wunsch* (wish), *Wine* or *Wini* meaning joy (cf. the names Winfried, Erwin), the Latin *venus* (love), the Old Indian *vanas* (desire, lust) and *vanati* (love).

This derivation of the word *Wahn* (delusion) thus already points to an element of striving and motivation, a desire to win or gain something (*gewinnen*), to assume something – cf. the contemporary pejorative form *Arg-wohn* (suspicion).

Delusion in a paranoid experience. *Paranoid* comes from the Greek παρά, νοῦς, νοός, i.e. mind, insight, reason. The term paranoid thus indicates a knowledge and an interpretation that ignores the generally shared common experience of the world and implies a disturbance of reality and sense of reference.

In English *Wahn* equals *delusion* – from the Latin *deludere, -lusi, lusum*, i.e. to play-act, to mislead. In delusion the patient, from the standpoint of his fellow men, sees an unreal world.

In Latin and in French *Wahn* is the equivalent of *delirium*, from *de lira ire*, 'to get out of the furrow' – to be pushed out (de-ranged) from the common world of men.

13.5 The gain in delusion (what is 'won' in *Wahn*) – concluding remarks

When we examine a delusion more closely in the context of the patient's life history, it becomes apparent that it can contain sense and answer a need. Many patients actually say this: as one said to Storch (1965), 'I build my own world, in order to surmount my misery.' Another said to Kretschmer (1963), apropos of reality, 'What do you want reality for? I think it is horrible'. Frau K (*Protocol 29*), talking about her beautiful delusional life, said 'That is my life, my freedom, my goal'.

It is not often, however, that the delusional world is more beautiful than the common world of man. At times the patient may succeed, often in part or intermittently, in achieving a happier world in his delusion, but at the cost of psychotic isolation. Sometimes ideas of exalted role status, noble descent, power, possessions, mandates, partnerships, or motherhood, bring the deluded patient a gain in terms of self-esteem. If such a delusion is to develop from his 'affective delusional need' (Bleuler, 1911), special conditions must already be present: for example, mental deficiency, dementia, an acute delusional episode with clouded consciousness, e.g. ecstatic inspiration in twilight state, or very acute disintegrative forms of psychosis.

In many forms of delusion a final interpretation of wish fulfilment does indeed suggest itself: delusions of noble descent, of healing, of being the Redeemer or reformer of the world, of being an inventor, of omnipotence, of love, of pregnancy, of motherhood, of riches, of mercy, of innocence. These can be viewed as examples of successful self-rescue through delusion (Kahn, 1929; O. Kant, 1927a, b, 1930), of flight into an autistic world apart, away from a reality that cannot be borne.

However, these are not the most common forms of delusion and the majority of delusional patients suffer great torment. How can we then arrive at any conclusive point of view? It is possible to take speculative interpretation much further, as for instance by advancing the view that the patient with delusions of persecution is experiencing an intense (if negative) benefit which brings him out of his isolation ('better to be persecuted than to be alone'),[4] or that the patient with Messianic or healing delusions can be altruistically concerned with other people, and that both these experiences increase his role status. The same logic can be applied to delusions of origin: 'I must be the child of another mother, because no real mother could behave as my mother did to me.'

In *delusional denial*, too, there is some finality, either positive or negative in form.

EXAMPLE

Protocol 29 (Delusional psychosis in epilepsy)

For this patient her mother, who died long ago, was still alive; she did not accept her death as real. At the same time she denied that she had a brother and refused to recognize him when he visited her, though she accepted the gift packages which he sent her.

Such conclusive interpretations can of course be attempted, but can hardly be corroborated by facts. It is easier at times to understand a delusion, especially in schizophrenia, as an attempt to overcome changes in self-experience (see p. 176). A first step in this direction might be to thematize and verbalize the delusion, attempting at least to establish the strange, worrying experience within an interpretation of self-experience. It can be no more than conjecture to suggest that further attempts to master the situation might develop into compensatory and over-compensatory ideas of the patient's experience, causing him to make a leap into the new delusional world. Anxiety acts as a 'compulsion to infer meaning' (E. Straus, quoted after v. Baeyer in: Schulte and Tolle, 1972, p. 2) and tends to lead to the attribution of meaning and significance. Out of the feeling 'I no longer understand myself and the world' comes the delusional belief 'I do understand' or perhaps even 'I understand better than before'. This is *delusion as a means of defence against the threat of the unfamiliar.*

Delusions of influence and delusions of persecution correspond to the extent to which the patient is affected and the extent to which he is dependent upon others. The reverse side of this is the notion of the dependence of others upon the patient, e.g. the inflation of the ego in omnipotence, in delusions of creating a new world, reforming the world, being a Redeemer, being an inventor. The overcoming of loneliness in delusions of persecution or in Messianic delusions and delusions of healing seem to bring the patient a new psychotic communion with his fellows. Denial or flight from the intolerable reality of his fate leads the patient to a semblance of freedom in delusion.

All this, of course, reveals nothing about why a man in an intolerable situation should succeed in creating a delusional world. Even if we can understand and can regard it as reasonable in the context of a patient's life history, this does not yet mean that we are in a position to explain the appearance of the delusion.

13.6   Causal associations of delusion

Delusions cannot be nosologically arranged according to their content and structure alone, i.e. without knowledge of their total psychopathological context.

Experimental situations

Some experimental situations, e.g. alterations of consciousness, sensory deprivation, the effects of hallucinogens, etc., may lead to delusional misinterpretation of the situation: 'reality' is then mis-identified and delusions of persecution or poisoning may appear. Similar effects may be produced accidentally (cf. p. 175).

Delusion as a reactive development

This is mostly a suspicious, paranoid, injured attitude in the face of the hearing difficulties, physical weakness, frustrations or deformities of old age.[5] Decrepitude and isolation provide the basis, and the ensuing *insecurity is thematized as delusion.* The injured attitude of the politically persecuted and of prisoners can also lead to delusion.

People removed to strange surroundings, where they do not understand the language, may come to adopt an attitude that is akin to the delusional, especially if they are immature and insecure. Should the native population be hostile, the reaction may become more pronounced (so-called exile's paranoia).

Prisoners, particularly in solitary confinement, may develop a paranoid prison psychosis characterized by delusions of destruction or of poisoning, e.g. gas being piped into the cell, perhaps accompanied by corresponding olfactory hallucinations or notions of food being poisoned. Another form of prisoners' delusion is the delusion of innocence or of mercy. More frequently there is a suspicious, paranoid, injured attitude.

Other forms of delusional reaction are the *sensitive delusions of reference and paranoia* (see the literature on special psychiatry). Kolle (1931) found a high incidence of schizophrenia in the relatives of patients with paranoid illness. The distinction between paranoia and paranoid schizophrenia is arbitrary.

Delusion in affective psychosis

Delusions in affective psychoses, especially depression, are more clearly 'morbogenic', i.e. attributable to the pathological mood (synthymic and holothymic) than is the case with schizophrenic delusions, where contemporary factors and the circumstances of the patient's life play a greater pathoplastic role and the change in affect is less clear and unambiguous – the so-called catathymic delusions.

Depression

Depressive mood and loss of feelings of vitality – with all the attendant insecurity, anxiety and feelings of inadequacy and guilt –

can lead to a depressive delusion in which the affective factor takes over and becomes the patient's world of reality.

With anxiety about physical well-being, hypochondriacal delusions and delusions of personal disaster may develop, the patients being convinced that they are ill, rotting, decaying, putrefying and ultimately ceasing to exist.

Delusions of financial ruin, of starvation, poverty, personal disaster ('I don't exist any more', 'I am just not alive') may be extended to the patient's immediate family, e.g. 'My wife and my children aren't living any more either', and ultimately to the whole world in *nihilistic delusions* (for the literature see Weber, 1938). In this depressively restricted and overwhelmed existence, the world is completely lost.

The experience of personal putrefaction, accompanied often by corresponding olfactory hallucinations like the smell of rottenness, corpses or the graveyard, can lead to *secondary delusions*, delusions of reference (e.g. 'I am rotting; they can smell it already; they are avoiding me; I can see they are shunning me, even the blackbird flew away from me.' 'I am a burden to everyone, the way I am').

These experiences may provoke or strengthen the impulse to commit suicide.

Other delusions include persecution (e.g. 'They want to destroy me'), or guilt, condemnation, damnation, in which ordinary little weaknesses, 'sins', offences against worldly or religious canons are magnified by the depressed patient into an intolerable, irredeemable burden. The patient is then tormented not only by self-reproach because his life seems to be a failure but also by a fear of punishment, execution or damnation in which he knows that his destiny is a lasting torment in hell.

Mania

In the affective psychosis of mania, delusions are rare. At times, however, exaggerated self-esteem and feelings of greatness and power can be magnified to the point of delusion – delusions of grandeur, megalomania. Here it is the manic expansive mood which entirely governs experience of the self and of the world. The existing affective mood takes over and becomes reality, assuming a delusional certainty. There is no firm boundary between delusional and non-delusional self-glorification. The distinction must be made on the basis of the manic patient's general mode of behaviour and therefore takes socio-cultural standards into account.

The content of simple manic delusions of grandeur includes enormous estates, a huge income, many attractive sexual partners, etc.

In the boundless expanse of his existence the manic patient may suffer from a vertiginous state akin to altitude vertigo, i.e. he may become insecure and worry about his 'high flying' – 'I have too much air in my head', 'There is too much air under my feet'. The patient may be concerned about whether to abandon his former rules and conditions of life and conduct.

Secondary delusions, e.g. of persecution or jealousy, may arise from this state and from the collision between manic self-esteem and espansiveness on the one hand and the real confines of everyday life on the other. The patient may believe that people grudge him his wealth, envy him for it, wish to steal it or to rob him.

Delusion in schizophrenia

The changes that occur in schizophrenia in respect of the self and the world and the loss of familiarity in states of alienation (derealization, depersonalization) constitute a delusional mood. At first this may still lack a theme ('Something is wrong, something is going to happen', etc.) and then, suddenly or gradually, its significance will dawn upon the patient who then develops a particular theme.

The delusional themes of schizophrenics are as varied as their life histories and depend upon the composition of their self-being (see *Ego-awareness*).

Delusion in psychoses of organic origin
Delusion in acute psychoses of organic origin

Delusional misidentification of situations and persons occurs in delirium and twilight states. A delirious patient thought that he was in his office, busily engaged in his professional work (so-called occupational delirium). A confused epileptic in a dream-like twilight state was entranced by his visual hallucinations and ecstatic inspirational experiences.

In alcoholic hallucinosis the patient often hears the threatening voices of people who are planning an attack on his life (delirious threats). In their anxiety patients with delusions of persecution sometimes flee blindly and may jump out of the window or otherwise harm themselves.

Delusions in chronic psychoses of organic origin

Delusions may occur in chronic organic psychoses of any aetiology. Delusions of reference and of injury arise in psycho-organic syndromes that foster insecurity and loneliness, often in old people living alone. Sometimes a delusion may develop before the amnestic psychosyndrome is even established. The true nature of the psychosis may then not be recognized, e.g. choreophrenia in Huntington's chorea, progressive paralysis.

A special group in which the most various forms of delusion occur consists in the *schizophrenia-like psychoses of epilepsy*.

Various forms of delusion are found in chronic *toxicomania* due to alcohol, amphetamine or cocaine.

In chronic *alcoholism* we may find an injured attitude developing, often predominantly concerned with sexual grievances (morbid jealousy).

In many progressive cerebral disorders, e.g. cerebral arteriosclerosis, a *dermatozoic* delusion may develop, with physical hallucinations of itching, prickling, crawling, etc.: the patient is convinced that his skin is crawling with little animals such as insects or worms. Sometimes this plague of ghostly creatures appears to enter the body – the bowels, sexual organs, bladder, etc., constituting an *enterozoic* delusion.

As the mind deteriorates in a psycho-organic syndrome and judgement becomes impaired, the way is sometimes open for delusions of grandeur, e.g. in Pick's or Alzheimer's cerebral atrophy, and in progressive paralysis.

EXAMPLE

See page 153.

In depressive illness of psycho-organic origin we may find *délire de négation* (delusional denial), ranging from *delusional smallness* (micromania) (for the literature see Cotard, 1882) to *general delusional nihilism* (q.v.). The opposite is the so-called *délire d'énormité*. For example, a patient did not defecate because he believed that the whole world would be flooded by his excrement and that everyone would be asphyxiated.

13.7 The course of delusion

The course of a delusion in the patient's subsequent life history depends entirely on the underlying illness, on the nosological category to which the delusion belongs and on the treatment administered.

Delusion in affective psychoses

The delusion subsides as the phase of affective psychosis subsides: it simply disappears and either there is no further talk about it or it is recognized as an erroneous fancy.

Delusion in psychoses of organic origin, e.g. in progressive paralysis, Pick's disease, etc.

The delusion may disappear as progressive cerebral disintegration leads to increasing dementia, though as judgement becomes more impaired it may first assume particularly grotesque forms.

However, even in psychoses of organic origin the delusion depends on the situation of the patient. If the patient feels that he is no longer alone and insecure, if he loses his feeling that it is no longer possible for him to understand or be understood, the delusion often disappears.

Delusion in special situations

A delusion can disappear when the special circumstances are removed.

Delusion in schizophrenia

This depends very much on the severity of the illness and on its treatment.

Acute psychotic episodes with transient, fairly unstructured delusions, often terminate spontaneously or quite quickly with psychotherapy or psychotropic drugs. In chronic illnesses the delusion may
persist for years. Patients may learn to live with their delusions: they
live 'in double registration' (Bleuler, 1911), delusional reality and
common reality existing side by side. Many learn to keep their sick
and normal experiences apart and no longer react to the sick
hallucinatory or delusional experience, often not telling anyone
about them any more.

In phasic illnesses the same delusion may keep recurring over the
years, disappearing as the morbid phase subsides. It is then switched
off, denied, forgotten, or perhaps still mentioned as a 'fancy', but it
no longer affects the patient's behaviour. Sometimes it may be dealt
with in a secondary way by rationalization, thus satisfying the
patient's need for causal connections.

Delusion as a reaction to life history and experience

Such delusions are often chronic and may in some circumstances last
a lifetime. The patient needs the structure of the delusion as a support
for his existence. A factor contributing to its persistence might also
be that an admission of its morbid nature would be too injurious to
the patient's self-esteem.

13.8 Effect of the delusion on the external world

Many patients living alone isolate themselves more and more in their
delusion and become completely withdrawn. In such cases the
delusion may go unrecognized for a long time, e.g. at their place of
work or among their neighbours.

EXAMPLE

During our family studies we heard of a deluded patient (in a rural
community) who had never been seen by a doctor. For years he had lived
alone in an attic, the doors of which were secured by bolts and bars. There
was only one old aunt to whom he sometimes said that at night in particular
he was afraid of persecutors, that he heard threatening voices and that he
was being tormented. Otherwise no one knew of his experience and he had
been going to work for years, often changing his job because he felt he was
being treated unfairly but never actually stating this at his place of work.

In many cases delusions may often go unrecognized for a long time by the patient's family, by friends, or by partners of lifelong standing. This depends very much on the patient's need to communicate and also on the theme of the delusion. For example, a delusion of persecution accompanied by defensive or protective measures, or morbid jealousy accompanied by accusations, are easier to notice than a hypochondriacal delusion or a delusion of guilt which the patient keeps for a long time to himself.

In general, a certain amount of odd, inexplicable or unacceptable behaviour is required before a family recognizes that one of its members is sick. Even then, depending on the behaviour of the patient, which is often changeable, the attitude towards him fluctuates between accepting the fact that he is sick, rejecting him, and excusing him on grounds of old age, overwork, difficulties at work or in personal relations.

A delusional illness in a member of the family or in a spouse is a heavy burden for the partner. Delusion is alien and uncanny and evokes anxiety and rejection; it often disturbs the community. Therapeutic help must often be made available to the partners of deluded patients too.

There are four main approaches that can be taken towards delusional patients (Schulte, 1972):

(1) To keep the patient at a distance.

Turning away from the patient leads to his increased isolation, separation and hospitalization.

(2) To accept the patient on his own terms.

Accepting the patient with full awareness of the nature of his illness makes it possible for him to remain within the community, even in a deluded state; it keeps open a way out of his delusion and may prevent re-admission to hospital. In cultures with a magical, religious outlook it is much easier for the patient to remain with his own people than in an urban industrialized civilization.

(3) To prolong the illness.

Sometimes the patient's partner may be more interested in prolonging the illness: as long as the patient remains ill, the partner maintains a more secure hold on him.

(4) To participate in the delusion.

Sometimes the delusion is shared, confirmed and even strengthened by the patient's relatives or life associates (shared delusion, see Baeyer, 1932). Very occasionally, against a background of hereditary predisposition and particularly binding psycho-dynamic factors, a *symbiontic psychosis* (Scharfetter, 1970) develops: one partner is 'induced' by the other, who is the first to fall ill, and participates to the extent that he himself becomes productively psychotic. These are rare cases in which the delusion itself is communicable.

13.9 Delusion from a transcultural point of view

Comparative psychiatry has enriched our knowledge of delusion (Murphy, 1967; Pfeiffer, 1970). The social and cultural relativity of this mode of experience and behaviour becomes clear in cross-sectional and historical comparative studies.

Delusion exists in every part of the world. Man seems basically liable to become deluded.

The socio-cultural status of the patient influences his proneness to delusion and thus the incidence of delusions; the content and theme of his delusion; the shaping and elaboration of his delusion; and the course and outcome.

Cultural influence on delusional liability

Different cultures exert different pressures to provide explanations for experience. The rational, technical outlook of urban industrialized cultures seems to be the most active in this direction. The explanations provided depend on cultural outlook, e.g. whether the culture recognizes a distinction between two worlds, an inner world and a transcendental one.

Paranoid schizophrenia seems to be more frequent in urban than in rural areas, where the inhabitants are more accustomed to the unfathomable and accept it as such. In Asiatic cultures, where there is less tendency to seek rational explanations, there are probably fewer deluded schizophrenics and more cases of schizophrenia simplex. People from cultures that believe in ubiquitous spirits develop fewer delusions, so long as they remain within their cultural community; however, they develop severe delusions when they are removed from their cultural setting.

Confrontation with the unknown can give rise to delusional elaboration, particularly if the individual is not prepared in advance for what is coming, e.g. the immigrant. Cultures with a strong bias towards the irrational and emotional show fewer individual delusions, because the entire community accepts the delusional conviction.

In cultures which are under pressure to change, paranoid reactions are in some circumstances an inevitable response to the situation.

Cultural influence on the content of delusions

While the main delusional themes – persecution, injury, religion, the end of the world, guilt, poverty, hypochondriasis – are to be found everywhere, the way in which they are elaborated depends partly on the patient's religious, partly on his political, background.

In primitive cultures we find belief in spirits and delusions of witchcraft; in the Judaeo-Christian culture we encounter delusions of guilt and of the end of the world, neither of which seems to occur frequently in Islamic and Buddhist societies. Local themes include, for example, delusions of marital infidelity in India and the delusion of being engaged or married in Ireland (Murphy, 1967).

The thematic elaboration of delusions is also influenced by the 'spirit of the age' and by the general state of knowledge (Kranz, 1955, 1967). Thus at the beginning of the century parapsychological and hypnotic influences were more frequent, whereas modern technology has given rise more to technical and physical influences, e.g. radiation, electric currents, radio. It is not yet clear how far hypochondriacal delusions have been affected by the spread of knowledge about atomic radiation.

Culture and the shaping of delusions

In European cultures, and particularly among persons of German descent, delusions tend to be more elaborate and there is a greater likelihood of their becoming chronic. In India there is little structural elaboration of delusions and it is often difficult to distinguish between delusion and the play of imagination and fantasy (Murphy, 1967).

Culture and the course of delusion

The pressure towards explanation and justification in European cultures causes delusions to become fixed and chronic. When a delusion is incorporated into collective beliefs, its acceptance as a case of witchcraft and its exorcism make it easier for the delusion to subside.

13.10   Hypotheses concerning delusion

Psycho-analysis

According to psycho-analytical theory delusion is brought about by projection. Freud saw projection as a defence mechanism which rids the mind of those contents, desires, aspirations, drives, people or objects from the external world that are unacceptable to the super-ego and cannot be assimilated by the ego. Unpleasantness and anxiety can thereby be avoided.

In the case of Schreber, Freud (1911) developed the following hypothesis: the homosexual impulse of 'I love him' has to be changed under the pressure of the super-ego into 'I hate him'; if this reversal is insufficient, projection changes the 'I hate him' into 'I am hated'.

The general sequence is as follows: Drives which cannot be assimilated release feelings of guilt; these are hard to tolerate and are warded off by projection; instead of the self-reproaches of a bad conscience there are threats and abuse or erotic proposals coming aloud from the external world in the form of voices, delusions of persecution or delusions of love. These are supposed to be easier to bear than self-accusation and shame.

According to this concept, delusion is a *necessary release which protects the patient against intolerable injury to his self-esteem, a fantasied fulfilment of infantile desires.* Every impulse which is intensively countered in this way may in certain life situations lead to delusion, if reality control is lacking, when judgement and critical faculties are weak, or when affective pressure is strongly developed from the pressure of unfulfilled desires or the conflict of drives.

Freud drew attention to the relationship between dreams and psychosis, especially delusion (*The interpretation of dreams; An*

*outline of psychoanalysis; Delusion and dreams in W. Jensen's
'Gradiva')* (see *Gesammelte Werke*). In delusion, as in dreams, we find
wish fulfilment. In delusions of persecution there is finally the
self-criticism of the super-ego projected on the external world. As far
as delusions of grandeur were concerned, Freud accepted Abraham's
interpretation (1908) of this delusion as a withdrawal of the libido
from the external world into the ego, which leads to inflation of the
ego. The process serves as a defensive measure against unconscious
feelings of inferiority and is a mirror of infantile omnipotence.

Freud more than once drew attention to the 'grain of historical
truth' in delusion and considered that 'by recognising the kernel of
truth' we can find 'a common ground on which to develop the work
of therapy'. (*Delusion and dreams in W. Jensen's 'Gradiva'*, p. 108;
Construction in analysis, p. 55). (For the literature see Abraham,
1908; Fenichel, 1971; Freud, 1906–1909, Nunberg, 1971).

Analytical psychology

Jung's concept of delusion is closely allied to those of Freud and
Bleuler. He deals with delusion in 'hysteria' and in schizophrenia.
Delusion, he maintains, arises from unconquered and affect-laden
complexes and through 'fixation of affects' (Neisser, 1897) (*On the
psychology of dementia praecox*). In a lecture in 1908 (*The content
of psychoses*) he put his final point of view more emphatically: 'the
unmistakable striving of patients to express something through and
in their delusions'. He thus seeks to take further Freud's concept of
fantasied satisfaction of infantile desires. Here too we find the first
mention of parallels between delusional content and mythological
themes, which were then further developed in *Changes in and symbols
of the libido*. The comparison between delusions and dreams was
taken up again in 1939 (*On the psychogenesis of schizophrenia*) and
carried further by his reference to the emergence of archetypical
symbols from the collective unconscious. In 1958 (*Schizophrenia*) he
returned to the same theme. In schizophrenia, 'material' emerges
from the collective unconscious; a violent repressed emotion calls
forth 'from the unconscious intensive phenomena of compensation
...These find expression in delusions and in dreams'.

In *The unconscious in psychopathology* Jung interprets the morbid jealousy of the alcoholic as an unconscious compensation for no longer loving the spouse. 'Love for his wife is not quite dead, it has only become unconscious. But it can now reappear from the unconscious only in the form of jealousy'. (For the literature, see Jung, 1968.)

Individual psychology

The ultimate viewpoint here is emphatic: *Delusion serves to mask defeat in life.* In delusions of persecution the difficulties are created by the patient himself and serve as a justification and an excuse for this defeat. (For the literature see Adler, 1920.)

Palaeopsychology

The Jacksonian law that cerebral injury uncovered regular, deeper, and phylogenetically older layers of cerebral functioning was renamed in palaeopsychology 'the law of phylogenetic regression in illness' (Heinrich, 1965). According to this view, delusion in organically based psychoses is the expression of a decline of differentiated functions to lower levels of functioning in the central nervous system. Paranoid experience of the world is a mythic-archaic life form which expresses all that the sick patient is still able to achieve in the way of cerebral activity.

Cerebral damage is accompanied by an additional 'thymogenic decompensation' caused by anxiety which, combined with the effect of psycho-organic impairment of the patient's critical faculty and his experience of his own inadequacy, leads to the manifestation of the psychosis.

The paranoid syndrome is characterized by a rigidly confined (encletic), self-centred attitude and by the restrained and formalized nature of the patients' reactions (for the literature see Bilz, 1967; Heinrich, 1965; Ploog, 1964; Storch, 1959, 1965).

Gestalt psychology

Conrad (1958) describes the following stages of delusional development as Gestalt changes in the schizophrenic experience.

Trema (fear and trembling)

Loss of the accustomed order of things leads to a feeling of change
either in oneself or in the external world, of alienation (depersonalization, derealization), of unfamiliarity, uncanniness and unrest; the
dominant mood is one of anxiety. This delusional mood still lacks
any definite theme.

*Apophenia (appearance of the phenomenon) and anastrophe
(change)*

The delusional mood of the trema phase gives rise to a new
physiognomy for the external world. Derealization, sensory illusions
and thought disorders, protopathic rather than epicritic, prepare the
way for the abnormal interpretations of delusion. In anastrophe
(change) the patient experiences himself as being at the centre of the
delusional world; he is imprisoned in a state of rigid egocentricity.
The theme of the delusion then takes form and the delusion is
eventually systematized. The patient isolates himself in an autistic-
derealized world, in which he can no longer reach any understanding
with his fellow men.

Apocalypse

In the apocalyptic stage, ego-experience crumbles, the Gestalts
disintegrate, with disorders of thought and affect and with catatonic
symptoms.

Conrad shows how the patient can no longer achieve the passage
(Binswanger, 1965) from delusional to non-delusional experience of
the world, how the 'Copernican change' is no longer possible (for
the literature see Conrad, 1958; Matussek, 1963).

Cybernetics

Central to this point of view is the concept of a defective filter or
defective regulator and a pathological state of over-vigilance.

The normal person lives in his environment in a state of constant
acceptance of probability. Low probabilities, i.e. unlikely outcomes,

are ignored, high probabilities are taken as assured, average probabilities are given consideration. The borderline between what is disregarded and what is given consideration is not rigid, it depends on external factors. On the one hand we may accept an improbability, or on the other hand we may ignore a probability. We recognize this according to the situation. In potentially dangerous situations even extreme probabilities are given consideration.

Our environment offers us many signs. Information from the external world is in inverse proportion to the probability we attach to what we are expecting, i.e. the occurrence of the unexpected brings an increase of information, as does the non-occurrence of something that was highly probable. If the regulation or filter is defective, much more information is accepted, because there is no weeding out of what is unimportant. A man whose regulation is defective is flooded with information which he can no longer organize and can no longer master. The external world then seems to him extraordinary, i.e. unexpected, uncanny and very full of significance. Inappropriate estimation of probability in everyday life leads us to read more into everything, with a correspondingly over-vigilant attention to external impressions (for the literature see Feer, 1970).

Neurophysiology

The starting point here derives from observations of experimental sensory deprivation. The nature and extent of the psychopathological experience encountered in sensory deprivation depends on the completeness and duration of the isolation, on the extent of the anxiety induced by it, and on the time of life at which the experiment is conducted. The more complete the isolation, and the longer the deprivation lasts, the less do delusion-like reactions depend on personality.

If it is to function normally, the nervous system must have an intact afferent system. If the input is disturbed, as by sensory deprivation or sensory impairment, mental disintegration may follow: hallucinations and delusions are viewed as the expression of disturbed reality control which is seen, but not explained, as a complex functioning of the total organism.

Multidimensional point of view

Gaupp (1920, 1938, 1947), using the example of the violent paranoia of his patient, Wagner, held that delusion develops when there is the requisite intermingling of psychoreactive and endogenous factors. Against the background of a hypothetical endogenous, hereditary predisposition or natural tendency, a particular kind of personality may, if the circumstances of life are also conducive, develop delusions. Wagner, who valued the respect of his fellow men, committed an act of sodomy and afterwards developed the delusion that the whole village knew of his lapse and was spreading evil tales about him. He decided to take his revenge and set fire to the village.

Kretschmer (1966), in his studies of sensitive delusions of reference, took this a stage further in his 'dynamics of typical reaction patterns' between character, environment and life experience (key experience). A sensitive personality, he argued, cannot get over the sting of wounded self-esteem once experienced and may then develop delusions in certain environmental conditions, e.g. being apart or alone (for the literature see Gaupp, 1920, 1938, 1947; Kretschmer, 1966).

Existential analysis (Existenzanalyse, Daseinsanalytik, Daseinsanalyse)

In phenomenological, hermeneutic (interpretative) studies of schizophrenic existence based on Heidegger's (1927) *Daseinsanalytik*, many authors have presented existential, i.e. no longer categorical, views of the life or being-in-the-world of schizophrenics (Binswanger, 1955, 1957, 1965; Blankenburg, 1967, 1971; Kuhn, 1963; Kunz, 1931, 1962, 1972; Laing, 1959; Storch, 1959, 1965). In delusional patients we find a disturbance of common human experience (*Mitweltlichkeit*), of feelings of sympathy in Max Scheler's sense (1913), a disturbance of communication (an imprisonment in ΐ θιος χόσμος = their own world). The schizophrenic's special experience of being-in-the-world, his split state, the fact that he has lost his way through life, his shattering of organized existence – all this may find expression in delusion as 'an explanation to himself of his schizophrenic existence' (Kunz).

This existential analysis by its nature does not lend itself to a brief review. It consists mainly of individual studies in depth. Its value lies chiefly in the demonstration it has provided of the total character of every human illness and the change such illness entails in the patient's world.

Daseinsanalyse (Boss, 1971, 1974), as an extension of the existential analysis that is based on Heidegger's philosophy, points to the *restriction* and *shut-in-ness* of the 'exquisitely sociological pheno-menon' of *schizophrenic existence:* in behaviour and responses there are two forms of the one impossibility – that of keeping one's own self-being free and receptive to one's own world. The consequence is a helpless apartness, a state of imprisonment and embarrassment, of being overwhelmed even by everyday life, with the development of delusions of persecution, delusions of influence and autism; a state of powerlessness in the face of the omnipotence of others. The restriction of his existence may lead the patient to expand and magnify his powers in delusion, to exaggerate his role. *Daseinsanalyse* has also provided guidelines for treatment.

So-called anthropological psychiatry

This point of view has been expounded in the German-speaking world by Zutt and Kulenkampff (1958), Zutt (1963) and Kulenkampff (1955, 1956). It regards psychosis as the result of a breakdown of the ordinary organization of the lived in, worldly body, characterized by loss of security, loss of boundary and loss of standing. At the centre of the paranoid experience, mainly concerned with delusions of persecution, is the notion of seeing and being seen.

DRIVE (BASIC ACTIVITY)

(Spontaneity, initiative, *Antrieb*)

14.1 Definition

Drive, or activity, in very general and imprecise terms, is the individual's basic mode of expression.

14.2 Function

Drive is a construct used to describe the hypothetical living force that makes possible all human mental and physical processes.[1] It determines liveliness, speed, alertness, general vitality, readiness for action and reaction, spontaneity and reactivity. It is a hypothetical foundation for attention, application, sympathy (in the affective sphere), interest, sensory and cognitive functioning in the broad sense, for thinking, decision-making and volitional functioning, for motor functioning and for instinctive behaviour.

Drive is not of itself a goal-setting activity. It becomes goal-directed through motivation, need, instinct and volition (q.v.).

Observations from human psychology and comparative ethology (Tinbergen, 1952; Lorenz, 1973; Eibl-Eibesfeldt, 1969, 1970) suggest that there may be a basic form of activity which is largely undirected and which, in the absence of any need-satisfying goals, seeks such goals in growing motor unrest (W. Craig's restless agitation and appetitive behaviour, 1918); once a goal is found, the activity takes thematic shape and discharges itself in volitional acts.

Every individual has his own characteristic form of active behaviour. His basic drive, agility and energy determine his personal tempo which, along with his basic mood, is an essential component of temperament. His basic activity also exemplifies man's dependence on his environment. If there is no external stimulation to evoke activity, boredom sets in (Bilz, 1960) and total activity is reduced to the point of sleepiness and yawning, with senseless, undirected, aimless movements which may at times be repeated monotonously (stereotypies). The importance of external stimulation for development may be seen from the clinical observation that children who lack adequate stimulation develop signs of institutionalism: their movements are slow, they are passive to the point of apathy, their facial expression is empty and their normal, interpersonal, emotional relationships are disturbed (Spitz, 1960).

14.3 Anatomical and physiological foundations

Basic activity is a construct which corresponds to no single activity that we can isolate. It should be thought of as the result of the organized interplay of all cerebreal functions and as such cannot be assigned exclusively to any one cerebral area, such as the substantia reticularis, the thalamus, the diencephalon and limbic system or the frontal lobes, the intact functioning of all of which render basic activity possible. In addition, the state of health and strength of the organism as a whole, its metabolic and hormonal balance, age, and in some circumstances circadian rhythm, all affect basic actdivity.

14.1 Possible methods of examining drive

Drive, or basic activity, can be studied through self-observation and by asking questions immediately concerned with the affective, cognitive, sensory, motor and other activities that depend on it. The nature of an individual's drive may be judged from cross-sectional and longitudinal observation of behaviour. Good indicators are liveliness, the richness of ideas and the fluency and speed of speech and emotional responses, as well as total motor behaviour.

14.5 The formal descriptive psychopathology of drive

Decrease in drive

Poverty of activity, lack of activity, inhibition of activity: the commonly employed distinction between poverty of activity and inhibition of activity is not an easy one to make and is therefore not pursued here. Poverty of activity is evidenced on examination by lack of spontaneity to the point of apathy, by paucity of movement, in some circumstances by slowness of movement, by dull, monotonous, monosyllabic speech, by poverty of ideas, by poor attention and by generally sluggish responses to stimulation. There is a characteristic unwillingness and inability to reach decisions, and lack of willpower (abulia). Left to themselves, individuals who are severely deficient in this respect sometimes sink into apathy and become benumbed in a mute and motionless stupor.

Increase in drive

Individuals with a raised basic activity deviate from their own characteristic behaviour: they are livelier than usual, possess more initiative and ideas; the quantity and speed of their speech increases; their movements are more frequent and more agile. Many of them also feel restless. They are constantly in motion, running around, wringing their hands, making scratching and wiping movements and drumming with their fingers. In severe cases this unrest may escalate into a state of severe general excitement and frenzy. The increased pressure of talk which often accompanies acceleration of speech is called logorrhoea.

14.6   Causal associations of anomalies of drive

Personality traits which characterize various levels of drive

Individuals with low drive are inert, limp, lacking in energy and vitality. They are dull, indifferent or phlegmatic, indecisive, passive and lacking in willpower. It is often impossible to draw a line here between psychopathic (native, constitutional) inertness and a neurotic development related to life events.

At the opposite pole we have the active hypomanics (Kretschmer, 1961), and hyperthymics, who are always energetically engaged, bustling and vigorous in performance.

Acquired disorders of drive

Decreased or increased (uninhibited) activity based on
  (*a*) general physical illness
  (*b*) endocrine disorders

(c) diffuse cerebral disease

(d) localized cerebral damage

(e) functional, so-called endogenous, psychoses

(f) psychoreactive, neurotic and psychopathic disorders of drive

(g) pharmacological influences.

(a) In all severe debilitating *physical illnesses* (e.g. infections, cancer, blood diseases), and in metabolic disorders (e.g. cirrhosis of the liver, renal failure), there is a lowering of the level of drive.

(b) In disorders of the *endocrine system* patients may develop the so-called endocrine psychosyndrome (Bleuler, E. and M., 1969; Bleuler, M., 1954, 1964): this is characterized not only by changes in affectivity (mood) but even more by changes in the level of activity, at times affecting also individual drives. In states of pituitary insufficiency, hypothyroidism, renal insufficiency (Addison's disease) and hypogonadism the level of activity falls. Hyperthyroidism leads to a rise in the level of activity and in some circumstances to a considerable degree of unrest.

(c) In *chronic diffuse cerebral disease* adult patients develop the so-called organic psychosyndrome (Bleuler) which in its advanced stage is characterised not only by memory disorders, the amnestic psychosyndrome, and poverty of thought but also, and most prominently, by disturbances of affect and a fall in the level of activity in the sense of lack of spontaneity, dullness and apathy, sometimes punctuated by episodic states of unrest. In the so-called apallic syndrome (Kretschmer, 1940) with akinetic mutism in cases of very severe general cerebral trauma, the patient finally loses all spontaneity.

Diffuse cerebral damage in childhood may lead to profound mental retardation, sometimes with severe and lasting hyperkinesis (an increase in motor activity) and a persistent state of excitement (erethismus). This may be called erethitic mental retardation. Erethismus can exist, however, without oligophrenia, in minimal brain damage. Other oligophrenics may be apathetic, dull and limp.

(d) In *localized cerebral damage* we may find Bleuler's so-called localized cerebral psychosyndrome: this, while outwardly resembling the endocrine psychosyndrome, with changes in mood and in individual drives, e.g. excessive eating, impulsive sexual activity, is also characterised by a rise or fall in the level of basic activity. It would seem that it is mainly disorders, e.g. tumours, haemorrhages and encephalitic nodes, in the basal area of the temporal lobes, in the mid-brain and hypothalamus, including the limbic system, that may lead to such disturbances of behaviour.

The extent to which disturbances in other cerebral areas may also give rise to specific and diagnostically valid psychopathological defects is debatable. Thus apathy, indifference, indolence and dullness of spirit have been described in cases of damage to the frontal cortex,[2] while lack of control, irritability, attacks of rage, a decline in ethical and aesthetic feelings, accompanied at times by silly, childish facetiousness (moria) have similarly been reported in cases of damage to the base of the brain. Damage to the mid-brain is characterized by phasic swings from normal to low activity, with maintenance of posture. Disorders of the basal ganglia, e.g. Parkinson's disease, Huntington's chorea, are also characterized in their advanced stages by low activity and dullness.

(*e*) In *functional psychoses* we find that in acute *schizophrenia* changes in the level of basic activity occur primarily in so-called catatonic schizophrenia. It is customary to distinguish between the akinetic-stuporose form and a hyperkinetic form, catatonic excitement. A low level of activity is also frequently found in chronic schizophrenia. Many authors have tried to see this lack of activity in chronic schizophrenics as a disturbance that is central to the schizophrenic process. Against this view it must always be borne in mind that a fall in level of activity may also be induced by a long stay in hospital in the protected, unstimulating milieu of an institution – the state of so-called institutionalization.

In the *affective* psychoses *mania* is characterized by excessive activity, a rise in feelings of vitality, an abundance of ideas, interested participation, an increase in the amount and speed of talk (logorrhoea) and at times also by severe excitement (manic frenzy). *Depression*, on the other hand, is characterized by a fall in the level of activity, decreased feelings of vitality, feelings of weakness, loss of initiative, indecisiveness, poverty of ideas and inhibition of thought, withdrawal of interest and poverty of movement to the point of so-called depressive stupor. So-called agitated depression manifests itself in a persistent state of excited, fidgety unrest. This empty, undirected increase in activity leads to stereotyped lamenting, groaning, sighing, digital exploration, pacing to and fro.

(*f*) *Psychoreactive and neurotic disturbances of activity:* even in the kind of sadness or grief that falls well within the bounds of normal psychology, there may often be a temporary loss of initiative. After severely traumatic life experiences, e.g. detention in a concentration camp (see Matussek, 1971; v. Baeyer *et al.*, 1964), and in neurotic development, particularly of a depressive kind, in obsessions (especially obsessional rumination) and in phobias, there is often a lowering of the level of activity. This may be particularly marked in so-called residual neurosis, i.e. chronic and to a large extent fixated neurosis (Ernst, 1959).

(*g*) *Pharmacological influences*, e.g. hypnotics or sleep-inducing drugs, induce a fall in the level of activity, tiredness, sleep. Caffeine in coffee, tea and nicotine are stimulants whose use is world wide. The so-called psycho-stimulants or psycho-energizers, e.g. amphetamine, methylphenidate, lead to a temporary increase in level of activity. Many antidepressants, e.g. imipramine, can likewise bring about a rise in level of activity. The so-called neuroleptics, on the other hand, reduce the level of activity and in higher doses can cause inertia.

15

AGGRESSION

15.1 Definition

Aggression (aggressive behaviour): a verbal or physical sttack on other living creatures or things.
Aggressivity: readiness to be aggressive, aggressiveness.

15.2 Function

By derivation aggression means to go up to, to 'go for', someone or something, an assault upon people or things carried out with a certain amount of energy and goal-directedness.

Aggression in this broad sense, which is by no means limited to the merely destructive, is an essential component of human behaviour. It is necessary for self-preservation and for maintenance of the species. Every living creature needs aggression in this broad sense in order to maintain his role in the group; his territory, domicile, den or retreat; the source of his food; his hunting-ground or pasture; or in order to win and keep his sexual partner via mating struggles.

Man also requires a certain amount of aggressiveness, a readiness to tackle people and things energetically, to enable him to get on in the world, to go his own way, to pursue his personal and professional career, to confront, seize and master all the opportunities, tasks and obstacles that may present themselves. Aggressiveness in this sense makes the individual ready to tackle and grapple with problems.

This concept of aggression is, however, completely engulfed in the broader concept of overall activity (readiness for action, initiative, see *Drive*). For ethological and psychopathological purposes, particularly where there are forensic implications, a narrower interpretation of the concept of aggression is to be preferred: to commit an act of aggression is to drive off, insult, damage, injure, destroy or kill a person, animal or thing. Aggressive behaviour is accompanied by the emotion of rage, anger, spite or fear; aggression can be a form of despair when one is driven into a corner.

There are essentially two alternative concepts of aggression which emerge from the literature.

(*a*) Aggression is an *innate drive*. This is the view, for example, of the Lorenz school (Lorenz, 1963, 1969; Eibl-Eibesfeld, 1969) and of psycho-analysis. Adler spoke of the aggressive instinct and Freud saw in it a derivative of the death instinct, thanatos. If this concept of aggression is accepted, the following argument applies to ways of overcoming it: aggression must, like all other instincts, be discharged or lived out, otherwise there will be disturbances, unless a process of repression or sublimation or something similar is successfully completed.

(*b*) Aggression is *acquired*, it is a *reaction* in accordance with the stimulus-reaction model. States of aggression have been aroused by learning, by experience and as a reaction to frustration, repression and above all to the aggression of others. Aggression is essentially seen as psycho-socio-genetic and is interpreted in terms of learning theory.

We may assume that a certain basic potential for aggressiveness is part of man's nature. The extent to which this aggression is expressed or has to be expressed, however, depends very much on environmental conditions. When the state of readiness is appropriate, a trifling cause is enough. It is not correct to speak of an aggressive instinct. Aggressiveness is on the contrary an underlying factor in behaviour and in many areas, including instinctive behaviour, it is a governing factor. Aggression can thus help to govern and shape many different instinctive acts.

15.3 Mechanisms of aggression in the central nervous system

It may be postulated that there are centres in the mid-brain the stimulation of which may release aggressive behaviour, attacking behaviour and rage, and other centres which can moderate such behaviour and repress it (see Delgado, 1967; Hess, 1962).

15.4 Examination

Aggressiveness can be judged from total behaviour. It is expressed in the motor system by movement, mimicry and gesture, and it announces itself audibly in cries, threats, abuse or curses.

15.5   Pathology

Increased aggressiveness

This leads to impulsive attacks (*raptus*) as in paroxysms of abuse, destructive rage, violence and attacks of frenzy.

Causal associations

(*a*) As a *habitual personality style*. In so-called excitable psychopaths the significance of aggression is chiefly forensic, since these people are liable to commit acts of violence. Alcohol may cause them to lose control, especially in certain social situations, e.g. making themselves conspicuous, or brawling in public houses.

(*b*) *Psycho-reactive*, expressed as rage, anger, fear or despair. One well-described form is the psychogenic reaction to imprisonment, the 'prison frenzy' of blind destructive rage, hitting out at random, and violence. Alcohol may lead to a loss of inhibition which encourages acts of aggression. Control is more readily lost by immature persons, who are at times also of lower than average intelligence, and by dements (see the *Organic psychosyndrome*).

(*c*) *Neurotic*. When life situations are worrying or when personal relationships are tense, a neurotic lack of balance may lead to increased aggressiveness, irritability and sensitivity.

(*d*) *Organic psychoses*. Aggressive impulses occur most frequently in alcoholism and epileptic twilight states. They may also arise in postencephalitic Parkinsonism associated with oculogyric crises, e.g. a desire to strangle others. In general brain damage (the psychoreactive syndrome) there is often a loss of control that leads to an increase in reactive aggression – irritability with impulsive violence. Localized cerebral psychosyndromes, e.g. after cranial trauma, may be accompanied by frenzied violence similar to that found in the endocrine psychosyndrome.

(*e*) *Mania*. A kind of frenzied violence may also be found in the excited form of mania.

(*f*) *Schizophrenia*. In catatonic excitement there is a risk of violent behaviour. In paranoid schizophrenics, especially those with delusions of persecution, verbal and physical attacks may occur as forms of defence or revenge.[1]

The interpretation of addiction as a form of increased self-aggression cannot be discussed here. Mention should be made, however, of the interpretation of suicide as a form of increased self-aggression and of impulsive self-mutilation. Both may occur in impulsive states.

(*g*) *Suicide.* When a state of *raptus melancholicus* has self-destruction as its goal, there may be brutal, ill-directed attempts at suicide which are ill-considered and therefore not always successful; these are sometimes extended to include near relatives, mostly spouses or children.

(*h*) *Impulsive self-mutilation* (automutilation) can occur, e.g. the self-castration or a schizophrenic on grounds of delusional, religiose inspiration. Another schizophrenic burnt his lips with lysol so as to avoid having to obey the command to gnaw his own mother with his teeth. An older woman cut off her own hand because she had used it in her youth for the sinful purpose of masturbation. Agitated depressives may make scratches all over their bodies. A mentally retarded patient tore out his own hair (trichotillomania).

In one of the many forms of the Münchhausen syndrome, which may be viewed as neurotic, patients injure themselves, e.g. by repeatedly sticking needles into their bodies, in order to be sent back again and again to hospital.

Decreased aggressiveness, inhibition of aggressiveness

(*a*) This is found as a *habitual personality style*, a neurotic-psychopathic life style (so-called neurotic lack of aggression) in individuals who are asthenic, limp and passive.

(*b*) It occurs in all *debilitating physical illnesses*.

(*c*) *Reactions to personal troubles*, grief and care may lead to this phenomenon.

(*d*) *Organic psychoses* with dementia are frequently, though by no means always, accompanied by a decrease in aggressiveness, which is part of a general decrease in activity accompanied by apathy.

(*e*) In almost all forms of *depression* aggressiveness is reduced (but see also the remarks on suicide and self-mutilation, above).

(*f*) In *chronic schizophrenia* the patient's behaviour is passive, limp, inactive, irresolute, and thus frequently lacking in aggressiveness.

THE MOTOR SYSTEM (MOTOR BEHAVIOUR)

16.1 Definition

Motor behaviour is the deportment, in rest and in movement, of man as an active being. His mimicry, gestures and deportment, his individual movements and the flow of his combined movements, express his whole being, his self-consciousness, his mood, his intelligence, his vigilance, his directedness, his volition and his drives.

16.2 Function

Motor behaviour, like other forms of behaviour, is a function of experience. We adopt a posture and we act, both of which are possible only with our entire being. Our whole existence is revealed in stolid or agitated, voluntary or involuntary behaviour, in our deportment at rest and in movement.

To isolate motor behaviour from the rest of human existence (from verbal, cognitive, gnostic, affective, conative and other behaviour) is an artificial exercise. Motor behaviour provides us with a picture of the living, active man, how he fares in his world, how he understands, interprets and responds to the demands made upon him by people and events.

Language is rich in informative expressions about motor behaviour. A person holds his head high, holds himself well, keeps himself in good countenance or loses countenance, stands firm on his own two feet, holds his own, stands up to life; or he may drag himself wearily through life, or he may ignore people and things by steering clear of obstacles; or he may set himself above others in an overbearing manner, or take difficulties in his stride. Another person crumbles in the face of adversity, falling apart or recoiling from a commitment, withdrawing or running away from a group. Another person confronts people and things directly, tackling anything, setting about things in a stormy or timid spirit but, right or wrong, getting on with the task in hand. One man is said to go through life erect (cf. Straus, 1960), another to be broken and bowed. He may cower, wriggle out of things, squirm. One person crawls in front of others, or lies down before them, bowing to their will. Someone who is embarrassed feels he is in a false position. Someone else is tense with excitement. Yet another is cranky, has taken a wrong turn, is warped in some way.

A child can be brought up well or badly. Someone who has himself well in hand knows how to keep a tight rein on himself. A proud man has his head in the air, his nose in the air. An unpractical man has his head in the clouds, or perhaps flies too high (see Binswanger, 1949, 1955), or moves by leaps and bounds. One individual may be quick-witted, hasty, rise to the occasion or pull himself together, another is limp, downtrodden, brought low. One man is stiff, clumsy, wooden; another is flabby, yet another is crooked, straight in neither movement nor thought. We put someone else into a certain position, and we find ourselves being put into a particular position. We sustain someone with comfort, we support him, prop him up. A wrongdoer, a criminal, trespasses upon others, forfeiting their trust. A ruffian with a cudgel lays about him. Someone grasps something easily, understands it, discovers something, discloses it. You have something at your fingertips, you can point to all its ramifications; you can put forward a point of view, deliver a judgement, lay on a spell or a curse. A stupid person's thinking is mixed up, he cannot draw clear distinctions. An unruffled man lets things happen; another gets excited or is smitten by something. For someone in a good frame of mind things go well; such a man can get over a great deal. A person may turn up his nose, pull a wry face, conceal his real expression, keep his eyes and his ears open, close his eyes to something. He may have his eye on something, or something may catch his eye. A man who stands loyally by his group is straight and true. A deviant, who separates himself from the group, must live apart or be considered deranged.

This brief, unsystematic and by no means complete set of examples serves to remind us of the all-embracing importance of the motor system in human behaviour.

A large proportion of motor behaviour is involuntary, taking place without any consideration, intention or effort. There are many skills which we acquire by practice and then perform automatically as complex acts, e.g. swimming, riding a bicycle, driving a car, without having to pay constant attention to the individual movements involved.

16.3 Foundations

The foundations of motor behaviour lie in the central nervous and peripheral motor systems: pyramidal pathways (voluntary motor behaviour), extrapyramidal system (involuntary motor behaviour), the interplay of afferent and efferent nerve conductors and of the motor apparatus of bones, joints, sinews and muscles.

Every person has his own innate and characteristic motor behaviour which is further developed in the course of his life in accordance with his own individuality and with the customs, norms and models of his group. It is affected by his overall frame of mind at any given time: we can recognize the worried, sad or jovial man not only by his words but even more by the sum of his expressive movements, by his mimicry and gestures, by the tempo and elasticity of his movement and by the bearing of his head and trunk (see also *Drive*).

Motor behaviour is learned early in life on the basis of inborn schemata and by imitation of the mother's facial mimicry, the act of touching, grasping, holding, etc. It is of decisive importance for the development of ego-consciousness (q.v.).

16.4 Examination

Observations of spontaneous movement and movement in response to instruction provide the physical findings obtained on neurological examination. In clinical psychiatry it is also important to observe patients outside the interview situation, in their contacts with other patients, with relatives, on walks, in holiday camps, in group gymnastics, at play, on festive occasions, and at work. This aspect of assessment is unfortunately often neglected.

For examples of how to describe motor behaviour, see under 16.2.

16.5 Pathology

The description of particular disorders of movement should not be allowed to mislead the investigator into looking at such abnormal phenomena in isolation. It is much more important always to see them for what they are: a proclamation of all the patient's modes of experience and behaviour. Even in their rarest forms they constitute a kind of message which must be understood if we are to deal justly with the reality of the patient's life.

In order to decide whether particular motor disorders are of psychopathological relevance, we must first learn to recognize *neurological* and *orthopaedic motor disturbances*. This enables us to distinguish between organic and psychogenic apraxias, paralyses, lameness and other motor abnormalities. We have to know the poverty of movement, the rigidity, and the basic posture of the patient with Parkinsonism, the coarse, involuntary, jerky movements of chorea, the slow, writhing movements of athetosis, and the twisting movements of torsion dystonia. The so-called *formes frustes* of early Huntington's chorea may be hard to distinguish from psychogenic disorders and may be wrongly diagnosed as tic-like psychogenic phenomena.

Torticollis, too, presents problems of differential diagnosis. It may occur in some forms of rheumatism, or as an abnormality of posture in psychosis, e.g. catatonia.

Patterns of regressive motor behaviour (Schablonen)

Differential diagnosis of motor disorders is particularly difficult when brain-damaged patients regress to earlier phylogenetic and ontogenetic patterns of movement (Kretschmer, 1953, 1958, the so-called motor stereotypies); chewing, swallowing, smacking the lips, gulping, sucking (so-called oral grasping), wiping, scratching, circling and kicking movements – these may occur in degenerative cerebral disorders of the most varied kind, e.g. in association with the amnestic syndrome, as well as in the so-called psychomotor attacks of temporal lobe epilepsy.

Tic

This is usually a repetitive, stereotyped movement in mimicry or gesture which, independent of mood and tension, is repeated in varying frequency and intensity, as if compulsively, i.e. it cannot be voluntarily suppressed. So-called writer's cramp may be regarded as a form of tic in this broad sense. This form of movement is regarded as a psychogenic (neurotic) disorder.

Gilles de la Tourette syndrome (Maladie des tics)

This syndrome includes tic-like motor disorders in mimicry (including grimacing) and gesture, shrugging the shoulders and throwing the arms around; in addition the patient utters inarticulate sounds, e.g. grunts and smacking of the lips and sometimes obscene words (cacolalia).

The syndrome occurs in association with various conditions, e.g. in degenerative cerebral disorders and in other psychoses including psychogenic reactions.

Hypokinesia, akinesia, stupor

Poverty of movement (hypokinesia) may reach the point of immobility (akinesia) in states of stupor. Spontaneous and reactive movements become less frequent, the patient showing little or no mimicry (hypomimesis, amimesis). When akinesia is complete, the patient is nearly always mute. Patients very often do not look at the observer, though they can look around them. The facial expression is often one of indifference, or at least is hard to interpret though at times it may express melancholy anguish, severe oppression or bewiderment. Patients in a state of stuporose anxiety seem to be particularly keyed up: it is as if they might at any moment suddenly assume a posture of attack or flight.

Sometimes the patient refused food and even drink, then requiring artificial feeding. Some of them still make such movements as are required to perform their bodily functions, others are incontinent. Alternatively, there may be retention of stool and urine, requiring the use of catheter and enema.

From the patient's appearance and the usually tense state of his musculature, it can be seen that he is still awake. It is often impossible to reach any firm conclusion about a patient's clarity of consciousness during stupor. However, after emerging from the stupor the patient may be able to talk about his experiences retrospectively and to furnish more information about them.

Stupor is not basically a new symptom: stuporose states can also occur in normal subjects when in situations of sudden terror, great anxiety and bewilderment, and in states of panic, cf. the simulated death reflex of hunted animals

Causal associations. As it is difficult or impossible to establish contact with patients in stupor, the differential diagnosis is exceedingly hard and at times impossible without a neurological examination, special investigations (EEG) and some knowledge of the case history.

Stupor in schizophrenia (catatonic stupor)

We may regard the catatonic schizophrenic as someone who is paralysed by anxiety, terror and bewilderment in the face of an extreme threat to his ego-consciousness in its various dimensions (q.v.). When a person no longer knows whether he is still alive, when he is no longer sure of himself as a living, acting being, when his own unity and separateness are no longer assured, or when he has lost the sense of his own identity, that individual may well become paralysed.

Everything which gives the patient a new assurance of his own ego-experience can therefore be of therapeutic benefit in catatonic stupor. Sometimes a patient who has lost his ego-identity is restored to himself when addressed freely by his own name, another can be helped back to ego-activity by joining in gymnastics or breathing exercises. It is clear that with such severely affected patients a purely verbal therapeutic approach is of itself not always enough. Treatment with neuroleptic drugs, or electroshock, is never by itself sufficient; a personal interest in the patient must always be exhibited.

Protocol 22 (Schizophrenia)

This young man was in a state of sub-stupor. When the examiner called out to him: 'Hello there, Werner', there was a long silence and then he whispered – 'Yes, if you call me that, now I know again who I am.'

The same patient was helped by touching his limbs one by one and naming them, since in his state of disintegrated ego-consistency he no longer knew how they all belonged together to form a whole. This simple measure gave him a renewed sense of himself; he found himself again.

Other patients may be more difficult to rouse from their stupor. Even if they show no visible reaction, however, it still does them good, as we learn subsequently, not to be left alone in this state, but to have someone stay with them and talk with them. Sometimes one will then succeed in taking a few paces with them: the first therapeutic step has then been achieved and the way is open for a return to the world of their fellow-beings.

Other patients in catatonic stupor may be under the overpowering influence of hallucinatory and delusional experiences, e.g. in states of ecstasy.

Stupor in severe inhibited melancholia: depressive stupor

Overpowering anxiety and guilt, devitalization and feelings of doom, great bewilderment and complete inability to reach a decision or undertake any activity can reach such a pitch that the patient is benumbed. Clinical experience shows that it is much more difficult to establish psychotherapeutic contact with a patient in a depressive stupor than with one whose stupor is catatonic.

Stupor as an immediate form of reaction: psychogenic stupor

In many cases stupor can occur as a reaction to severe shock, terror or panic: the patient is paralysed with fright. This happens in catastrophes, on receipt of overwhelmingly bad news, e.g. death of a child, or being deserted, as well as, for example, before and during examinations (so-called examination stupor).

Stupor-like states in the acute exogenous reaction type

Examples include toxic reactions (pharmacogenic stupor, neuroleptica), encephalitis and epilepsy.

It is precisely this kind of stupor which brings home to us the need for exhaustive neurological and physical examination of every stuporose patient.

Stupor may last for minutes, hours, or weeks, depending on its nature, its severity and the possibility of finding the appropriate treatment.

Hyperkinesis, catatonic excitement, raptus

Catatonic patients may sometimes move suddenly from stupor to a state of extreme excitement (raptus) in which they rush around, storm, scream, run against the walls and windows or attack anyone who happens to be present.

Other signs of excitement are running to and fro, jumping, fingering, tying things up, wringing the hands, scratching themselves (which is sometimes seen also in agitated depressives), sighing, scolding and loud inappropriate laughter.

Many symptoms of excitement may be seen in erethitic mental defectives. Self-mutilation may also occur.

A *catatonic burst of excitement* may be regarded as an expression of anxiety: it is a desperate bid on the patient's part to recover his sense of being himself, to assure himself that it is still possible for him to pursue his own activity (see *Ego-consciousness*). It is important to remember this when psychopharmacological remedies are being considered. Neuroleptics may make matters worse: the patient's despair is increased and his excitement then calls for maximal doses. It is better, if possible, to direct the excitement into other channels, e.g. gymnastics. Sometimes the patient may flee in panic from hallucinatory pursuers or make a sudden switch from flight to attack.

Grimaces, grotesque facial contortions, paramimesis

These are mostly exhibited in catatonic schizophrenia. Some of the symptoms, like many instances of hyperkinesis and stereoptypy, may be related to disturbed ego-consciousness: the patient no longer has a sure sense of his own being and fights frantically against this awareness. Other possible interpretations which suggest themselves are the mimicry of individuals who are embarrassed, crushed, inhibited, bewildered, thunderstruck, anguished, and those who simper, are indecisive or ambivalent.

Fixed postures (catalepsy), stereotyped postures

These are unnatural postures, rigidly maintained, in which the patients persist for a long time. They are present almost exclusively when the patient is receiving insufficient care and attention. Sometimes the patients will remain for a long time in a posture into which they have been passively placed, behaving as if their limbs were made of wax, resembling automatons (waxy flexibility, *flexibilitas cerea*). These symptoms are an expression of disturbed ego-activity. 'Communal activity' (Bleuler) in gymnastics, play and work provide the most important form of treatment.

Causal associations are found mostly in catatonic schizophrenia.

Negativism

Many patients resist every movements which they are asked to make or which others try to impose on them. Negativism may be passive (refusal) or active (doing the opposite of what is requested). It may be postulated that this is often based on a threatened consciousness of ego-activity, every movement urged upon the patient being experienced as a form of subjugation and evoking resistance.

Motor stereotypies

These uniform, repetitive movements of the most varied kind may be simple, e.g. wiping or scratching, or they may consist of a complicated series of movements.

Simple stereotypies like snuffling, wiping or knocking, occur most frequently in brain-damaged patients, e.g. cerebral atrophy, cerebral arteriosclerosis, encephalitis. They are found in association with a psycho-organic syndrome, with an acute exogenous reaction type and at times also with neurological focal phenomena.

Complicated stereotypies occur chiefly in acute catatonic schizophrenia. It is worth while trying to understand them, though this may
not always succeed, by enquiring into the patient's life and
experience.

EXAMPLE

Protocol 22 (Schizophrenia)

This young man in his sub-stuporose state kept making the same slow
circular movements with his hands held out before him. When asked why he
did this, he finally said: 'Then I know that I can still move'. This stereotyped
movement made it possible for him to reassure himself of his own being in
the face of threatened ego-activity. The repeated movement allowed him
repeated reassurance.

Sometimes this patient hyperventilated for several minutes (forced
breathing). He did this so that he would know that he was still alive. The most
elemental function of inspiration and expiration was violently repeated as
a form of self-reassurance.

Catatonic patients are often seen to make stereotyped movements
of the hands, at the same time staring at their hands. Since the hands
and the face are of particular importance for ego-consciousness, it
may be suggested that such movements also serve to reassure the
patients of their own capacity for activity, of their own identity. This
assumption is confirmed by the often surprising effectiveness of
spontaneously touching the patient's hands: this may be done by the
therapist or in communal exercises (movement therapy).

Chronic, ingrained stereotyped movements may sometimes be
maintained for years if treatment is inadequate.

EXAMPLE

Protocol 169 (Schizophrenia)

The patient had been almost speechless for years, with no intelligible
communication, though he carried out his work industriously. Every time
someone greeted him, he raised his hand in greeting and made three complete
turns on his own axis. After more than three decades his neologistic secret
language was decoded: he was able to communicate again and to say what
compelled him to these remarkable parakineses. He stated that he always
had to turn 360 degrees to the right: when he greeted anyone, when he went
to bed or when he sat down, having first turned his eating utensils in the
same way. He also had to make any movement backwards and upwards:

with his trunk and head and raised arm, or at least in a rudimentary fashion with his head, with his eyebrows and with his nose, at the same time expelling air and closing his eyes. This complicated avoidance ritual had the following meaning: turning to the right prevented deviation to the left (left for him was the equivalent of 'bad', 'no longer existing', 'being broken', 'being injured'. If a left turn was made 'time did not go any more', i.e. life stood still, his existence was no longer located in time. His world was full of negative signs which 'caught his eye' and did him 'harm'. The backward and upward movements enabled him to avoid this danger.

His stereotyped movements also included a constant pacing up and down, like the tramping of a wild animal trapped in a cage. This is hardly ever seen now in well-run hospitals. Sometimes, of course, this pacing up and down is also intended to mark off the patient's own preserve. Other stereotypies may be defence measures against bodily hallucinations, others again may be movements of embarrassment or of wiping things away (Kläsi, 1922).

The speech (verbigeration), writing, drawing and painting of many schizophrenics can also be stereotyped.

Echopraxia (*imitation of posture and movement*)

The patient copies like an automaton or echo any movement that is made before him, especially movements of the limbs. Sometimes he also repeats words or sentences (echolalia).

The symptom occurs most frequently in schizophrenics and is associated with disturbed ego-activity (q.v.): when a man no longer experiences himself as acting intentionally, he is inclined to copy the movements of others (*echo symptoms*) or to repeat movements once he has begun to make them (stereotypy) or to resist movements that are forced upon him (*negativism*).

EXAMPLE

Protocol 21 (Schizophrenia)

'When I see other people and hear them speak, then it can happen that I say just the same things and make just the same movements – and then I am afraid that I am the other people. I know it isn't so, but I still have this fear. When someone else limps, then I have to walk more slowly.'

Echo symptoms occur when the experience of ego-activity and ego-identity are threatened.

Bizarre and inadequate behaviour

This is the name given to unusual and inappropriate behaviour which deviates from the culturally and socially determined standard. It includes so-called indecent behaviour, e.g. spitting, belching, passing flatus, vulgar talk, overfamiliar and impertinent behaviour.

Posturing refers to the adopting and maintenance of bodily postures which are not in keeping with social custom.

Mannerisms, studied, stylized and often affected, may be seen also in style of speech, writing, drawing and painting.

Many patients break off in the middle of a movement, for example withdrawing their hand when it has carried the spoon halfway to their mouth, or stopping halfway (inhibition of intention, ambivalence, alien influence, see *Ego-actvity*).

OBSESSIONS AND PHOBIAS

Synonyms:
  Obsession = anankasmus; anankastic, obsessional-compulsive symptoms.
  Phobias = compulsive fears; phobic states, phobic avoidance, situational anxiety.

Obsessions and phobias are discussed together because they have much in common. Both show a loss of freedom of action and in both a self-examining attitude is maintained. Many obsessional acts take place on a basis of definite fears. Obsessions and phobias are also found, often in association, in similar personalities, e.g. anankastic and phobic (q.v.).

17.1 Obsessions

Definition

Obsessions are imperative experiences, accompanied by a feeling of inevitability and of the futility of struggling against them, which force themselves upon the patient in spite of his resistance and in spite of the fact that on reflection he recognizes the compulsions to be absurd and incongruous, i.e. based on no rational grounds. Obsessions may take the form of thoughts, ideas, questions, speech or counting, or may consist of certain actions that have to be carried out or avoided.

The patient knows that the obsession is something which he himself generates, in contrast to the orders and alien influences that occur in schizophrenia. He does not like the obsession, he rejects it, he tries to protect himself from it, but in so doing he becomes aware of the futility of his resistance. The experiences and acts of the obsessional patient thus preserve their ego-quality, but he does not feel free in his thoughts, decision and actions.

Obsessions are not necessarily of themselves absurd in content. What is experienced as absurd or unjustified, however, is their persistence and penetration and their tendency to constant, monotonous repetition.

Classification of obsessions

Obsessional thinking: obsessionally persisting thought content

Obsessional ideas, thoughts, images, memories, questions, or rumi-
nations often appear as counter-impulses directed against a situation:
for example, the compulsive obtrusion of obscene pictures, or the
blasphemous thoughts in church during the sermon. Obsessional
rumination may raise persistent questions, e.g. why is the tree just
there?, why does the world exist?, why do I exist?

Obsessional impulses

These are impulses to perform certain actions that obtrude compulsively upon the patient in spite of his resistance. By way of
examples: the impulse to check something, obsessional checking,
entails always having to check again and again whether the door is
locked, whether the light or the gas or the tap is turned off; the
impulse to utter obscene words (coprolalia), or to count or to do
sums (arithmomania). Such impulses do not necessarily lead to
action.

Obsessional impulses of a more disturbing kind, e.g. to knife one's
own child, to throw it out of the window, to take the breadknife and
stab the woman sitting opposite at table, to throw oneself out of
the window or off the bridge, are hardly ever translated into action.
They can, however, trouble the patient greatly and all his energy is
used up in resisting them.

Obsessional acts

Acts of an obsessional nature are usually carried out on the basis of
obsessional impulses or fears (see phobias). A common example is
obsessional cleaning and washing, for example because of a morbid
fear of dirt and bacteria. Many obsessional acts are concerned with
bodily functions, e.g. defaecation and micturition, or with care of the
body, the acts in question having to be accompanied by certain
precautionary measures, rituals or avoidances.

Obsessional acts are usually accompanied by a ritual which points
to the magical, apotropaic (averting) nature of the action. The ritual
follows a precise and prescribed form and often has to be repeated

a certain number of times. After it has been completed, doubts often arise as to whether it was performed correctly in the prescribed manner. This can lead to endless repetition of obsessional rituals.

Obsessional acts seriously interfere with the patient's freedom and may take complete possession of him for years, so that he becomes incapable of working (because he has constantly to attend to his 'duties'), cannot look after his family, or does himself harm, e.g. in the form of eczema or abrasions of the skin due to excessive washing or use of disinfectants.

17.2 Phobias

Definition

Phobias are obsessional fears which arise in connection with certain situations or objects, although these situations and objects do not obviously and in the common view justify such fears. Phobias can be distinguished from the usual symptoms of anxiety by the fact that the compelling and overpowering nature of the fears, which is what leads to their classification alongside obsessional symptoms, is combined with complete, partial or intermittent intellectual insight into their irrationality from an objective point of view and with an experience of inner resistance to them. Phobias compel people to perform certain actions which are sometimes given specific names, e.g. compulsive washing, or force them into compulsive omissions or avoidances.

Types of phobia

Obsessional fears are often inflicted with special names according to the object or situation which gives rise to them. The neologistic powers of psychiatrists in this field are seemingly infinite. There is no point in listing all these names and accordingly we give here only a few examples:

Acarophobia (fear of parasites in the skin)
Agoraphobia (fear of open places, streets, etc.)
Aichmophobia (fear of sharp objects, or of injuring oneself or others with them)

Acrophobia (fear of heights)
Aquaphobia (fear of stretches of water, or running water)[1]
Bacteriophobia (fear of germs)
Claustrophobia (fear of enclosed spaces)
Erythrophobia (fear of blushing)
Ceraunophobia (fear of lightning)
Coprophobia (fear of contamination by excreta, dust, etc.)
Mysophobia (fear of being touched, dirtied)
Nyctophobia (fear of the night)
Panphobia (fear of many things, many situations, etc.)
Phobophobia (fear of fear)
Zoophobia (fear of animals)

17.3 Causal associations of obsessions and phobias

Clinically we may distinguish between the occurrence of individual obsessions or phobias as *symptoms* accompanying different psychiatric illnesses and so-called *obsessional illness* which, with its predominant symptoms of fears and phobias, can have a very damaging effect on the patient's life.

Individual obsessional symptoms

These may in certain circumstances occur in normal persons, for example in boredom (obsessional counting), in states of fatigue or exhaustion (obsessional thoughts), in sleep disorders (obsessional rumination, obsessional memories). Obsessional symptoms which accompany *organic psychoses* are of particular clinical significance, e.g. after encephalitis, where obsessional impulses are specially important; they also occur in endogenous psychoses and may accompany *schizophrenia* or appear long before that illness is diagnosed. Patients with endogenous *depression* are not infrequently tormented by obsessions and obsessional fears which disappear when the depressive phase subsides (so-called anankastic depression).

Obsessional illness

This is also called obsessional neurosis, obsessional compulsive states. For a long time, perhaps even throughout his entire life, the patient is constantly or intermittently at the mercy of obsessions and fears of every kind and of every degree of intensity.

Epidemiology

The prevalence of obsessional illness in the general population is estimated at 0.5 per cent. Women are more frequently affected than men (50–70 per cent of cases). The majority of patients are of good socio-economic status.

Personality

Most obsessional patients are of a particular personality type (anankastic, obsessional personalities). Of good intelligence, they are often rigid and perfectionist, have high ethical standards, and scrupulous, over-conscientious and anxious regard to the mainten- ance of order in their external life and in their ethical and moral dealings; they are pedants or sticklers. On the other side of the coin, they are also inclined to be jealous, covetous, petty and grudging and to lack affection in the exercise of their authority, e.g. in bringing up children; they are characterized by the contrast between their strong instinctive drives (the id) and their strict conscience (the super-ego).

Course and outcome

Obsessional illness begins at an early age – about half of all cases become manifest soon after the age of ten and up to the age of twenty – and is usually gradual in onset, often with no recognizable cause, sometimes after a trying experience, e.g. the death of a relative. The illness may become slowly worse, may continue unchanged for many years or may fluctuate. About a third of all obsessional patients retain their symptoms unchanged throughout their lifes, a third improve with age and a third deteriorate.

Symptoms

Obsessional illness is characterized by the most varied compulsions and compulsive fears (for examples, see p. 228) and is often accompanied by general anxiety with associated vegetative phenomena (autonomic anxiety) or by hypochondriacal fears, e.g. fears of cardiac disease, depressive moods and sometimes symptoms of depersonalization

Aetiology

Family studies (see Zerbin-Rüdin, 1953) lend weight to the assumption that there is an inherited factor which helps to determine the obsessional personality type and with it the general diathesis.

According to our own unpublished review of the literature in 1970, out of 38 pairs of monozygotic twins, 27 (71 per cent) were concordant and 11 (29 per cent) discordant.

Life experience plays a decisive part in determining when, how and with what content obsessional illness manifests itself.

Psycho-dynamic theories:

(a) *Psycho-analytical.* Psycho-analytical interpretation points to the contrast between a strong instinctual pressure and a strict conscience, and thus to a conflict between the id and the excessively powerful super-ego. According to this theory obsessional symptoms correspond to rejected unconscious desires which the super-ego has not been able to suppress completely. These desires can then be satisfied only if they present themselves forcibly as alien, that is to say as something not belonging to the personality. Particular emphasis is laid on the defence against anal-erotic and sado-masochistic tendencies. Individual obsessional symptoms are interpreted as acts of defence or atonement. Thus, for example, obsessional washing is a defence against sexual contamination, e.g. by masturbation (Freud, 1906–1909).

(b) *Analytical psychology* (Jung): This psycho-dynamic view of obsessions is similar to Freud's psycho-analytical view. A huge shadow, e.g. of sexuality or of aggression, cannot be adequately suppressed and has then a disruptive effect, leading to the obsessional symptom.

(*c*) *Existential-* and Dasein-*analytical:* This does not offer an explanation but rather an analysis of the obsessional patient's existence, emphasising the restriction of his freedom and the narrowing of his existence. A phenomenological approach is used to examine the intrinsic factors that manifest themselves in obsessional symptoms or phobias (for the literature see Boss, 1971). For example, what is manifested in agoraphobia is the fear of rootlessness, of losing direction and standing in the world; the claustrophobic constricted existence is seen as a form of defence against degrading onself.

In line with this phenomenological point of view we have also the unbiased, theoretically uncommitted inquiry into what is revealed by the patient's symptoms and life history.

EXAMPLES

Fear of asphyxiation

An obese, dysplastic girl of about 22 complained of severe difficulties in breathing associated with fear of dying. Biographical inquiry revealed that she was not allowed to leave home and become a nurse, as she very much wanted to do, but had to go into a factory and earn money. The girl, oppressed by an unhappy and restrictive home, left on her own because of her appearance and without friends of either sex, could only watch jealously while other girls of her age went around with their friends. As a last straw she had to work in a factory making condoms, spending the whole day testing the thickness of the sheaths by blowing them up. This position, which apparently offered no hope of escape and which only accentuated her own life situation, led to the phobic syndrome.

Compulsive cleaning

A hitherto healthy woman developed in middle age a cleaning obsession which on closer inquiry turned out to be a compulsive wiping away of gold dust which she thought she saw everywhere. The obsessions had developed when the woman after many years met a friend of her youth whom she still loved and who in these early days used to call her 'his gold'. This renewed acquaintance produced a severe crisis of conscience in regard to her husband and her children. She wanted to wipe away the experience. (Example taken from Weitbrecht, 1963, p. 117.)

Protocol 39 (Compulsive swallowing)

A young depressive man, a cocaine addict, complained of persistent compulsive swallowing. During psycho-analytical treatment he revived the memory of the beginning of the obsession: when he was six and his mother was urging him to say his prayers, instead of praying he thought: 'my mother – the cow'. His compulsive swallowing then started and was interpreted as a continual swallowing of the forbidden expression.

Agoraphobia has been reported as a defence against an inclination to be a prostitute.

Treatment of phobias and obsessions

Psycho-analytic therapy seeks to secure release from the obsession by uncovering the mechanisms of repression.

Psychagogic treatment aims at teaching the patient to live with his obsessions and not to allow them to assume overpowering significance.

Frankl's logotherapy (1956) reports some success using the so-called paradoxical intention, in which the patients are, to their surprise, advised to follow their compulsive drives, e.g. to throw themselves out of the window. In successful cases the patient is nonplussed by this (it produces an 'antireflex') and renounces his impulse.

Behaviour therapy, having first worked out a hierarchy of fears, is directed purely at symptoms and, using verbal and practical measures of desensitization and flooding, seeks to achieve the patient's deconditioning.

At the same time patients can be made generally more relaxed and less anxious by the use of psychotropic drugs, e.g. tranquillizers, neuroleptics, antidepressants, and by autogenic training and graduated active hypnosis.

In the most severe cases, which respond to no other form of treatment, leucotomy is sometimes performed, nowadays using a stereotactic approach.

18

IMPULSIVE ACTS

18.1 Definition

These are acts executed forcefully with no deliberation or reflection, under the influence of a compelling pressure that restricts the subject's freedom of will. Since reflective control or consideration is lacking, the consequences of such acts are not thought out or taken into consideration. Voluntary inhibitions either do not exist or cannot withstand the pressure.

Many such impulsive acts seem to be preceded by a far-reaching, aimless and undirected (amorphous) tendency to explosive action.

18.2 Pathology

Impulsive acts are aetiologically heterogeneous, occurring in the most varied illnesses, reactions and developments, e.g. in brain-damaged patients suffering from epilepsy or encephalitis, in patients with endocrine disorders, in depressives, in schizophrenics and in so-called psychopaths.

Fugues (poriomania, dromomania)

Fuges include sudden, compulsive acts of running away and aimless wandering. They occur in mood disorders of endogenous-psychotic, psychopathic, epileptic origin and in children and young people as a reaction to conflicts at home or at school.

Hoarding

This involves amassing collections of useless objects, e.g. paper-clips, cigarette stubs. It occurs at times in chronic schizophrenics who are not being well cared for, in the mentally retarded, in dements and in some eccentrics.

Pyromania

This impulsive fire-raising may be psychopathic in origin, may occur in epilepsy or in schizophrenics as a result of inspiration and delusional arguments, or may be the result of hatred, defiance or revenge on the part of people of low intelligence who have a sense of grievance. (For the literature see De Boor, 1955; Többen, 1971, and also Göppinger and Witter, 1972.)

Kleptomania

A sudden and usually recurrent impulse to steal objects which are not needed and are often of no value. It is interpreted in various ways: as a wager to do something that is forbidden; as displaced sexual gratification from stealing; as revenge for emotional or material deprivation in childhood; as aggression against society. Occasional stealing by fetishists (q.v.) is, on the other hand, directed at obtaining a particular object which exercises a fetishistic fascination (for the litgerature see Bräutigam, 1973).

Dipsomania

Impulsive modes of behaviour are sometimes taken to include dipsomania (periodic drunkenness) which refers to recurrent bouts of compulsive drinking in those who are otherwise not chronic alcoholics. It occurs in mood disorders, mostly depressive or discontented, of a reactive, psychopathic, affective-psychotic or epileptic kind. The excessive drinking which sometimes takes place on pay-days should not be included here.

AFFECTIVITY, AFFECT, EMOTION

19.1 Definitions

Affectivity

Affectivity (synonym: emotionality, temperament) denotes a man's entire emotional life or temperament, in respect of its predominant nature, i.e. the intensity, responsiveness and durability of his basic mood. Affectivity in this sense, taken together with basic activity or drive, provides an indication of personality. Thus we say, for example, that a man has a happy nature or is of a melancholy turn of mind.

Affect, emotion, feeling, mood[1]

These terms refer to the current frame of mind, the mood, the feelings of the moment; for example, a person is happy, or is in a cheerful mood. Ordinary speech covers a wide range of experiences which are expressed in emotional terms: this reflects not only a lack of precision in speech but also the realization that every experience contains an element of affect and, even if it seems to be neutral, is set within a certain frame of mind. We are always in some kind of mood vis-à-vis our world.

It is important to distinguish between the following:

(a) Localized bodily perceptions (protopathic, proprioceptive sensations) which affect our total mood: physical feelings of hunger, thirst, pain, the need to perform bodily functions, or sexual excitement, are experienced not only locally but as part of the whole mood, e.g. of unrest or tension.

(b) General physical perceptions, general feelings, feelings of vitality or zoe-aesthesia, which sustain the quality of mood and the basic activity or drive. They determine how an individual feels, rendering him lively, active, vigorous, brisk, excited, well, healthy, calm or relaxed. When he feels warmth or cold, each individual does so within his own frame of mind. When general feelings, feelings of vitality, are negative, the individual may express himself as feeling tired, limp, depressed, downcast, weak, ill, restless, etc.

(*c*) The less physically based frames of mind or spirits which permeate and govern the whole of experience and behaviour, e.g. joy, cheerfulness, high spirits, ill humour, vexation, anger, grief and anxiety, and from which the general feelings mentioned under (*b*) above cannot be sharply distinguished.

(*d*) Less structured, protopathic experiences of the self and the environment which can lead to presentiments[2] or misgivings that evoke a mood of ominous foreboding, with suspicion and distrust: for example, something menacing seems about to happen, someone is about to let us down, one may feel threatened (cf. delusional mood).

19.2 Neurophysiological foundations

Central nervous system

If the play of our emotions is to be normal, the brain as a whole must be unimpaired. There is also some reason to believe that the anterior brain stem, the thalamus and the *limbic system*, as well as the frontal thalamic pathways, are of particular importance in emotional experiences.

We know that disturbance in these areas from tumours or focal inflammation, or lesions deliberately produced as in leucotomy, can lead to changes in affectivity – poverty of affect, apathy, reduced sensitivity to pain.

Autonomic nervous system (*vegetative system*)

The centres of this system are closely associated with the cerebral areas mentioned above. Every affective state is accompanied by vegetative and, in particular, by sympathetic excitation which varies in extent according to the strength and acuity of the feeling aroused and according to individual reactivity: this determines the physical accompaniments of emotions: sweating, blushing, increased blood flow, awareness of heart-beat, rise or fall in blood pressure, hyperventilation, frequency of micturition, diarrhoea, etc. This brings us close to the so-called psychosomatic disorders.

When affective states are very strong, in violent fear, panic, rage, etc., we may get the so-called regressive motor patterns (Kretschmer, 1953, 1958): phylogenetically determined forms of behaviour, e.g. loss of consciousness, simulated death, crises of motor excitement, including running away or committing acts of violence.

Endocrine system

Hormonal changes are likewise closely associated with central nervous processes and with the functioning of the vegetative nervous system: the endocrine system plays an essential role, particularly in emergency reactions (pituitary ACTH, adrenal cortex-adrenaline, thyroid gland, etc.) and in instinctive behaviour.

19.3 Classification of emotions

The synopsis presented below represents a brief review of the relevant vocabulary and in no sense covers the endless multiplicity of the emotions.

States of emotion (spirits, moods)

The feelings listed below are those whose effect is predominantly upon the individual's own frame of mind. There is, however, only an artificial distinction between them and the emotions which affect all men in a more uniform manner.

(a) *Emotional states that are experienced almost physically* (feelings of vitality)

Pleasant; briskness, buoyancy, high spirits, well-being, light-heartedness, elation.

Unpleasant: weariness, feeling out of sorts, jitters, exhaustion, limpness, weakness, feeling ill, unrest.

(b) *Emotional states that are experienced less physically*

Pleasant: joy, cheerfulness, happiness, jubilation, peacefulness, merriness, contentment, confidence.

Unpleasant: sorrow, worry, grief, fear, anxiety, uneasiness, uncanniness, despondency, helplessness, homesickness, hopelessness, being harrowed, despair, horror, terror, emptiness, irritation, vexation, anger, rage, envy, jealousy.

(c) *Feelings that accompany the experience of self-evaluation* can hardly be separated from the above.

Positive: power, pride, superiority, triumph, vanity, defiance.

Negative: feelings of inadequacy, shame, guilt, remorse, embarrassment.

Feelings in regard to others

Positive: love, liking, trust, empathy, sympathy, esteem, interest, approval, gratitude, respect, admiration, worship.

Negative: hatred, dislike, mistrust, scorn, hostility, mockery, antipathy, indignation.

19.4   Examination

For clinical purposes enough information can be obtained from observation of the patient's behaviour and from his speech.

19.5   Pathology of the emotions

Summary:

Individual concepts

In clinical psychiatry certain characteristic changes in affect emerge as important:

Ambivalence

Parathymia

Poverty of affect

Feeling of emotional emptiness

Rigidity of affect

Tenacity of affect

Lability of affect

Incontinence of affect

(See below)

Affective states or syndromes

Clusters of symptoms in which changes of mood are the central feature are grouped together under the name of affective syndromes.

Depressive state or syndrome

Manic state or syndrome

Schizo-affective state or syndrome

Anxiety state or syndrome

Dysphoria, dysphoric state or syndrome

Hypochondriacal state or syndrome

(See below)

Primitive reactions (impersonal affective reactions)

(See below)

Persistent mood disorders

(See below)

Individual concepts in the psychopathology of the emotions
Ambivalence

Ambivalence (Bleuler, 1911) denotes the co-existence of positive and negative feelings, moods and strivings, a synchronism of Yes and No. The following categories may be distinguished:

Ambivalence of affect is the simultaneous existence of contradictory feelings towards a particular object, idea or experience. For example, love and hatred of the same person may exist simultaneously, without cancelling each other out – this is not the same as alternating emotions.

Ambivalence of intention and inclination covers the simultaneous existence of contradictory aspirations. For example, a patient who wants at one and the same time to eat and not to eat, may in consequence become frozen in a stupor-like state, the spoon halted halfway to his mouth.

Intellectual ambivalence is the existence of contradictory ideas, emotions and behaviour. For example, a patient stated: 'I am a human being like you and I am not a human being like you'.

Causal associations. Ambivalence is extensively encountered in normal psychology, when it is partially overcome by reflection and by feelings. In the sphere of religious psychology ambivalence is ubiquitous: the spirits and the gods are simultaneously loved and feared. An ancestral spirit, or a totem, arouses simultaneous fear and veneration. It is also widespread among depressives with their brooding indecisiveness and bewilderment, as well as among obsessional patients and at times in mixed states of manic-depression. Schizophrenics in particular suffer from severe ambivalence, arising from their deep sense of inner conflict, of lack of cohesion, of splitting and of inadequacy, and in addition from a sense of no longer being able to feel anything. For example, a schizophrenic mother killed the child she loved and then exhibited no affect of any kind; she 'switched off'.

Ambivalence can sometimes be overcome by excessive forms of behaviour: in drinking, in ecstasy, in panic, in forced and manic overacting.

Parathymia (inappropriate affect)

The patient's emotions do not match in a natural way the content of his current experience, either qualitatively in colouring and tone or quantitatively in intensity (cf. *Ego-consciousness*). Parathymia is seen chiefly in schizophrenics.

EXAMPLES

A patient reported that in the previous night he had again been tortured in the most terrible way, but he laughed while talking about it.

Another was pleased to receive a present, but complained about it (paramimia).

Another stated in a carefree matter-of-fact way that his intestines had been turned into ashes.

Another schizophrenic reported calmly that his insides were made entirely of gold and that every night he was sawn lengthwise into strips.

Poverty of affect

An individual is said to show poverty of affect, to be emotionally crippled, emotionally flat or emotionally barren, when there is a lack or loss of affective response and variety, when there is emotional indifference. Such people can develop no feelings for others; they seem to be cold and indifferent, to lack love, to be unsympathetic or at times callous, brutal, cold-hearted (the moral insanity of earlier psychiatric parlance). Poverty of affect may extend to feelings of self-worth. Such people are incapable of experiencing feelings of guilt, remorse, shame or pride.

Causal associations are:

(a) Constitutional, on a psychopathic-neurotic basis

(b) In the organic cerebral psychosyndrome, e.g. post-traumatic or alcoholic

(c) As a secondary development in addicts, e.g. alcoholics or heroin addicts

(d) An emotional barrenness sometimes also occurs as a residual symptom after schizophrenic illnesses

Feelings of emotional emptiness

Many depressed patients complain of an emotional void, stating that their feelings have withered and they can no longer experience joy, love or sorrow. This is usually associated with a severe decline in feelings of vitality.

For example: 'I am quite dead inside, I can't feel anything any more; everything in me is dead and empty; I can't take pleasure in anything, or be sad about anything; nothing moves me any more; everything is numb and desolate, as if it had turned to stone.'

Causal associations are found:

(a) Predominantly in endogenous depression

(b) At times also as an affective 'black-out' in neurotic and reactive depression

Rigidity of affect, stiffness of affect

This denotes a loss of the capacity for affective modulation. Unlike those with poverty of affect, the patients retain certain emotions, but their moods or affective states are set and do not vary with the external situation or with the topic under discussion.

For example, during a long conversation touching on various themes a patient will maintain the same heated hostility or mistrustful rejection.

Causal associations are found:

(a) In the organic psychosyndrome

(b) In many schizophrenics

(c) Sometimes in chronic excited mania

(d) In many depressives

Tenacity of affect (persistence of affect)

This is similar to rigidity of affect. Once a particular affect is established, it continues and colours the patient's mood for an inordinate length of time, e.g. in some epileptics, in the 'sticky' moods encountered in mental retardation sometimes, and also among depressive psychopaths.

Lability of affect

Here there are swift changes of mood and an increased distractibility of affect. Usually such emotions do not last for long: they show many swings or change their direction. For example, during interview a patient was very moved and became upset when asked about his home, his relatives and his dog. On the other hand, however, he very quickly brightened up again as he remembered something pleasant and his mood switched into exactly the opposite.

Causal associations are:

(*a*) The organic psychosyndrome

(*b*) Habitually in labile personalities; so-called explosive psychopaths show a particular lability in the direction of intemperate outbursts and aggressiveness

(*c*) Children and adults with infantile personalities

(*d*) Mental retardation

Incontinence of affect

By this terms is meant lack of emotional control so that emotions spring up with excessive suddenness, are excessively strong and cannot be mastered. For example, when asked his wife's name, a senile dement began to weep bitterly.

Causal associations are:

(*a*) In the organic psychosyndrome

(*b*) In psycho-labile personalities

N.B. The sudden and excessive outbursts of laughing and crying that occur in incontinence of affect should not be confused with the so-called *pathological laughing and crying*, formerly known as compulsive laughing and crying, that can be seen in many cerebral disorders, for example in post-encephalitic Parkinsonism: this is only mimicry of laughing and crying and there is no accompanying affective change.

Individual affective syndromes

Depressive state or syndrome

Particularly good introductions to this theme are to be found in Kielholz (1971), Binswanger (1960), Petrilowitsch and Baer (1970). *Psychopathological features* are listed below.

(1) Affect. The phenomena include sadness, dejection, misery, cheerlessness, a sense that all feeling is lacking (that emotion can no longer be felt); emptiness, numbness; a feeling that everything is a burden and that one's vitality is low; depression, despondency, hopelessness, pessimism, despair, feelings of guilt, anxiety, unworthiness, inferiority and suicidal impulses.

(2) *Hypochondriasis* (see Hypochondriacal state, Hyponchondriasis, below). The patient fears, imagines or suspects that he is ill. The bodily functions are anxiously observed, with increasing and often exaggerated attention.

(3) *Thinking.* Thoughts move in circles, with brooding, obsessional rumination, lack of ideation, emptiness and poverty of thinking, an inability to think and to decide or come to conclusions, an inhibition of thought and lack of will-power.

(4) *Depersonalization* (see page 50).

(5) *Derealization* (see pages 50, 135).

(6) *Experience of time* (see page 90): Time moves very slowly or even stands still. On the other hand, it can also seem to race.

(7) *Delusions.* The patient's whole experienced is coloured by his depressed mood, which leads also to delusional fears and convictions:

(*a*) Of physical illness, decay, dying (hypochondriacal delusion, delusion of perishing), e.g. 'I am rotten, I'm rotting away, I have fallen to pieces inside'. This may be extended to become a *nihilistic delusion*: 'I'm not alive any more'.

(*b*) Of guilt, sin, damnation. Here one finds delusions of guilt which may refer to infringement of worldly law, or of moral or religious canons.

(*c*) Of economic ruin, poverty. When suffering from delusions of poverty a patient said: 'I've got nothing left...I will have to starve...' (see also the chapter on *Delusion*).

(8) *Perception.* Everything is grey, faded, bleak, lifeless. The patient himself feels lifeless and unreal (depersonalization) and the world around him may look like this too (derealization). This reduced intensity of perceptual experience can affect all sensory modalities.

(9) *Hallucinations.* In severe depression hallucinations are not uncommon, often partaking of the nature of pseudo-hallucinations. The patient sees shadowy figures of death, of the devil, of a skeleton. Olfactory hallucinations are also fairly common, e.g. 'I smell of decay and pus'. 'It smells like a cemetery or a morgue'. Occasionally there are auditory hallucinations, e.g. voices making accusations of guilt.

(10) *Motor system.* On the one hand there may be motor inhibitions – slowness, rigidity to the point of stupor and mutism. Alternatively the patients may be agitated, excited, troubled by constant unrest; they may rush to and fro, scratch themselves, and utter stereotyped moans. The clinical picture may therefore be one of either inhibited or agitated depression.

(11) *Physical symptoms.* These are in keeping with the low vitality and include loss of drive and liveliness, tiredness, limpness, lack of strength, disturbed sleep, poor appetite, reduced flow of saliva with dryness of the mouth, constipation, loss of weight. Patients also look older, their skin is slack and their hair becomes dry and rough. Loss of libido and cessation of menstruation may occur.

(12) *Bodily ailments.* These are variegated and may include pains in the head, neck and back, a feeling of constriction in the neck, pressure on the chest, pains around the heart, heavy breathing, sighs, pressure in the stomach, a feeling of fullness and a feeling that the body is blown up.

Causal associations are:

(*a*) So-called endogenous depression: within a framework of monopolar endogenous depression, involutional depression or manic-depressive illness

(*b*) Depression in schizo-affective mixed psychoses

(*c*) Depression in schizophrenia

(*d*) Organic depression in structural cerebral damage

(*e*) Symptomatic depression accompanying various physical illnesses, including metabolic disorders and pharmacogenic depression, e.g. associated with reserpine

(*f*) Neurotic depression

(g) Depression in persistent affective states (fatigue depression, exhaustion depression)

(h) Psychoreactive depression (depressive reaction to life experience), an immediate reaction to a painful experience; a reaction of abnormally long duration (for details see the literature on special psychiatry).

Manic states

For the literature see Binswanger, 1945, 1960; Petrilowitsch and Baer, 1970; Rümke, 1924.

Psychopathological features are listed below.

(1) *Affect.* The basic mood ranges from cheerfulness to euphoria. The patient experiences feelings of power, elation, great capabilities, self-confidence, a spirit of enterprise leading to excessive and unrealistic planning and scheming with no critical self-awareness, confidence and optimism. There is also an excited-dysphoric variant of mania.

(2) *Thinking.* This is characterized by a wealth of ideas and associations, many plans and flight of thoughts and ideas.

(3) *Motor system.* There is an increase in the basic patterns of motor behaviour, with much bustle and hyperactivity, ranging from restlessness to manic excitement and frenzy.

(4) *Perception.* Sometimes there is an increase in the intensity of perception. Perceptual experiences are more vivid and penetrating.

(5) *Delusions.* These are rare on the whole. Sometimes there are expansive delusions of grandeur and self-aggrandizement.

Causal associations are:

(a) Endogenous mania within a framework of manic-depressive illness. It is not certain whether a monopolar form of endogenous mania exists.

(b) Manic state in schizo-affective mixed psychoses

(c) Manic state in schizophrenia

(d) Manic state in cerebral diseases, e.g. general paresis, or in general physical illness, e.g. manic states which accompany the acute exogenous reaction type

(e) Manic states in neuroses and in psychoreactive disorders are on the whole rare. At times, however, labile neurotic patients may show a temporary switch to manic overactivity

Affective changes in schizophrenia

(For the literature see Bleuler, 1911.) Many schizophrenics show poverty of affect, heightened affect and rigidity of affect, as well as tension. The patients are then abnormally attentive, expectant, excited and ready for action. A tense patient gives the impression that he might at any moment react in a surprising way, start attacking someone, become dangerous or abusive, or fly off the handle; there may be a perceptible readiness to attack.

A further characteristic of many schizophrenics is their emotional inaccessibility, their parathymia. This is not to say, however, that all schizophrenics show such affective abnormalities. There are also some who are sensitive and warm-hearted. Depressive and manic states also occur in schizophrenics and are accompanied by corresponding and considerable affective changes.

Anxiety state

For the literature see Battegay, 1970; Eysenck, 1957; Freud, 1894, 1926; v. Gebsattel, 1959; Kielholz, 1967; Lader, 1969; Lewis, 1967; Riemann, 1961; Wolpe, 1952.

Psychopathological features are listed below.

(1) *Mood.* The patient feels restricted, uncertain, restless, exposed, driven into a corner; his breath seems to have been taken away, he feels choked, frightened, worried about his physical health (hypochondriasis), conscious-stricken (guilt), 'afraid of life' (*Protocol 54*), etc. There are transitional stages between this and depressive states in which there is also always some element of anxiety.

(2) *Basic activity or drive.* The patient may appear tense, restless, excited, panic-stricken or benumbed.

(3) *Consciousness, perception, thinking.* There is a reduced capacity for reflection, for reviewing the situation, for consideration, with a narrowing of the field of perception.

(4) *Physical symptoms.* These include oppressive headache, palpitations, constricted throat, cardiac pains, tremors, giddiness, respiratory disorders, impotence and frigidity.

(5) *'Vegetative' symptoms. Sympathetic* excitement is accompanied by wide pupils, a raised pulse rate and blood pressure, a dryness of

the mouth, sweating and increased muscular tonus. *Parasympathetic* excitement is accompanied by nausea, vomiting, frequency of micturition and diarrhoea.

Anxiety states as such follow a typical pattern of behaviour but of course also show many other diverse characteristics which vary with the individual.

Causal associations are:

(*a*) General: this would include anxiety in the face of dangerous situations, e.g. serious physical disease, and anxiety associated with profound doubt, e.g. philosophical and religious doubt.

(*b*) Neurotic anxiety (see Freud's anxiety neurosis) denotes anxiety which is free floating, with no clearly recognizable cause, or which arises in response to objects or situations that in common experience are not dangerous, or only slightly so (phobias, situational anxiety, phobic avoidance). This is the province of psychotherapy in the broad sense and of the minor tranquillizers, the 'anxiolytics'.

(*c*) Anxiety in so-called *endogenous psychoses* is much more deeply rooted. Here it is a question of maintaining a hold on life (a state of devitalization), of ego-activity, ego-consistency, ego-demarcation, and ego-identity (see *Ego-consciousness*). This form of anxiety cannot usually be alleviated by minor tranquillizers, though it can often be helped by the use of neuroleptics and antidepressants. For other forms of treatment, see *Ego-consciousness*.

(*d*) Anxiety occurs in *mental disorders associated with physical illnesses*, both acute, e.g. delirium, alcoholic hallucinosis, and chronic, e.g. dementia. It is often also encountered in metabolic and endocrine disorders, e.g. hypoglycaemia, hyperthyroidism, phaeochromocytoma.

Dysphoria, dysphoric state

(Synonym: dysphoric = morose.)[3] Dysphoria is partly identical with hostility.

Psychopathological features. The patient is bad-tempered, surly, irritable, grizzly, crabbed, filled with stubborn anger, at times mistrustful and hostile. He is irritated by every stimulus, e.g. noise or being spoken to, and is often grimly pessimistic, a real misery who sees and paints everything in sombre colours. He is sometimes abusive, flaring up in a venomous manner; he can be carping, indulging in petty faultfinding and at times blustering and threatening, aggressive and violent. He blames others rather than himself and is broody and retiring, with occasional outbursts of irritation or greater excitement and aggressiveness; he may wander off or run away (poriomania), lock himself in his room, and indulge in paroxysms of abuse or violent acts of senseless destruction.

Causal associations:

(a) Ordinary bad temper in states of irritation and tension

(b) As a morose variant of depressive mood, in the premenstrual phase of the menstrual cycle

(c) As a permanent personality style of the bully or ill-tempered loner

(d) The influence of drugs, e.g. drunkenness, amphetamines

(e) In diffuse or more localized cerebral disorders, e.g. cerebral arteriosclerosis, cranial trauma

(f) In epileptics, as a spontaneous or reactive mood disorder

(g) In the mentally retarded

(h) As variants of depressive mood disorders of the most diverse aetiology (Weitbrecht's 'endoreactive dysthymia' (1968) partly belongs here

(i) In schizophrenics with feelings of persecution or grievance, or hallucinations (being pestered).

Hypochondriacal state, hypochondriasis

For the literature see Bräutigam, 1956; Feldman, 1972; Fischer-Homberger, 1970; Häfner, 1959; Janzarik, 1957, 1959; Kohn, 1958/59; Kulenkampff & Bauer, 1960; Ladee, 1966; Plügge, 1958, 1960; Ruffin, 1959; Weitbrecht, 1951; Wulff, 1958.

Psychopathology. Hypochondria is a fear, assumption or suspicion that one is ill or will become ill, for which there are insufficient 'objective' grounds (nosophobia). The hypochondriac has lost confidence in the functioning of his body, which he no longer takes for granted. He has no faith in his physical well-being and watches himself anxiously, paying excessive attention to his bodily functioning. He keeps feeling all manner of peculiar sensations and pains which provide him with constant warnings and renew his fears.

Hypochondriasis often begins in association with one of the many varieties of depressive mood disorder and is then part of the whole depressive state (q.v.). Within the framework of the depressive state with its diverse nosological implications, hypochondriacal fears of illness and destruction can also be associated with suicidal impulses.

Hypochondriacal delusion. If the hypochondriac's concern increases to the point of a delusional conviction, a delusional certainty that he is critically and incurably ill, that he is destined to be a chronic invalid or to die, this is called a hypochondriacal delusion (see chapter on *Delusion*).

Content of hypochondriacal fears. These cover basically every kind of physical and mental illness. The most common are: fear of cancer of the brain, the breast, the abdomen, the bowels, the liver, fear of dying of leukaemia, of multiple sclerosis, of syphilis, of consumption, of a heart attack. Sometimes there is a fear of being mentally ill, which can also occur as a well-grounded fear in the early stages of schizophrenia. The content of the fear may have family associations, e.g. a relative with or having died of cancer, or may carry social connections, e.g. the illness of a prominent figure in society. In India, as a transcultural variant of hypochondriacal fears, one encounters the delusional fear that the penis is shrinking and will disappear.

Causal associations are to be found:

(*a*) In *endogenous depression*, where hypochondriasis may be the dominant state and may be reflected in a variety of ways by all the other symptoms, especially obsessions, phobias and feelings of guilt and poverty. There are also expansive variants of delusional hypochondriasis: the patient thinks he is so ill, so foul, so rotten, so poisonous that the whole world, or his fellow patients, are being harmed by him and will have to perish because of their contact with him.

(*b*) In *schizophrenics* in whom hypochondriasis is associated with localized bodily sensations (somatic hallucinations) or with disturbances of all the patient's physical sensations (general or coenaesthetic sensations). Physical ruin, decay, illness are expressions of the disturbed and threatened ego-experiences (q.v.), though the complaints are not always experienced as emanating from outside the patient, as being 'done to him' by other people.

(*c*) In chronic *organically based psychoses* where a hypochondriacal state may occur in association with a psycho-organic state.

(*d*) In *neurotic illness* where hypochondriasis is an expression of weakness in coping with life, the world or personal relationships. It occurs in generally insecure, anxious, anankastic personalities, especially around puberty and then again at the beginning of old age, though it may also persist throughout life. It is often then associated with obsessions and phobias, with moods of anxiety and depression, and it may lead to a restricted style of life.

At times, too, neurotic hypochondriasis may be 'telephrenic', i.e. purposive, directed towards achieving the benefits of ill-health, in order to escape from the private and professional demands of life, to arouse sympathy, or to gain control over the family.

Neurotic hypochondriasis also includes hypochondriacal psychosomatic disorders, such as cardiac phobias (Kulenkampff and Bauer, 1960).

Primitive reactions (impersonal affective reactions)

These include the so-called *affective hysterical states* which begin with strong affective accompaniments: twilight states, confusional states, clouded consciousness, as well as explosive outbursts of rage (*raptus*) with accompanying physical (motor and vegetative) changes. *Affective stupor* denotes a switching off in states of great emotion, rage, grief and reaction to catastrophes (simulated death reflex, storm of motor excitement). In these primitive reactions (Kretschmer, 1958, 1971) the individual is so overpowered by emotion that his reaction no longer bears the stamp of his own personality.

Persistent mood disorders

These are lasting states of emotion that amount to changes in personality, to abnormal reactive developments resulting from persistent emotional pressure. They include bitterness, mistrust, querulance, chronic feelings of inadequacy and resentment. Such developments are found, for example, in persons who have undergone very harrowing experiences, e.g. in a concentration camp (Baeyer *et al.*, 1964; Eitinger, 1964; Matussek, 1971) or suffered insurmountable injury in the personal or professional sphere.

CONATIVE FUNCTIONS (DRIVES)

This term (Latin: *conatus* = striving) is used to cover such functions
as are not included in cognitive, affective and motor functioning, i.e.

Need
Drive
Instinct
Motivation
Will, intention

20.1 Definitions

These functions are often ill-defined and the terms lack consistency.
Their nature is often not made sufficiently clear, i.e. whether they
denote phenomena that can be experienced (e.g. a need) or are
constructs, such as drive or instinct. At times the concepts cover
something that is directly identifiable, e.g. actions prompted by drives
or instincts; at other times they cover states of mind, e.g. needs, that
are accessible to self-observation, can be learned from direct
conversation, or can be inferred from behaviour. For the present
purpose we interpret the various concepts as follows:

Need (a phenomenological concept): a striving towards a particular
object, state or action, that is experienced as a desire.

Drive (a construct): an inclination to satisfy certain primary, i.e.
innate, needs.

Instinct (a construct): an innate pattern of behaviour which leads
to drive-satisfaction.

Motivation: (*a*) as a phenomenological concept: a more or less
clearly experienced mood or affect which is governed by needs
and which moves us to actions which satisfy these needs; (*b*) as
a construct: a hypothetical activating factor.

Will (a phenomenological concept): a goal-directed striving or
intention based on cognitively planned motivation.

20.2   Review and classification

Review of needs (and actions which satisfy needs)

Primary needs: innate, not learned. These needs correspond to an essential requirement of life, essential for the maintenance of homeostasis, i.e. for survival: they are fixed, brook no postponement and are little affected by acquired or learned characteristics:

Hunger (appetite)
Thirst
Breathing
Urination and defaecation
Sleep
Self-preservation

Other needs are not essential for survival: they can be postponed, more scope can be allowed to satisfy them, they are more affected by acquired, as opposed to instinctively controlled, patterns of behaviour:

Sexual drive
Social or community drive
Drive to care for one's young
Drive to movement and play
Exploratory drive (curiosity)

Secondary needs. Acquired or conditioned needs are very numerous and vary with the individual, e.g. variants of appetite, smoking.

The clinical and practical classification of drives

For practical purposes the vital drives may still be divided into the traditional two broad classes, according to the functions which they mainly subserve:

Individual survival
  Hunger
  Thirst
  Sleep
  Self-preservation (defence or flight)
Survival of the species
  Sexual drive
  Drive to care for one's young

20.3 Foundations and determinants

Anatomical localization

On the basis of experimental stereotactic studies in neurophysiology it has been postulated that drives are localized in centres in the midbrain (hypothalamus) which also partly govern their inhibition and release (Hess, 1962). The findings suggest an anatomical and physiological basis for the polar structure of drives (activity and inhibition).

Hormonal and metabolic aspects

Insulin and blood sugar, together with the filling and evacuation of the intestinal tract, regulate hunger and satiety; sex hormones, *inter alia*, regulate the sexual drive, while various hormones affect water and electrolyte balance, thereby influencing thirst amongst other drives.

Sensory afference

Total sensory afference helps to determine conative tension. In other words, all the acoustic, visual, olfactory and tactile stimuli that impinge on the individual exercise a positive or negative, inhibitory effect on his different needs. This underlines, of course, the importance of social influences, which may have either a strengthening or an inhibitory effect.

Learning processes

The learning processes and ingrained habits of the individual and of his society help to determine the emergence of his primary needs and, above all, of the actions which satisfy these needs.

20.4 Examination

No special measures are normally required, information being obtained in conversation and from observation of relevant conative behaviour.

Comments on the expression of conative functions. Conative behaviour, as revealed in the observation of others, can be theoretically viewed as the product of drive strength and inhibition. So-called instinctual behaviour need not be the expression of an excessively strong drive, but may result from lack of control or the relaxation of inhibition. Weak instinctual behaviour may be the expression of excessive, anxious control, inhibiting drives that are possibly of normal strength. Instinctive psychopaths are persons who immediately give way to impulses and often also to drives in the narrower sense over which they have no control. Such individuals thus yield more easily to temptation when opportunity presents itself, e.g. sexual crimes. In mania, with its framework of generally heightened vitality and lack of control, impulsive behaviour is naturally more marked. In depression, total basic activity (q.v.) decreases and with it all individual drives. In severe and debilitating physical illnesses activity (q.v.) and individual drives also decrease sharply in force.

20.5 Pathology

Hunger (appetite)
Quantitative anomalies

These fall into two categories:
(1) Excessive appetite, (bulimia, polyphagia). Excessive appetite and excessive eating, leading often to obesity (adiposity).
   Causal associations are:
   (*a*) Organic. Bulimia is encountered in disorders of the hypothalamus, at times also in diffuse cerebral damage, e.g. cerebral arteriosclerosis.
   (*b*) Psychogenic-neurotic. Excessive consumption of food, especially sweets, occurs as a substitute gratification in chronic emotional frustration, in chronic conflict and tension (to settle the nerves, stress fatness).
   (*c*) Psychotic. Bulimia is sometimes found in schizophrenics but is rare in psychotic states.
(2) Decrease or loss of appetite (anorexia).
   Causal associations are:
   (*a*) Organic. Anorexia occurs in severe physical illnesses, exhaus-

tion, fever, and particularly in many and varied disorders of the central nervous system.

(*b*) Psychogenic-neurotic. Anorexia is often found in depressive mood disorders, grief or worry. Anorexia nervosa, occurring usually in young girls, is a psychogenic disorder of appetite (reduced intake of food, alternating with ravenous hunger, which has been interpreted as a kind of boggling at growing up, an outcome of anxiety when faced by the role and demands of womanhood (or manhood) (for the literature see Jores, 1954; Kuhn, 1951, 1953; Meyer, 1965; Thomä, 1961; Zutt, 1948).

(*c*) Psychotic. Endogenous depressives usually lose all appetite. Many negativistic schizophrenics, or schizophrenics suffering from delusions of poisoning, may also refuse to eat.

Qualitative anomalies of hunger

Anomalies of appetite take various forms. Special cravings (known as pica) are sometimes found in pregnant women, or in psychotic or mentally retarded patients. Psychopaths, psychotics and mentally retarded patients sometimes eat unpalatable things, e.g. coprophagia (eating faeces), necrophagia and anthropophagia (eating corpses, cannibalism). Some neurotic and psychopathic individuals swallow nails and spoons, seeking thereby to gain admission to hospital (so-called Münchhausen syndrome). Convicted prisoners sometimes try in this way to get out of prison and into a hospital from which it is easier to escape.

Thirst

Excessive thirst (polydipsia) (for the literature see Berning *et al.*, 1972; Peters *et al.* 1974).

Causal associations are:

(*a*) Organic. Polydipsia occurs in pituitary or renal diabetes insipidus. Because of antidiuretic hormone deficiency, the kidneys do not reabsorb enough water and therefore pass too much liquid, thus causing a chronic thirst. Renal diseases, as well as certain drugs, can also cause excessive thirst.

(*b*) Psychogenic-neurotic. Polydipsia is often interpreted as a substitute oral gratification or as a form of purification (washing clean).

(c) Psychotic. Excessive thirst occurs sometimes as a habit in schizophrenics, who then may also use abnormal sources for their fluids, e.g. drinking water from the lavatory bowl.

N.B. In dipsomania we find an abnormal, periodic thirst for alcohol. This represents less of a real thirst than a need for alcohol. Many dipsomaniacs suffer basically from a periodic endogenous or reactive mood disorder.

There is no such thing as loss of thirst, though some patients who refuse in general to eat will also refuse to drink, e.g. catatonics.

Self-preservation

At times patients may fail to follow the natural self-preserving instinct of defence or flight, e.g. severely retarded patients and schizophrenics with a very low activity level and severe autism. On the other hand, danger may also shock a schizophrenic out of his autistic state.

21

SEXUALITY

21.1 Definition

Sexuality denotes experience and behaviour which is based on the male–female sex differentiation. It includes consciousness of sex, one's own and the opposite sex, sexual desire, sex-instinct, libido, and sexual behaviour.

21.2 Foundations

For the literature see Dörner (1972); Giese (1971); Masters and Johnson (1966); Orthner (1971a, b); Sigusch (1972).

(1) Sex chromosomes determine *genetic* (gonosomal) sex: male = XY, female = XX.

(2) Gonads determine *gonadal* sex. The Y-chromosome leads to differential development of the testes through the action of the hormone androgen on the sexual centre in the midbrain at an early stage of foetal development. Two X-chromosomes determine the development of the ovaries.

(3) Development of the gonads during the specific and sensitive phases of foetal organisation leads to the development of *somatic sex* by the hormonal action of androgens, oestrogens and gestagens: the internal and external sexual parts are developed as primary sex characteristics, the secondary sex characteristics being formed at the same time.

(4) Genetic, gonadal and somatic sex together form the basis which enables *psychological sex* to develop under the most varied psychosocial post-natal conditions: understanding of one's own sex (sexual consciousness), sexual desire (sex instinct) and sexual behaviour. Sex hormones determine the strength of sexual drives, but not their direction which depends on the total development of the individual within his community.

21.3 Development

Firmly established facts about the development of sexuality are still meagre, even in regard to the age at which it is possible to speak of a child's sexual feelings (Klein, 1932; Rutter, 1971; Stoller, 1973). The onset of menstruation (12–14 years) and ejaculation (13–14 years) signify only the beginning of the period of fertility: the ages given apply to the mid-European area.

If sexual consciousness and sexual feelings are to develop normally, it is essential for a child to have a healthy psychosocial environment in which to mature, including the relationship with the mother and the rest of the family, especially brothers and sisters, as well as with playmates of both sexes. Apart from the somatic prerequisites already mentioned, which operate in their own special phases, the following influences also affect personality development, which is inseparable from sexuality: social factors, including the ethical, religious and cultural background, as well as the individual's entire life-history, experience and situation (Schelsky, 1955). Sexuality evolves in the course of this development and is at the same time founded on social education, on the development of a sense of 'us', an *Intention des Du* (Frankl, 1959). Sexuality as a form of behaviour involves the entire soma and the whole field of human relationships, and becomes centred on sexual areas only with the growth of sexual stimulation.

Freud's concept of sexuality has been the most influential and is reproduced here because of its widespread dissemination and its significance for the interpretation of sexual deviations (Freud, 1924; Abraham, 1971) (Table 9).

According to Freud the libido may be arrested at any of its stages of development, by conditioning, fixation or regression; this leads to perversions. Freud assumed a 'polymorphous perverse sexuality' in children.

Early childhood and puberty appear to be particularly sensitive phases in human sexuality. The capacity for forming normal relationships and developing normal sexuality comes into being only in the society of one's own kind and in the timely and playful exercise of human intercourse, by example and verbal instruction as well as by learning to conquer anxiety and pain.

Table 9. *Psycho-analytical schema of psychosexual development*

Age	Organization of the libido	Object love	Associated abnormalities
6 months	1. Oral stage (sucking) oral passive	None Auto-erotism	Auto-erotism
1st year	2. Oral stage (biting, eating) oral aggressive	(polymorphous perverse) Narcissism Object incorporation pre-ambivalent	Oralism
2nd year	1. Anal stage (pleasure in defecation) eliminative	ambivalent Partial love (polymorphous perverse	Masochism
3rd year	2. Anal stage (pleasure in retaining faeces) retentive	(polymorphous perverse)	Sadism
3rd year	Early genital stage Urethral stage (pleasure in urinating)	(polymorphous perverse)	Urethralism
4th year	Early genital stage Phallic stage	Object love excluding the sexual organs	Exhibitionism
5th year	(pleasure in manipulating own sexual organs)	Masturbation	
6th year	Early genital stage	Object love (oedipal)	Homosexuality Disorders of potency
12th year	Latency period		Frigidity
Puberty Adult-hood	Late (mature) genital stage	Mature hetero-sexual genital sexuality (post-oedipal)	

21.4   The problem of normality

Any judgement of what constitutes normal sexuality is very much affected by social, cultural and religious circumstances, by the context of time, place and civilization, and by traditional, moral and ethical ideas. Judgements are thus subject to great variation and are often dogmatic. The early Central European *Psychopathia sexualis* (Krafft-Ebing, 1918; Hirschfeld, 1926; etc.) has been overtaken by the findings of ethologists like Malinowsky (1962) and Mead (1949, 1959) and of systematic, statistical research based on interviews and questionnaires (Kinsey, 1948, 1953). This liberation of sex from dogma opened up new pathways of research. (For a review of the literature on forms of sexuality, see Ford and Beach, 1968; Marshall and Suggs, 1971.)

Mating or coitus (copulation, cohabitation) is central to the sexual behaviour of the sexually mature individual. Coital behaviour may be defined as *normal when it takes place with a partner of the opposite sex in such a way that there is a possibility of fertilization, and that neither partner suffers from it or is damaged by it.*

Non-coital sexual behaviour on the part of sexually mature individuals may be called abnormal only when it is practised not just as an introduction to or accompaniment of coitus but, despite opportunities for coitus, as the exclusive or preferred form of behaviour. Then only can we speak of *sexual deviations*. The further such behaviour is removed from normal coital behaviour, the more immature it is, the more rigid its performance, the more passionate dependence there is on it, the more justifiable it is to use the term *perversion*.

N.B. Sexuality is one dimension of interpersonal relationships. All sexual disturbances should be regarded as signs of disturbed relationships reaching far beyond the narrow sexual field.

21.5   Pathology

This schematic classification of sex disorders takes no account of the severity of the deviation. There is frequent overlapping, particularly between (1) and (2) below

(1) Abnormal sex object
   Homosexuality (sexual partner of the same sex)
   Primary homosexuality
   Secondary homosexuality

Psychotic homosexuality
Paedophilia (child as sexual partner)
Gerontophilia (elderly person as sexual partner)
Bestiality (animal as sexual partner)
Autosexuality (sexual activity without a partner)
Necrophilia (corpse as sex object)
Fetishism (non-genital object)

(2) Abnormal sexual practices (abnormal way of achieving sexual excitement/satisfaction)
Oralism (mouth)
Coprophilia (faeces), coprophagia, urolagnia (urine), necrophagia
Analism (anus)
Urethralism (urinary tract)
Sadism (pleasure in inflicting pain)
Masochism (pleasure in suffering pain)
Scoptophilia (voyeurism, peeping)
Exhibitionism
Frotteurism (extragenital rubbing)
Transvestism (wearing the clothes of the opposite sex)

(3) Abnormal sexual identity
Transsexualism

(4) Abnormal intensity of sex drive
Hypersexuality
Hyposexuality

(5) Disorders of potency
Impotence, frigidity
Organic
Psychotic
Neurotic-psychogenic
Psychogenic impotence in the male
Psychogenic impotence in the female

Three theories of perversion deserve mention (Boss, 1966):

(*a*) *Psychoanalytical theory of perversion* (Freud, 1904–5, 1920, 1924, 1925–1932; Fenichel, 1931). This postulates 'polymorphous perversion' as a normal transitional stage in sexual development. Repressions due to castration and Oedipus complexes, learning processes and character stamp, lead to the dominance of partial drives and to their fixation as perversions in the adult. The psychoanalytical causal-genetic theory of perversions does not furnish an understandable presentation of the perverted, unsuccessful relationships encountered in the 'omnipotence of love' (Freud, 1904–1905). For a critique of this theory see Boss (1966).

(*b*) *'Anthropological' theory of perversion* (see v. Gebsattel, 1929;

Straus, 1930; Kunz, 1942). According to this view, perversions represent a 'destructive mutilation and fragmentation of the erotic sense of love'; destructive impulses prevail; the normal direction of love is reversed. But this, too, fails to provide an understanding of the perversions and deformations that mar love's striving for 'a unification and augmentation of existence' (Boss, 1966). For a critique of this theory see Boss (1966).

(c) *Existential theory of perversion* (*daseinsanalytische Perversions-theorie*). Boss (1966) interprets the 'sense and content' of sexual perversions as concrete, ontological forms of interpersonal behaviour within the context of the fundamental ontological stipulation of 'being-in-the-world' (*In-der-Welt-sein*) and 'being-with' (*Mitsein*) in the sense of Heidegger's *Daseinsanalyse*. This theory makes it possible to apply a biographical historical understanding to these special and deformed ways of loving and to explain them in their essential nature as limitations of existence (for details see the perversions).

Abnormal sex object
Homosexuality

Synonyms are sexual inversion, contrary sexual feeling, homophilia. (For the literature see Feldman and McCulloch, 1971; Freud, 1969; Giese, 1958; Wolff, 1973.) It is defined as erotic attraction, sexual excitement and possibly sexual gratification from association with partners of the same sex.

Not every attraction between persons of the same sex should be classed as homosexual, e.g. friendship. The concept of unequivocal homosexuality, in inclination or practice, should moreover be kept distinct from the psycho-analytical concept of latent homosexuality. *Difficulties of delineation* lie essentially in the *bisexual predisposition* which it is possible for an individual to possess. Between homosexuality and heterosexuality there is a broad spectrum with a central band of bisexuality that may last a lifetime. Moreover, towards the end of puberty there is in normal psychological development a transitional stage of homoerotic inclination (*developmental homosexuality*) that precedes the final stage of heterosexual adjustment. Difficulties in delineation are also caused by *homosexuality from need*, that is to say when heterosexual contacts are not available to men who are not homosexually inclined, e.g. in prison, at sea, in military service; this is an example of the way in which situations can affect sexual behaviour. In many societies homosexual practices, mostly between men and boys before their initiation, exist side by side with heterosexual practices (Malinowski, 1962; Ford and Beach, 1968).

Occurrence. Persistent and exclusive homosexual practices are found in about 4 per cent of men and about 2 per cent of women. Homosexual experience, however, is much more frequent. Kinsey *et al.* (1954) found that homosexual contacts to the point of orgasm had been experienced at one time or another by about 37 per cent of adult males and about 13 per cent of adult females.

Genesis of homosexuality. This is not known. It would now seem certain that there are no regularly occurring macroscopic or microscopic organic changes in 'homosexuals' in general, nor are there biochemical, hormonal or other pathophysiological deviations. On the other hand, however, there is no satisfactory evidence of a pure and exclusive psychogenesis that applies to all cases of homosexuality. *Homosexuality is heterogeneous in origin* and is heterogeneous also in regard to the readiness to put homosexual inclinations into practice, to ways of doing this, to any desire to be therapeutically liberated from such inclinations, and to therapeutic accessibility.

There are essentially two current and conflicting hypotheses concerning the origin of homosexuality.

(*a*) Biological. In biological terms homosexuality becomes an inborn variant of sexuality and is somatic in origin. This argument is supported by the family constellation of homosexuality that is occasionally found and by the higher concordance found in monozygotic as compared with dizygotic twins.

(*b*) Psychological. According to both the psycho-analytical and behaviourist concepts, homosexuality is an acquired disorder of psychosexual maturation. It is learned, imprinted and fixated in certain psychosocial conditions. It is the expression of a comprehensive disturbance of interpersonal relations.

According to the psychogenetic interpretation, neurotic homosexuality is produced by strong, overprolonged emotional ties, either positive or negative, with one or both parents. There are four possibilities to consider (Allen, 1969).

(1) Hostility towards the mother. In male homosexuals, hostility

towards the mother prevents the individual from making an emotional transfer from the mother to other women: fear and hostility towards the mother become generalized in a rejection of all women. Hostility towards women means that erotic attraction is then limited to men. In female homosexuals hostility towards the mother makes it impossible to assume a female role in relation to others, especially in relation to men.

(2) Strong positive ties with the mother. This leads in men to a lasting fixation on mother and blocks the way to maturity. No mature relationship is thus possible with other women, and at the same time there is a childish devotion – 'remaining true to mother'. In girls an excessive and persistent attachment to the mother may be generalized into a lasting, erotic attraction to other women. Such excessive attachment to the mother is not always entirely due to the mother. It may occur also if there is no father, e.g. as the result of such factors as divorce or war, or if the father is not 'emotionally involved' in the family.

(3) Hostility towards the father. This prevents a man from assuming a masculine role, while in a woman it becomes hostility towards men in general.

(4) Strong attachment to the father. A strong positive attachment to and internalized identification with a father who is effeminate in the sense that he does not adopt the traditional role of leading partner – for example, when he is dominated by his partner or when he is divorced – and who is forced to take over what are usually regarded as women's functions in regard to his son, may prevent the son from developing a mature masculine relationship with women, thus preparing the way for homosexuality.

The possibilities listed above are examples of an attempt at explanation and interpretation which is only partly borne out by experience and which may be valid for many homosexuals without necessarily excluding the contribution made by other circumstances. In particular, it is not clear how such disturbed relationships necessarily lead to homosexuality, since obviously by no means every son who feels hostility towards his mother, for example, becomes a homosexual. There must also be other factors which play a part, for example a subsequent seduction or some such event, but it is not clear whether, and if so to what extent, homosexual seduction in adolescence affects the development of homosexuality. There are strong grounds, derived in particular from ethnology, for assuming it to be of no significance if there is not already an inclination in this direction. There are no clear indications of the causes of the supposed hostility. It would seem that the hatred may stem from actual experience, e.g. oppression, brutality, alcoholism, weakness, but that it can also have its roots in the imagination.

On the basis of their therapeutic experience many authors have distinguished three kinds of homosexuality (Boss, 1966; Bräutigam, 1972; Feldman and McCulloch, 1971).

(1) Primary homosexuality. This is assumed to be constitutional, based on predisposition. No reliable data exist about its cause and genesis. The cause is presumably biological. In the dreams of primary homosexuals, heterosexual elements never appear. Nor do such homosexuals show any desire to be freed from their inclination. They are not in this sense treatable. If they get into personal or social difficulties, therapy is more concerned with helping them to recognize their own inclination and with removing any feelings of inferiority.

(2) Secondary homosexuality. This is associated with fear of heterosexuality based on a variety of factors. Secondary or *inhibitory homosexuality* is thus to be regarded as a substitute form of behaviour for heterosexuality, which is repressed because of fear. In the dreams of such homosexuals heterosexual elements appear again and again, i.e. such people can experience heterosexual relationships in their dreams. Many such homosexuals are immature. They are afraid of sexuality in general: of their own sexuality because on the basis of earlier experience they equate it with brutality, and of female sexuality because they are unsure of themselves in their sexual role. These homosexuals often suffer because of their preference; they want to be successfully treated for it, and are more easily accessible to therapy.

(3) Psychotic homosexuality. Boss (1966) defines this as the homosexuality which may arise in a schizophrenic whose shrinking existence leads to increasing restriction in the possibilities of forming interpersonal relationships.

The social problems of homosexuals. Homosexuals suffer greatly from society's scorn and prohibition of their inclinations. They are often outcasts, leading clandestine and lonely lives, especially in old age. Many develop a chronic attitude of resentment against society and develop chronic depressive states. This may lead to secondary alcoholism and other forms of addiction, such as drug addiction, and also to suicide.

Forensic implications. Homosexual acts between consenting adults do *not* constitute a punishable offence in Europe, apart from Finland and Austria, so long as they do not take place in public. Homosexual activity with minors is a punishable offence.

Society's ban on homosexuality can lead to blackmail. Fear of discovery can become a cause of murder. Theft or robbery, as encountered in the heterosexual milieu of prostitution, is also common among homosexuals of a particular circle.

There is also a form of homosexual prostitution by boy prostitutes, often involving individuals who themselves have no clear homosexual tendencies.

Treatment should be attempted only where there is a desire for treatment.

(*a*) Analytical psychotherapy. The aim here is to achieve psycho-sexual maturity. Only neurotic homosexuality is likely to be cured by treatment. There are no unequivocal reports of the results of treatment.

(*b*) Behaviour therapy. This is used in many forms e.g. aversion therapy, deconditioning. There are virtually no convincing statistics of successful therapy, supported by case histories.

(*c*) Supportive, advisory therapy. The aim is acceptance of homo-sexuality as a variant of human sexuality, with removal of feelings of inferiority and resentment, treatment of secondary depression and preventive measures against suicide.

Paedophilia (*sexuality with children*)

This is defined as sexual desire and sexual gratification from sexual contact with sexually immature individuals. Paedophilia occurs in homosexual and in heterosexual forms (about 75 per cent). It is found usually in inhibited individuals who are poor at making interpersonal contacts and can find no access to adult sexual partners. It may also occur in psychopaths, alcoholics, the mentally retarded and at times in old people. Sexual activity mostly takes the form of masturbation.

Forensic implications. Paedophilia is a criminal offence. The children involved, who are usually girls, are not often injured by paedophilic acts. Detrimental effects on their subsequent psychosexual development have not been confirmed, and inviting behaviour on the part of the victim is not infrequent.

Apart from encouraging contacts and giving supportive therapy, therapeutic measures include preventive castration or suppression of sexual desire by the use of drugs.

Gerontophilia

This is defined as sexual desire and perhaps sexual gratification from contact with elderly people. It is extremely rare and of little practical significance. Both heterosexual and homosexual variants have been described.

Bestiality

Bestiality (synonyms: zooerasty, sodomy) is the use of an animal as sex object. Existing data on occurrence are very vague, as most cases do not come under observation. According to Kinsey, 8 per cent of men and about 3.6 per cent of women in the U.S.A. had had some sort of bestial experience. Zooerasty would seem to occur primarily in situations favouring the act and is found among shepherds, peasant boys and sometimes in the mentally retarded. Brutal men, especially when drunk, may commit acts of bestiality. Such acts are often combined with sadism, e.g. putting the handle of a fork into the vagina of a deer or a mare (see v. Hentig, 1962).

Bestiality has more implications in forensic and veterinary medicine, e.g. cruelty to animals and injury to animals, than in therapeutic psychiatry. In Europe it is not a criminal offence, though as cruelty to animals it may be indictable.

Autosexuality

Autosexuality (synonyms: sexual 'ipsism', self-gratification) is any sexual act performed on one's own person. The most frequent form of autosexuality is *masturbation* (onanism). *Masturbation is abnormal only if it is practised by adults as the only form of sexual activity that is desired and practised when possibilities of normal sexual activity exist.* It follows from this that manipulation of the genitals in childhood, or masturbation in puberty or by adults who have no heterosexual contacts (onanism from need) should not be regarded as abnormal. Masturbation is abnormal when it is carried out in an addictive-neurotic way, often less to satisfy sexual needs than as a means of relieving tension, e.g. to counteract nervousness, or induce sleep. Masturbation was formerly and erroneously blamed as the cause of many physical and mental illnesses, not least the psychoses. Depressive, hypochondriacal or paranoid elaboration of onanism in early life is not uncommon even today.

The danger and ill-effects of masturbation as the sole form of sexual activity lie in the extensive narcissistic encapsulation which ensues, and in a sexual self-sufficiency which leads further and further away from the adoption of normal heterosexual contacts. Pathological autosexuality occurs in many variants: as masochistic autosexuality, as auto-analism, or as auto-urethralism.

Necrophilia

This use of a dead body as sexual object is very rare, and usually occurs in association with other perversions, e.g. sadism, fellatio. Necrophilia has been described in both men and women. Necrophiliacs are clearly abnormal in many ways: individuals who are mentally retarded, mentally ill or otherwise handicapped and who for whatever reason cannot attain satisfactory sexual relations with living human beings. Necrophilia has forensic implications, e.g. the desecration of corpses, and has been known to lead to murder, cf. necrophagia. (For the literature see Spoerri, 1959.)

Fetishism

Fetishism is sexual excitement and gratification from substitute objects which are unsuitable for normal sexual pursuits. These include extra-genital parts of the body, e.g. feet and hair, and various objects such as linen, articles of clothing, stockings, showed, fur, rubber teats and wigs.

Fetishism occurs mostly in men, in heterosexual and homosexual forms. There is also a paedophilic variety, e.g. nappy fetishism. The fetish not only represents the human partner, but effaces him. The fetishist is too much afraid of his partner, especially of his genitals, and therefore avoids him by seeking a substitute (see in particular Boss's existential interpretation, 1966). According to the psychoanalytical interpretation fetishism is an aberration that arises at the pre-genital stage as a fixation on the first love object, the mother's breast. There is often an additional sadistic element: the fetish is often violently handled and destroyed. Fetishism is chiefly of forensic significance, as it may lead to theft (kleptomania), assault and robbery.

Abnormal sexual practices

(Abnormal ways of achieving sexual excitement/gratification)

Oralism

Oralism (synonyms: penilingus (fellatio) = oral stimulation of the penis; coitus *per os*; and cunnilingus = oral/sexual stimulation of the female genitals) is defined as sexual gratification from oral stimulation of the sexual organs, e.g. sucking, licking, biting. It may be heterosexual or homosexual, active or passive and is a frequent and in no sense abnormal practice with both sexes. It becomes a perversion only when an individual is fixated on oralism as his or her exclusive form of sexual activity and the only one which brings satisfaction.

Oralism can be viewed as the sexual practice which is governed by the child sucking at the mother's nipple. Oralism is thus interpreted as a fixation at an early libidinous (oral) stage of development. Oralism is also interpreted as a sign of immature, incomplete, arrested psychosocial development.

Coprophilia, coprophagia, urolagnia, necrophagia

Necrophagia is sexual excitement derived from eating victims one has killed; often only the genitals are eaten. Necrophagia is on the whole rare and seems to be a crime committed by very seriously abnormal personalities. There appears to be a relationship between this and coprophilia (see Boss's interpretation, 1966) urolagnia (sexual excitement gained from faeces, urine, spittle) and coprophagia (sexual pleasure in eating such substances).

Analism

Analism (synonyms: anal intercourse, coitus *per anum*, paederasty, sodomy, buggery) is the use of the anus for sexual stimulation and gratification. It is more a homosexual than a heterosexual practice and comprises about 20 per cent of the sexual practices of homosexuals. It may be active or passive. Auto-analism is more rare – obtaining sexual stimulation from the introduction of an instrument, e.g. a bottle, into the anus. In some cultures, e.g. in New Guinea, anal intercourse is a regular occurrence between men and boys, in the magic belief that this alone allows boys to mature into men.

   The psycho-analytical interpretation of analism speaks of fixation and regression to an anal stage of development. It is also considered that the anus may become a substitute for the vagina either by natural inclination (*Prägung*) or by conditioning.

Urethralism

The use of the urethra for sexual stimulation and gratification occurs mostly as auto-urethralism: the introduction of objects into the urethra and thence often also into the bladder. According to casuistic reports, all manner of animate and inanimate objects enter the bladder in this way, e.g. thermometers.

Sadism

Sadism (synonyms: active algolagnia, love of torture) is sexual stimulation and gratification derived from the infliction of pain. No reliable data exist on the frequency of sadism, which appears to occur predominantly in men. Sadism may occur in conjunction with all kinds of other perversions. Not only may it be heterosexual and homosexual, but it can also be combined with paedophilia or bestiality, or it may be polymorphous. The sadist's methods are chiefly beating, cutting or biting of the breast, buttocks and genitals. Sadism is principally of forensic significance since it can lead to injury to the sex object or even to murder. It is doubtful whether there are transitional stages between sexual sadism and sexual cruelty or brutality. The sexual sadist can express his feelings towards his fellows only by cruelty. He is dangerous only to those whom he would love if he were normal. He is usually impotent and can release his sexual tension only by sadistic acts.

Theories on the origin of sadism. Sadism represents a violent attempt on the part of an immured man seeking love (Boss, 1966) to break out by inflicting pain, often upon himself as well (sado-masochism). Theories concerning its genesis depend upon the theories held about aggression.

Freud (1920–1924, *Beyond the Pleasure Principle*) put forward the following hypotheses: (1) The death instinct (Thanatos) is directed against one's own self; (2) Sexual pleasure in killing arises from a combination of libido (Eros, love instinct) and Thanatos: this first produces masochism; (3) Masochism is then inverted and externalized as sadism. Other authors (e.g. Allen, 1969) take as their starting point a lack of mother love, an early childhood frustration, which leads to hatred of and aggression against the mother. The theoretical rather than empirical way in which this then leads to heterosexual and homosexual sadism may be seen in the diagram (Fig. 7).

Masochism

Masochism (synonym: passive algolagnia) i.e. sexual stimulation and gratification from suffering pain, may be heterosexual or homosexual or take the form of automasochism.

Masochism in the male. Methods: torture, sometimes self-inflicted, by beating, chaining, strangulation, electric shock, tying a cord round the penis. It can lead to injury and even to self-inflicted fatalities.

Masochism has been interpreted as follows (Allen, 1969):

Heterosexual masochism. (1) A desire to inflict pain on the mother, a hatred of the mother, is postulated. (2) This desire is inverted into a desire to suffer pain at the hands of the mother. (3) This in turn becomes a generalized desire to suffer pain at the hands of other women.

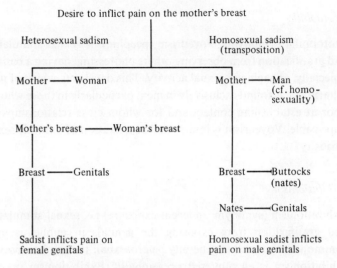

Fig. 7. Psycho-dynamic construct of the genesis of heterosexual
and homosexual sadism (after Allen, 1969).

Homosexual masochism. (1) and (2) as above. (3) Transposition
from the mother to males in general (see *Homosexuality*). (4) This
results in a desire to suffer pain at the hands of a man.

Automasochism. (1) A desire to injure the hated father. (2) The
sexualization of this desire. (3) The inability to reach the father,
because, for example, he is too powerful. This leads to inversion,
when the hatred is turned against the individual himself.

Masochism in the female. This can also be heterosexual or homosexual or can take the form of automasochism. The methods are
similar to those employed by the male. In automasochism objects
may be introduced into the genitals, into the urinary passage
(masochistic urethralism), into the bladder or into the rectum
(masochistic analism). Surgical intervention may be called for.

Female masochism is interpreted as follows: (1) Hatred of the
father. The individual's aggressive impulses are directed against the
father because he is experienced as restrictive. (2) Hatred of the
father cannot be effectively expressed and is transformed into self-
hatred.

Scotophilia

Scotophilia (synonyms: voyeurism, peeping), is sexual stimulation and gratification from observing others undressing, having a bath or, especially, engaging in sexual activity. This deviation, which of itself is harmless, is found exclusively in men, particularly in those who are poor at establishing contact and for whom close relationships are impossible. Voyeurism is interpreted as a fixation of infantile sexual curiosity.

Exhibitionism

Exhibitionism (synonym: indecent exposure) i.e. sexual stimulation and gratification from exposing the genitals in public, is most common in men and is generally heterosexual, though homosexual exhibitionism is encountered occasionally. Exhibitionism may be viewed as a fear of inadequate sex appeal. Psycho-analytically it is seen as a fixation of the gratification of infantile sexual exposure. Exhibitionism has forensic implications, being the most frequent sexual offence. It has no harmful effect on adults, and in the majority of cases seems also to have little traumatic effect on children.

Frotteurism

This sexual stimulation and gratification from rubbing, squeezing oneself, pressing against other people, occurs mostly in crowds, e.g. cinemas, public gatherings, public transport, and is often associated with other perversions such a exhibitionism and fetishism. Frotteurism has been interpreted as an arrest of development (fixation) at the infantile stage of making close bodily contact with the mother.

Transvestism

Transvestism (synonym: eonism), is sexual pleasure from wearing the clothes of the oposite sex. There appears to be a complete change of sex but this extends only to the wearing of clothes and is accompanied by pleasure in such a change of dress. Often the change is limited to underwear. Transvestism is often only intermittent, e.g. under the influence of alcohol. It is found equally in the heterosexually and the homosexually inclined, and more frequently in men than in women. The causes are not known. Transvestism has forensic implications because it is often combined with theft of clothing, with exhibitionism and with fetishism.

Abnormal sexual identity

Transsexualism (Green and Money, 1969) applies to individuals who show normal sex differentiation but are convinced that they belong to the opposite sex (contrary sexual identity). Many transsexuals are not homosexual, but have little desire for sexual activity. Their conviction leads to a desire for a change of sex in all its aspects, physical, social and professional. Transsexualism occurs mostly in men who want to be women. The male–female ratio is 3 to 1. The frequency is about 1.5 per 100,000. Transsexualism or inverse sexual identity in the male has been interpreted as pathological female identification in individuals who have an excessively strong attachment to the mother, a tendency to identify with her, and a desire for self-castration.

N.B. Transsexualism is not the same as hermaphroditism or intersexuality, when the individual usually adopts the sex role he has learned and not the biological role (see Overzier, 1961).

Treatment:

(1) Psychotherapy is often rejected and cannot therefore be carried out.

(2) Change of sex by operation is employed, usually from male to female: techniques include castration, amputation of penis, plastic surgery of vagina.

(3) Castration and administration of female hormones has also been used in male transsexuals.

Abnormal intensity of drive

The concepts of hypersexuality and hyposexuality hardly lend themselves to precise definition, since the average sexual desire or sexual activity in an individual case can hardly be assessed, apart from the statistical norm, and since there are so many factors which affect sexuality, e.g. physical health, the state of relaxation or exhaustion, age, stimulation, the positive response of a partner, the opportunity for sexual activity, the emotional state and temperament.

Hypersexuality (erotomania) is also known in the male as satyriasis, and in the female as nymphomania. Possible foundations of hypersexuality include:

(*a*) Psychological grounds which are many and varied. For example, impulsivity and general lack of inhibition play a special part in the expression of sexual desires. Hypersexual behaviour can often be understood as a form of self-reassurance by renewed sexual conquests. It may, however, also partly reflect an antipathy to the parent of the opposite sex which appears as a generalized hatred of the other sex, with a desire to conquer it, to triumph over it again and again, to subjugate it.

(*b*) Psychotic basis. In organic psychoses we may find a relaxation of inhibitions, a lack of self control, while in endogenous psychoses also, e.g. in mania, there may occur a similar relaxation of control, though there may also be a genuine increase in sexual needs as a result of the general heightening of vitality. In mania there is often consequently an indiscriminate promiscuity or sexual abandon that may result in venereal disease or pregnancy. Sexuality in schizophrenics is on the whole less predictable than in manic patients. Sometimes there is apparent hypersexuality resulting from a lack of inhibition and defective control in schizophrenic women, but at times this should be regarded more as an expression of rebellious self-assertion than as a genuine increase in sexual desire. Many disorders of the central nervous system, e.g. the midbrain, the epiphysis, the temporal lobes, seem to lead sometimes to hypersexuality.

(*c*) Hormonal. Administration of male sexual hormones leads to an increase in sexuality in both men, especially those who are themselves deficient in this regard, and women.

(*d*) Drugs. Most of the stimulant action of the so-called aphrodisiacs is centred locally on the blood flow of the sexual organs. Yohimbin is the best known of these substances.

Hyposexuality (synonym: asexuality, anerotic) is encountered in general infantilism (physical and mental) in neurotically inhibited, anxious individuals (see *Impotence*). Endogenous depression is almost always accompanied by a lack of sexuality. Schizophrenia, with its disturbed human relationships, is also often associated with a decline in sexual contacts of every kind.

Hormonal hyposexuality is found in hypogonadism and agonadism (abnormally low gonadal functioning or lack of gonadal activity), in castrated individuals and after administration of anti-androgenous substances, e.g. cypoteronazetate.

Organic hyposexuality may occur in general debilitating diseases, in all extensive diseases of the central nervous system and also in sex chromosomal abnormalities. The neuroleptics have a lowering effect on sexuality and in smaller doses may delay ejaculation.

Disorders of potency

Sexual potency is the capacity to achieve sexual intercourse in a form which could potentially lead to impregnation. A disturbance of this function is generally called impotence. It is important to distinguish between the concept of *infertility* (sterility, inability to procreate, *impotentia generandi*) and *inability to achieve coitus* due to a disordered performance of the sexual act (*impotentia coeundi* or, more briefly, impotence. In the male this includes a reduction in or lack of libido, inability to achieve erection (*impotentia erigendi*), disorders of ejaculation (*impotentia ejaculandi, ejaculatio praecox* and *ejaculatio retardata*). In the female it includes lack of sexual desire, sexual anaesthesia or *frigidity* (sexual coldness), lack of orgasm (anorgasmia), muscular tensions (*adductor spasmus*) and *vaginismus* (vaginal cramp) as well as painful sexual intercourse (*dyspareunia*).

Causal associations of disorders of potency

A general review is given below.

Organic. Diseases of the central nervous system (brain and spine), severe general illnesses, e.g. of the liver, and urological disorders of varied kinds can all lead to impotence. In addition, higher doses of certain drugs, e.g. neuroleptics, anti-androgens, can reduce libido to such an extent as to induce impotence.

Psychotic. A complete lack of libido renders endogeneous depressives impotent.

Neurotic-psychogenic. Anxiety is usually the central dynamic factor. Erection and ejaculation are particularly liable to be disturbed in the male and libido and orgasm in the female (Masters and Johnson, 1970; Matussek, 1959).

(*a*) Psychogenic impotence in the male includes all non-organic coital difficulties. Disturbances of erection and *ejaculatio praecox* are of particular practical importance.

In every case it is necessary first to ascertain whether the impotence is intermittent or whether it is consistently present, and whether it occurs with one sexual partner or with different partners. Detailed biographical and situational histories must always be obtained, so that even relatively banal situational factors should not be overlooked. Many such factors exist, for example, fatigue, the effect of alcohol, a tense life situation, the general behaviour of the partner and not merely their sexual technique, frigidity in the female partner with a clear indication of her lack of involvement; the place where intercourse occurs – a room that allows easy disturbance, with thin walls, where neighbours or members of the family may perhaps be listening exemplifies such environmental factors.

Neurotic impotence may be the expression of a general disturbance in interpersonal relationships, or of special difficulties in the relationship with the particular partner: the extra-erotic relationship may be a complicated one and charged with conflict. There may be some kind of restraint, e.g. because of reservations about the partner, about his or her earlier life, about something that has been said or some form of behaviour.

Anxiety often arises as a form of reaction to a challenge, sexual potency becoming a kind of test performance. This may arise directly from the situation, e.g. impotence on the wedding night, impotence in a brothel; it may be generated by the partner, or by the patient himself if he sees his own sexuality being put to the test and turned into a challenge, if he is anxiously watching himself in case of accidental failure, or if he is watching for a decline in sexuality with age; if sexuality has become a matter of neurotic self-assertion or of mastering the partner, impotence may also be the result. But even a forced determination to equate sexuality with pleasure may adversely affect potency. Many sexual neuroses arise from an identification of sexual technique with sex life as an expression of

personal love life. Anxious self-observation born of reading explanatory sex literature is also an important factor affecting sexual
performance due to excessive reflection and the bibliogenic anxiety
of anticipation.

The psycho-analytical point of view stresses the possibiity of an
unconscious fear of fulfilling infantile sexual goals (Oedipal situations,
incest), unconscious pathological attachment to the mother and fear
of being unfaithful to her, a fear of castration and a general fear of
being swallowed up. Feelings of inferiority, hostility, guilt and
resentment may lead to marital and extra-marital disturbances of
potency.

In *ejaculatio praecox*, or premature ejaculation, many of the
above-mentioned factors also apply. It often occurs in cases of very
strong sexual stimulation after a long period of sexual abstention, and
may develop into impotence if it leads to anxious self-observation.
On the other hand, it may also be the expression of a lack of desire
or a refusal to give of oneself. *Ejaculatio retardata* is more rarely
psychogenic and is clearly more often organic in origin. When it is
psychogenic it is often regarded as a refusal to give of oneself.

(*b*) Disturbances of potency in the female: for practical purposes
the most important disorders are *frigidity* or sexual coldness, *vaginismus* and *dyspareunia* (Schätzing, 1959).

In frigidity, as in all disorders of potency, it is first necessary to
establish the degree of the disturbance, i.e. whether it is permanent
or temporary, whether it is associated with a particular situation,
whether there has always been a history of frigidity. Here too
situational factors are important: cramped living quarters, children
sleeping in the room and relations nearby, particularly the mother;
in addition, frigidity may be due to the general stresses of life, a heavy
burden of responsibility, various kinds of depression, fear of pain,
or fear of the scandal of a pregnancy. The psycho-analytical point
of view emphasizes unconscious fears of ego-loss in orgasm. Frigidity
often depends on the partner, the woman from experience being
usually more dependent than the man on her relationship with the
partner and on a total commitment to and emotional involvement
with him.

When a sensitive woman has relations with a man who is thinking
only of his own sexual pleasure, she may become frigid. False

expectations also often play a part, for example that an orgasm should be experienced every time coitus takes place (according to Kinsey (1953) it is not until after the age of about 29 that women achieve a higher than average rate of orgasm); and that vaginal orgasm as distinct from clitoral orgasm will occur. Feelings of shame engendered by upbringing or by the confessional, may also lead to frigidity – the denial of the pleasures of the flesh.

Treatment of impotence is directed at such causes as can be ascertained. Specialist examination – urological, andrological, gynaecological – is of particular importance. Psychotherapeutic procedures depend entirely on the personal circumstances and do not lend themselves to schematization. In some cases analytical psychotherapy is to be recommended, in others behaviour therapy (Kockott and Dittmar, 1973). In many other instances it is enough to clarify relationships, to allay fears, and in some circumstances to recommend temporary sexual abstinence with de-conditioning (de-reflexion).

21.6 Incest

This is of concern to psychiatrists in so far as it usually occurs in the lowest social classes, often in families with a history of mental retardation, psychopathy, sociopathy or alcoholism. The most frequent incestuous relationship is between father and daughter, then between brother and sister: incest between mother and son is less common. Damage may be done when paedophilia is practised. Apart from this, there are no consistent views about injurious effects.

21.7 Prostitution and sexual promiscuity

This, too, is of marginal interest to psychiatrists. In sexually promiscuous young girls one should always be on the look-out for early signs of endogenous mania as a part of a manic-depressive illness. Among prostitutes there is a higher than average incidence of low intelligence, character disorders and addictions to nicotine, alcohol, drugs and medicaments of various kinds. There are conflicting reports about the sexuality of prostitutes. It would seem certain that many of them are capable of sustaining a normal sexual relationship with a personal male friend, while remaining frigid with their clients.

In isolated cases hypersexuality may provide a motive for prostitution. In psychiatric case histories it is necessary to look out for dealings with prostitutes, since they may be sources of venereal disease where prostitution is not under the control of police and health authorities.

BIBLIOGRAPHY

1. PREFACE AND INTRODUCTION

Abraham, K. 1908. Die psychosexuellen Differenzen der Hysterie und der Dementia praecox. *Zbl. ges. Neurol. Psychiat.*, **31** (NF 19), 521–33

Alanen, Y. O. 1966. The family in the pathogenesis of schizophrenic and neurotic disorders. *Acta psychiat. scand.*, Copenhagen, Suppl. **189**

1970. The families of schizophrenic patients. *Proc. roy. Soc. Med.*, **63**, 227–30

Arbeitsgemeinschaft für Methodik und Dokumentation in der Psychiatrie (AMP). 1972. *Das AMP-System. Manual zur Dokumentation psychiatrischer Befunde*. 2nd edn. rev. and ed. Ch. Scharfetter. Berlin: Springer

Argelander, H. 1970. *Das Erstinterview in der Psychotherapie*. Darmstadt: Wissenschaftliche Buchgesellschaft, Darmstadt

Arieti, S. 1955. *Interpretation of Schizophrenia*. New York: Brunner

1971. The origins and development of the psychopathology of schizophrenia. In *Die Entstehung der Schizophrenie*, ed. M. Bleuler and J. Angst. Berne: Huber

Baltes, P. B. and Schaie, K. W. 1973. *Lifespan Development Psychology. Personality and Socialization*. New York: Academic Press

Bash, K. W. 1955. *Lehrbuch der allgemeinen Psychopathologie*. Stuttgart: Thieme

Bateson, G., Jackson, D. D., Haley, J. and Weakland, J. W. 1956. Towards a theory of schizophrenia. *Behav. Sci.*, **1**, 251–64

Baumann, U. 1974. Diagnostische Differenzierungsfähigkeit von Psychopathologie Skalen. *Arch. Psychiat. Nervenkr.*, **219**, 89–103

Benedetti, G. 1973. *Psyche und Biologie*. Stuttgart: Hippokrates-Verlag

1975. *Psychiatrische Aspekte des Schöpferischen und schöpferische Aspekte der Schizophrenie*. Göttingen–Zürich: Vandenhoeck & Ruprecht

Bleuler, E. 1911. Dementia praecox oder Gruppe der Schizophrenien.

In *Handbuch der Psychiatrie*, part 4, ed. G. Aschaffenburg. Vienna: Deuticke

1926. Zur Unterscheidung des Physiogenen und des Psychogenen bei der Schizophrenie. *Allg. Z. Psychiat.*, **84**, 22–37

1930. Primäre und sekundäre Symptome der Schizophrenia. *Zbl. ges. Neurol. Psychiat.*, **124**, 607–46

1969. *Lehrbuch der Psychiatrie.* 11th edn. rev. M. Bleuler, pp. 99–104. Berlin: Springer

Bleuler, M. 1954. *Endokrinologische Psychiatrie.* Stuttgart: Thieme

1964. Endokrinologische Psychiatrie. In *Psychiatrie der Gegenwart,* 1st edn., vol. I/1b, ed. H. W. Gruhle, R. Jung, W. Mayer-Gross, and M. Müller, pp. 161–252

Bochenski, I. M. 1954. *Die zeitgenössischen Denkmethoden.* 5th edn. Munich: Francke

Bonhoeffer, K. 1910. *Die symptomatischen Psychosen.* Leipzig–Vienna: Deuticke

Boss, M. 1971. *Grundriß der Medizin.* Berne: Huber

Bräutigam, W. 1974. Anthropologie der Neurose. In *Neue Anthropologie,* ed. H.-G. Gadamer and P. Vogler, vol. VI, pp. 114–37. Stuttgart: Thieme

Brickenkamp, R. 1975. *Handbuch psychologischer und pädogogischer Tests.* Göttingen, Hogrefe

Chalmers, N., Crawley, R., and Rose, S. P. R. 1971. *The Biological Bases of Behaviour.* London: Oxford University Press

Cohen, R. and Meyer-Osterkamp, S. 1974. Experimentalpsychologische Untersuchungen in der psychopathologischen Forschung. In *Klinische Psychologie,* ed. W. G. Schraml and U. Baumann, vol. II. Berne: Huber

Conrad, K. 1958. *Die beginnende Schizophrenie* (1st edn.) 3rd edn. 1971. Stuttgart: Thieme

Cooper, D. 1971. *Psychiatrie und Antipsychiatrie.* Frankfurt/M: Suhrkamp

Cooper, J. E. 1970. The use of a procedure for standardising psychiatric diagnosis. In *Psychiatric Epidemiology,* ed. E. H. Hare and J. K. Wing, pp. 108–31. London: Oxford University Press

Curtius, F. 1959. *Individuum und Krankheit.* Berlin: Springer

Delay, J. and Pichot, P. 1966. *Medizinische Psychologie,* 4th edn. 1973. Stuttgart: Thieme

Devereux, G. 1974. *Normal und abnormal. Aufsätze zur allgemeinen Ethnopsychiatrie.* Frankfurt/M: Suhrkamp

Dörner, K. 1969. *Bürger und Irre*. Frankfurt/M: Ennup

1974. Wohin sollen wir den Krankheitsbegriff in der Psychiatrie entwickeln? *Psychiat. Prax.*, 1, 123–9

Eccles, J. C. 1970. *Facing Reality*. Berlin: Springer (German version: *Wehrheit und Wirklichkeit*. 1975)

Eibl-Eibesfeldt, I. 1969. *Grundriß der vergleichenden Verhaltensforschung*. 2nd edn. Munich: Piper

1972. Stammesgeschichtliche Anpassung im Verhalten des Menschen. In *Neue Anthropologie*, ed. H.-G. Gadamer and P. Vogler, vol. II. Stuttgart: Thieme

Ellenberger, H. F. 1970. *The Discovery of the Unconscious*. New York: Basic Books

Erikson, E. 1959. *Identity and the Life Cycle*. New York: International University Press

Ey, H. 1967. *Das Bewußtsein*. Berlin: de Gruyter. (French edn. 1963)

Eysenck, H. J. 1973. *Handbook of Abnormal Psychology*. 2nd edn. London: Pitman

Feer, H. 1970. *Kybernetik in der Psychiatrie*. Basle: Karger

Fenichel, O. 1971. *The Psychoanalytic Theory of Neurosis*. London: Routledge & Kegan Paul

Fischer-Homberger, E. 1970. Der Begriff Krankheit als Funktion außermedizinischer Gegebenheiten. *Sudhoffs Arch. Gesch. Med.*, **54**, 225–41

Freud, S. 1894. Die Abwehrneuropsychosen. Weitere Bermerkungen über die Abwehrneuropsychosen (1896). *Gesammelte Werke*, vol. I. Frankfurt/M: Fischer, 1968

1911. Psychoanalytische Bemerkungen über einen autobiographisch beschriebenen Fall von Paranoia (Dementia paranoides). *Gesammelte Werke*, vol. VIII. Frankfurt/M: Fischer, 1968

1914. Zur Einführung des Narzißmus. *Gesammelte Werke*, vol. XI. Frankfurt/M: Fischer, 1968

1916–1917. Vorlesungen zur Einführung in die Psychoanalyse. *Gesammelte Werke*, vol. XI. Frankfurt/M: Fischer, 1968

1924. Das Ich and das Es. *Gesammelte Werke*, vol. XIII. Frankfurt/M: Fischer, 1968

Fromm-Reichmann, F. 1950. *Principles of intensive psychotherapy*. Chicago: University of Chicago Press

Gadamer, H.-G. 1972. *Wahrheit und Methode*. 3rd edn. Tübingen: Mohr

Gadamer, H.-G. and Vogler, P. 1974. *Neue Anthropologie*, vol. VI. Stuttgart: Thieme

Garfinkel, H. 1956. Conditions of successful degradation ceremonies. *Amer. J. Sociol.*, **61**, 420–4

Gauron, E. F. and Dickinson, J. K. 1966. Diagnostic decision making in psychiatry. *Arch. gen. Psychiat.*, **14**, 225–37

Glatzel, J. 1972. Zum Begriff des Symptoms in der Psychopathologie. *Nervenarzt*, **43**, 33–6

Goethe, J. W. 1952. Beobachten und Denken. *Gedenkausgabe der Werke, Briefe und Gespräche*, vol. XVII, p. 723. Zürich: Artemis

Goffman, E. 1967. *Stigma – über Techniken der Bewältigung beschädigter Identität.* (German version) Frankfurt/M: Suhrkamp

Goldberg, D. P., Cooper, B., Eastwood, M. R., Kedward, H. B. and Shepherd, M. 1970. A standardized psychiatric interview for use in community surveys. *Brit. J. prev. soc. Med.*, **24**, 18–23

Göppinger, H. and Witter, H. 1972. *Handbuch der forensischen Psychiatrie.* Berlin: Springer

Gottschaldt, K., Lersch, Ph., Sander, F. and Thomae, H. 1966. *Handbuch der Psychologie.* Göttingen: Hogrefe

Habermas, J. 1973. *Erkenntnis und Interesse.* Frankfurt/M: Suhrkamp

Hallowell, A. I. 1955. *Culture and Experience.* Philadelphia, University of Pennsylvania Press

Hassler, R. 1967. Funktionelle Neuroanatomie und Psychiatrie. In *Psychiatrie der Gegenwart*, ed. H. W. Gruhle, R. Jung, W. Mayer-Gross and M. Müller, 1st edn., vol. I/1a, pp. 152–285, Berlin: Springer

Heidegger, M. 1959. *Gelassenheit.* Pfullingen: Neske
1972. *Sein und Zeit.* (1st edn. 1927) Tübingen: Niemeyer

Hess, W. R. 1962. *Psychologie in biologischer Sicht* (2nd edn. 1968). Stuttgart: Thieme

Heston, L. L. 1966. Psychiatric disorders of foster home reared children of schizophrenic mothers. *Brit. J. Psychiat.*, **112**, 819–25

Hocking, F. 1970. Extreme environmental stress and its significance for psychopathology. *Amer. J. Psychother.*, **24**, 4–26

Holt, R. R. and Luborsky, L. 1958. *Personality Patterns of Psychiatrists. A Study of Methods for Selecting Residents.* New York: Basic Books

Holzhey, H. 1970. *Kants Erfahrungsbegriff.* Basle: Schwabe
1974. *Wissenschaft/Wissenschaften. Interdisziplinäre Arbeit und Wissenschaftstheorie.* Basle: Schwabe

Hunger, J. 1973. Zum Krankheits- Normen- und Verantwortungs-

282   Bibliography

begriff in der psychiatrischen Begutachtung. *Psychiat. clin.*, **6**, 211–25

Husserl, E. 1913. *Ideen zu einer reinen Phänomenologie und phänomenologischen Philosophie*. 1st edn. The Hague: Nijthoff, 1950

Jackson, H. 1932. Croonian lectures, 1884–1887. In *Selected Writings*. London: Hodder & Stoughton

Jacob, H. 1962. Wandlungen, Möglichkeiten und Grenzen der klinisch-psychiatrischen Exploration. In *Festschrift zum 65. Geburtstag von H. Bürger-Prinz. Randzonen menschlichen Verhaltens. Beiträge zur Psychiatrie und Neurologie*, pp. 62–75. Stuttgart: Enke

Jaspers, K. 1925. *Psychologie der Weltanschauungen*. 3rd edn. Berlin: Springer
1959. *Allgemeine Psychopathologie*. 7th edn. (9th edn. 1973) Berlin: Springer

Jensen, A. E. 1951. *Mythos und Kultur Bei Naturvölkern*. Wiesbaden: Steiner

Jung, R. 1967. Neurophysiologie und Psychiatrie. In *Psychiatrie der Gegenwart*, ed. H. W. Gruhle, R. Jung, W. Mayer-Gross and M. Müller, vol. I/a , pp. 325–928. Berlin: Springer

Kaplan, B. 1964. *The Inner World of Mental Illness*. New York: Harper & Row

Karlson, J. L. 1966. *The Biologic Basis of Schizophrenia*. Springfield, Ill.: Thomas
1974. Inheritance of schizophrenia. *Acta psychiat. scand.*, Suppl. **247**

Keller, W. 1975. Philosophische Anthropologie – Psychologie-Transzendez. In *Neue Anthropologie*, ed. H.-G. Gadamer and P. Vogler, vol. VI, pp. 3–42. Stuttgart: Thieme

Kerekjarto, M. v. and Lienert, G. A. 1970. Depressionskalen als Forschungsmittel in der Psychopathologie. *Pharmakospsychiat.*, **3**, 1–21

Keupp, H. 1972a. *Der Krankheitsmythos in der Psychopathologie*. Munich: Urban & Schwarzenberg
1972b. *Psychische Störungen als abweichendes Verhalten*. Munich: Urban & Schwarzenberg

Kiev, A. 1972. *Transcultural Psychiatry*. New York: Free Press & Collier Macmillan International

Kind, H. 1973. *Leitfaden für die psychiatrische Untersuchung*. Berlin: Springer

Kreitman, N. 1961. The reliability of psychiatric diagnosis. *J. ment. Sci.*, **107**, 876–86

Kretschmer, E. 1948. *Geniale Menschen*. Heidelberg: Springer

   1953. *Der Begriff der motorischen Schablonen und ihre Rolle in normalen und pathologischen Lebenvorgängen*. *Arch. Psychiat. Nervenkr.*, **190**, 1–3

   1958. *Hysterie, Reflex und Instinkt*. 6th edn. (7th edn. 1974) Stuttgart: Thieme

Kuhn, Th. S. 1973. *Die Struktur wissenschaftlicher Revolutionen*. Frankfurt/M: Suhrkamp

Kunz, H. 1930. *Die existentielle Bedeutung der Psychoanalyse in ihrer Konsequenz für deren Kritik*. *Nervenarzt*, **3**, 657–68

   1954/55. *Zur Frage nach dem Wesen der Norm*. *Psyche, Heidelberg*, **8**, 241–71

   1956. *Die latente Anthropologie der Psychoanalyse*. *Schweiz. Z. Psychol.*, **15**, 84–102

   1975a. *Grundfragen der psychoanalytischen Anthropologie*. Göttingen: Vandenhoeck & Ruprecht

   1975b. *Die Erweiterung des Menschenbildes in der Psychoanalyse Sigmund Freuds*. In *Neue Anthropologie*, ed. H.-G. Gadamer and P. Vogler, vol.. VI, pp. 44–113

Laing, R. D. 1967. *Phänomenologie der Erfahrung*. Frankfurt/M: Suhrkamp

Laing, R. D. and Esterson, E. 1964. *Sanity, Madness and the Family*. London: Tavistock

Lange-Eichbaum, W. and Kurth, W. 1967. *Genie, Irrsinn und Ruhm*. 6th edn. Munich: Reinhardt

Lebra, W. P. 1972. *Transcultural Research in Mental Health*. Honolulu: University Press of Hawaii

Lewis, A. 1971. 'Endogenous' and 'exogenous': a useful dichotomy? *Psychol. Med.*, **1**, 191–6

Lidz, Th. 1973. *The Origin and Treatment of Schizophrenic Disorders*. New York: Basic Books

Lidz, Th., Cornelison, A., Fleck, St. and Terry D. 1957. Marital schism and marital skew. *Amer. J. Psychiat.*, **114**, 241–8

Lorenz, K. 1963. *Das sogenannte Böse*. Vienna: Borotha-Schoeler

   1973. *Die Rückseite des Spiegels*. Munich: Piper

Lorenzer, A. 1973. *Über den Gegenstand der Psychoanalyse oder: Sprache und Interaktion*. Frankfurt/M: Suhrkamp

   1974. Die Wahrheit der psychoanalytischen Erkenntnis. Frankfurt/M: Suhrkamp

Lorr, M. 1966. *Explorations in Typing Psychotics*. Oxford: Pergamon Press

Lorr, M. and Klett, C. J. 1967. *Inpatient Multidimensional Psychiatric Scale (IMPS)*. Palo Alto: Consulting Psychologists Press

Lorr, M., Klett, C. J. and McNair, D. M. 1963. *Syndromes of Psychosis*. Oxford: Pergamon Press

McKinnon, R. A. and Michels, R. 1971. *The Psychiatric Interview in Clinical Practice*. Philadelphia: Saunders

Maxwell, A. E. 1971. Agreement among raters. *Brit. J. Psychiat.*, **118**, 659–62

Meerwein, F. 1965. *Psychiatrie und Psychoanalyse in der psychiatrischen Klinik*. Basle: Karger

1974. *Das ärztliche Gespräch*. 2nd edn. Berne: Huber

Meyer-Osterkamp, S. and Cohen, R. 1973. *Zur Größenkonstanz bei Schizophrenen*. Berlin: Springer

Mombour, W. 1972. Verfahren zue Standardisierung des psychopathologischen Befundes. *Psychiat. clin.*, **5**, 73–120, 137–57

1974. Syndrome bei psychiatrischen Erkrankungen. *Arch. Psychiat. Nervenkr.*, **219**, 331–50

Mombour, W., Gammel, G., von Zerssen, D. and Heyse, H. 1973. Die Objektivierung psychiatrischer Syndrome durch multifaktorielle Analyse des psychopathologischen Befundes. *Nervenarzt*, **44**, 352–8

Nathan, P. E. 1967. *Cues, Decision and Diagnoses*. New York: Academic Press

Nietzsche, F. 1955. Zur Genealogie der Moral (1887). *Werke*, ed. K. Schlechta, vol. II, p. 975. Munich: Hanser

Nunberg, H. 1959. *Allgemeine Neurosenlehre*. (1st edn. 1932) Berne, Stuttgart, Vienna: Huber

Perret, E. 1973. *Gehirn und Verhalten. Neuropsychologie des Menschen*. Berne: Huber

Perrez, M. 1972. *Ist die Psychoanalyse eine Wissenschaft?* Berne: Huber

Peters, M. 1967. Neuropathologie und Psychiatrie. In *Psychiatrie der Gegenwart*, ed. H. W. Gruhle, R. Jung, W. Mayer-Gross and M. Müller, 1st edn., vol. I/1a, pp. 286–324. Berlin: Springer

Pfeiffer, W. M. 1970. *Transkulturelle Psychiatrie*. Stuttgart: Thieme

Piaget, J. 1972. *Erkenntnistheorie der Wissenschaften vom Menschen*. Frankfurt/M: Ullstein

Pichot, P. and Olivier-Martin, R. 1974. Psychological measurements in psychopharmacology. In *Modern Problems of Pharmacopsychiatry*, ed. Th. Ban, F. A. Freyhan, P. Pichot and W. Pöldinger, vol. VII. Basle: Karger

Pohlen, M. 1969. *Schizophrene Psychosen. Ein Beitrag zur Strukturlehre des Ich.* Berne: Huber

Pophal, R. 1925. *Der Krankheitsbegriff in der Körpermedizin und Psychiatrie.* Berlin: Karger

Popper, K. 1959. *The Logic of Scientific Discovery.* 5th edn. New York: Basic Books

1963. *Conjectures and Refutations. The Growth of Scientific Knowledge.* New York: Basic Books

1973. *Objektive Erkenntnis. Ein evolutionärer Entwurf.* Hamburg: Hoffmann & Campe. (English: 1972. *Objective Knowledge,* Oxford: Clarendon Press)

Rapaport, D. 1970. *Die Struktur der psychoanalytischen Theorie.* 2nd edn. Stuttgart: Klett

Richter, H. E. 1972. *Patient Familie.* Hamburg: Rowohlt

Rosenthal, D. 1970. *Genetic Theory and Abnormal Behavior.* New York: McGraw-Hill

Rosenthal, D., Wender, P. H., Kety, S. S., Schulsinger, F., Welner, J. and Ostergaard, L. 1968. Schizophrenics' offspring reared in adoptive homes. In *The Transmission of Schizophrenia,* ed. D. Rosenthal and S. S. Kety, pp. 377–91. Oxford: Pergamon Press

Saint-Exupéry, Antoine de. 1950. *Der kleine Prinz.* Zürich: Die Arche

Sartorius, N., Brooke, E. M. and Lin, T. 1970. Reliability of psychiatric assessment in international research. In *Psychiatric Epidemiology,* ed. E. H. Hare and J. K. Wing, pp. 133–47. London: Oxford University Press

Savigny, E. v. 1974. *Die Philosophie der normalen Sprache.* Frankfurt/M: Suhrkamp

Scharfetter, Ch. 1973. Psychiatrie als Wissenschaft und Praxis. *Nervenarzt.,* **44**, 255–61

1974. Die Wissenschaft und die Medizin mit besonderer Berücksichtigung der Psychiatrie. In *Wissenschaft/Wissenschaften. Interdisziplinäre Arbeit und Wissenschaftstheorie; Philosophie aktuell,* vol. III ed. H. Holzhey. Basle: Schwabe

Scheff, Th. 1973. *Das Etikett 'Geisteskrankheit'.* Frankfurt/M: Fischer

Schilder, P. 1973. *Entwurf zu einer Psychiatrie auf psychoanalytischer Grundlage* (1st edn. 1925). Frankfurt/M: Suhrkamp

Schmitz, H. 1964–69. *Der leibliche Raum. System der Philosophie,* vol. III/1. Bonn: Bouvier

1972. *Nihilismus als Schicksal?* Bonn: Bouvier

Schneider, C. 1942. *Die schizophrenen Symptomverbände.* Berlin: Springer

286 *Bibliography*

Schneider, K. 1967. *Klinische Psychopathologie*, 8th edn. (10 edn. 1973) Stuttgart: Thieme

Schooler, C. and Feldman, S. E. 1967. *Experimental Studies of Schizophrenia*. Galeta/Calif.: Psychonomic Press

Schraml, W. J. and Baumann, U. 1974. *Klinische Psychologie*, vol. II. Berne: Huber

1975. *Klinische Psychologie*, vol. I, 3rd edn. Berne: Huber

Seiffert, H. 1971. *Einführung in die Wissenschaftestheorie*. Munich: Beck

Shepherd, M., Brooke, E. M., Cooper, J. E. and Lin, T. 1968. An experimental approach to psychiatric diagnosis. *Acta psychiat. scand.*, Suppl. **201**

Siegler, M. and Osmond, H. 1974. *Models of Madness, Models of Medicine*. New York/London: Macmillan & Collier

Slater, E. 1972. The psychiatrist in search of a science. *Brit. J. Psychiat.*, **121**, 591–8

1973. *Brit. J. Psychiat.*, **122**, 625–36

1975. The psychiatrist in search of a science. III – The depth psychologies. *Brit. J. Psychiat.*, **126**, 205–24

Sommer, R. and Osmond, H. 1960. Autobiographies of former mental patients. *J. ment. Sci.*, **106**, 1030–2

1961. *J. ment. Sci.*, **107**, 648–62

Spitzer, R. L. and Endicott, J. 1969. Diagno II: Further developments in a computer program for psychiatric diagnosis. *Amer. J. Psychiat.* Suppl. **125/I**, 12–20

Stevenson, I. 1971. *The Diagnostic Interview*. 2nd edn. New York: Harper & Row

Stierlin, H. 1975. *Von der Psychoanalyse zur Familientherapie*. Stuttgart: Klett

Storch, A. 1923. Bewußtseinsebenen und Wirklichkeitsbereiche in der Schizophrenie. *Zbl. ges. Neurol. Psychiat.*, **82**, 321–41

Sullivan, H. S. 1953. *The interpersonal theory of psychiatry*. New York: Norton

1955. *The Psychiatric Interview*. London: Tavistock

Szasz, Th. 1961a. The uses of naming and the origin of the myth of mental illness. *Amer. J. Psychol.*, **16**, 59–65

1961b. *The Myth of Mental Illness*. New York: Harper & Row. (German: *Geisteskrankheit – ein moderner Mythos?* 1972. Olten–Freiburg i. Br.: Walter)

1970. *The Manufacture of Madness, a Comparative Study of the Inquisition and the Mental Health Movement*. Szasz, Trustee

Tart, C. T. 1969 *Altered States of Consciousness.* New York: Wiley

Tellenbach, H. 1974. Die Begründung psychiatrischer Erfahrung und psychiatrischer Methoden in philosophischen Konzeptionen vom Wesen des Menschen. In *Neue Anthropologie,* ed. H.-G. Gadamer and P. Vogler, vol. VI, pp. 138–81. Stuttgart: Thieme

Watzlawik, P., Beavin, J. H. and Jackson, D. D. 1967. *Pragmatics of Human Communication.* New York: Norton

WHO 1971. *International Classification of Diseases.* 8th edn. Geneva: World Health Organization

1973. *Report of the International Pilot Study of Schizophrenia.* Geneva: World Health Organization

1974. *Glossary of Mental Disorders and Guide to their Classification.* Geneva: World Health Organization (German: Diagnosenschlüssel und Glossar psychiatrischer Krankheiten, übersetzt von W. Mombour and G. Kockott. 1971. Berlin: Springer)

Wieck, H. H. 1967. *Lehrbuch der Psychiatrie.* Stuttgart. Schattauer

Wing, H. H. 1970. Standardisation of Clinical Assessment. In *Psychiatric Eipdemiology,* ed. E. H. Hare and J. K. Wing, pp. 91–108. London: Oxford University Press

Wing, J. K. and Brown, G. W. 1970., *Institutionalism and Schizophrenia.* London: Cambridge University Press

Wing J. K., Cooper, J. E. and Sartorius, N. 1974. *Measurement and Classification of Psychiatric Symptoms. An Instruction Manual for the PSE and Catego Programme.* London: Cambridge University Press

Wulff, E. 1972. *Psychiatrie und Klassengesellschaft.* Frankfurt/M: Fischer

Wynne, L. C., Day, J. and Ryckoff, I. M. 1959. Maintenance of stereotype roles in the family of schizophrenics. *Arch. gen. Psychiat.,* **1,** 109–14

Wynne, L. C., Ryckoff, I. M., Day, J. and Hirsch, S. I. 1958. Pseudomutuality in the family relations of schizophrenics. *Psychiatry,* **21,** 205–20

Wyss, D. 1970. *Die tiefenpsychologischen Schulen von den Anfängen bis zur Gegenwart.* 3rd edn. Göttingen: Vandenhoeck & Ruprecht

1971. *Lehrbuch der medizinischen Psychologie und Psychotherapie.* Göttingen: Vandenhoeck & Ruprecht

1973. *Beziehung und Gestalt.* Göttingen: Vandenhoeck & Ruprecht

288 Bibliography

Zerssen, D. v. 1973. Diagnose. in *Lexikon der Psychiatrie*, ed. C. Müller. Berlin: Springer

Zimmerli, W. 1974. *Wissenschaftskrise und Wissenschaftskritik.* Basle: Schwabe

Zubek, J. P. 1969. *Sensory Deprivation: Fifteen Years of Research.* New York: Meredith

Zubin, J. 1967. Classification of the behaviour disorders. *Ann. Rev. Psychol.*, **18**, 373–401

Zubin, J. and Hunt, H. F. 1967. *Comparative Psychopathology.* New York: Grune & Stratton

2. CONSCIOUSNESS

Cobb, S. 1957. Awareness, Attention, and Physiology of the Brain Stem. Experiments in Psychopathology. *Proc. Amer. psychopath. Assoc.*, 45th meeting, 194–204

Ebbecke, U. 1959. *Physiologie des Bewußtseins in entwicklungsgeschichtlicher Betrachtung.* Stuttgart: Thieme

Ey, H. 1967. *Das Bewußtsein.* (French edition 1963) Berlin: de Gruyter

Graumann, C.-F. 1966. Bewußtsein und Bewußtheit. Probleme und Befunde der psychologischen Bewußtseinsforschung. In *Handbuch der Psychologie*, ed. K. Gottschaldt, Ph. Lersch, F. Sander and H. Thomae, vol. I, 1st half-vol., pp. 79–127. Göttingen: Hogrefe

Jaspers, K. 1959. *Allgemeine Psychologie.* 7th edn. (9th edn. 1973) Berlin: Springer

Jung, R. 1967. Neurophysiologie und Psychiatrie. In *Psychiatrie der Gegenwart*, ed. H. W. Gruhle, R. Jung, W. Mayer-Gross and M. Müller, 1st edn. vol. I/a, pp. 325–928. Berlin: Springer

Kretschmer, E. 1940. Das apallische Syndrom. *Z. ges. Neurol. Psychiat.*, **169**, 576–9

Scharfetter, Ch. and Scharfetter, F. 1968. Über das apallische Syndrom. *Dtsch. med. Wschr.*, **93**, 2131–3

Störring, G. E. 1953. *Besinnung und Bewußtsein.* Stuttgart. Thieme

Wyrsch, J. 1958. Über den Zustand des Bewußtseins bei Schizophrenen. *Wien. Z. Nervenheilk.*, **14**, 121–35

3. EGO-CONSCIOUSNESS

Ackner, B. 1954. Depersonalisation. I. Aetiology and phenomenology. II. Clinical syndromes. *J. ment. Sci.*, **100**, 838–72.

Ammon, G. 1973. *Dynamische Psychiatrie. – Grundlagen und Probleme einer Reform der Psychiatrie.* Neuwied/Rhein:
Luchterhand

Balint, M. 1952. *Primary Love and Psychoanalytic Technique.*
London: Hogarth Press
1973. *Therapeutische Aspekte der Regression.* Hamburg: Rowohlt

Bellak, L., Hurvich, M. and Gediman, H. K. 1973. *Ego Functions
in Schizophrenics, Neurotics and Normals.* New York: Wiley

Benedetti, G. 1964. *Der psychisch Leidende und seine Welt.* Stuttgart:
Hippokrates-Verlag

Berze, J. and Gruhle, H. W. 1929. *Psychologie der Schizophrenie.*
Berlin: Springer

Blanck, G. and Blanck, R. 1974. *Ego Psychology: Theory and
Practice.* New York: Columbia University Press

Blankenburg, W. 1971. *Der Verlust der natürlichen Selbstverständlichkeit; ein Beitrag zur Psychopathologie symptomarmer
Schizophrenien.* Stuttgart: Enke

Bleuler, E. 1908. Die Prognose der Dementia praecox (Schizophre-
niegruppe). *Allg. Z. Psychiat.*, **65**, 436–64
1911. Dementia praecox oder Gruppe der Schizophrenien. In
Handbuch der Psychiatrie, ed. G. Aschaffenburg, spec. pt. 4.
Vienna: Deuticke

Brauer, R. 1970. Depersonalisation phenomena in psychiatric
patients. *Brit. J. Psychiat.*, **117**, 509–15

Burger, J. O. 1910. Zur Psychologie der Organgefühle und Fremd-
heitsgefühle. *Z. ges. Neurol. Psychiat.*, **1**, 230–41

Collett, P. 1972. Structure and content in cross-cultural studies of
self esteem. *Int. J. Psychol.*, **7**, 169–80

Cutler, B. and Reed, J. 1975. Multiple personality. *Psychol. Med.*,
5, 18–26

Drews, S. and Brecht, K. 1975. *Psychoanalytische Ich-Psychologie.*
Frankfurt/M: Suhrkamp

Engel, G. L. 1962. *Psychological Development in Health and Disease.*
Philadelphia: Saunders

Erikson, E. H. 1950. *Childhood and Society.* New York: Norton
1966. *Identität und Lebenszyklus.* Frankfurt/M: Suhrkamp. (English version: 1959. *Identity and the Life Cycle.* New York:
International University Press)

1974. *Jugend und Krise.* 2nd edn. Stuttgart: Klett (English version: 1968. *Identity – Youth and Crisis*)

Eysenck, H. J. 1967. *The Biological Basis of Personality.* Springfield/Ill.: Thomas

Federn, P. 1956. *Ich-Psychologie und die Psychosen.* Berne: Huber (English: 1952. *Ego Psychology and the Psychoses.* New York: Basic Books)

Fenichel, O. 1946 (1st edn.), 1971. *The Psychoanalytic Theory of Neurosis.* London: Routledge & Kegan Paul

Freeman, Th., Cameron, J. L. and McGhie, A. 1965. *Studies on Psychosis.* London: Tavistock

Freud, Anna 1936. *Das Ich und die Abwehrmechanismen.* Munich: Kindler

Freud, S. 1911. Psychoanalytische Bemerkungen über einen autobiographisch beschriebenen Fall von Paranoia (Dementia paranoides). *Gesammelte Werke,* vol. VIII. Frankfurt/M: Fischer 1968

1924a. Das Ich und das Es. *Gesammelte Werke,* vol. XIII. Frankfurt/M: Fischer 1968

1924b. Neurose und Psychose. *Gesammelte Werke,* vol. XIII. Frankfurt/M: Fischer 1968

1938. Die Ich-Spaltung im Abwehrvorgang. *Gesammelte Werke,* vol. XVII. Frankfurt/M: Fischer 1968

Gebsattel, V. F. v. 1937. Zur Frage der Depersonalisation. *Nervenarzt,* **10,** 169–78

Gill, M. 1967. *The Collected Papers of David Rapaport.* New York: Basic Books

Glatzel, J. 1971. Über das Entfremdungserlebnis. *Z. Psychother. med. Psychol.,* **21,** 89–99

Glover, E., 1943. The concept of dissociation. In *On the Early Development of the Mind.* New York: International University Press

Göppert, H. 1960. *Zwangskrankheit und Depersonalisation.* Basle: Karger

Gruhle, H. W. 1956. *Verstehende Psychologie-Erlebnislehre.* 2nd edn. Stuttgart: Thieme

Hallowell, A. I. 1955. *Culture and Experience.* Philadelphia: University of Pennsylvania Press

Hartmann, H. 1953. Contribution to the meta-psychology of schizophrenia. In *The Psychoanalytic Study of the Child,* vol. VIII. New York: International University Press

1939. Ich-Psychologie und Anpassungsproblem. New edn. 1960 in *Psyche*, **14**, 81–164

1964a. *Essays on Ego Psychology.* New York: International University Press

1964b. Zur psychoanalytischen Theorie des Ich (7 Aufsätze). *Psyche*, **18**, 330–474

1972: *Die Grundlagen der Psychoanalyse* (Leipzig: 1st edn. 1927). Stuttgart: Klett

Hartmann, H., Kris, E. and Loewenstein, R. M. 1946. Comments on the formation of psychic structure. In *The Psychoanalytic Study of the Child*, vol. II, pp. 11–38. New York: International University Press

Hegel, G. W. F. 1970. *Phänomenologie des Geistes* (1st edn. 1807). Frankfurt/M: Ullstein

Jacobson, E. 1964. *The Self and the Object World.* New York: International University Press

Jaspers, K. 1959. *Allgemeine Psychopathologie.* 7th edn. (9th edn. 1973). Berlin: Springer

Jung, C. G. 1952. Die Schizophrenie. *Schweiz. Arch. Neurol. Psychiat.*, **81**, 163–77

Kernberg, O. F. 1967. Borderline personality organization. *J. Amer. psychoanal. Ass.*, **15**, 641–85

1970. Factors in the psychoanalytic treatment of narcissistic personalities. *J. Amer. psychoanal. Ass.*, **18**, 51–85

1972. Early ego integration and object relations. *Ann. N.Y. Acad. Sci.*, **193**, 233–47

Kimura, B. 1965. Vergleichende Untersuchungen über depressive Erkrankungen in Japan und in Deutschland. *Fortschr. Neurol. Psychiat.*, **33**, 202–15

1967. Phänomenologie des Schulderlebnisses in einer vergleichenden psychiatrischen Sicht. In *Beiträge zur vergleichenden Psychiatrie*, vol. 16, *Aktuelle Fragen der Psychiatrie und Neurologie*. ed. N. Petrilowitsch, pp. 54–65. Basle: Karger

1969. Zur Wesensfrage der Schizophrenie im Lichte der japanischen Sprache. In *Jahrbuch für Psychologie, Psychotherapie und medizinische Anthropologie*, ed. V. E. v. Gebsattel, P. Christian, W. J. Revers, and H. Tellenbach, pp. 28–37. Freiburg: Alber

Kisker, K. P. 1964. Kernschizophrenie und Egopathien. Bemerkungen zum heutigen Stand der Forschungen und zur Methodologie. *Nervenarzt*, **35**, 286–94

1968. Der Egopath. *Soc. Psychiat.*, **3**, 19–23

Kohut, H. 1971 *The Analysis of the Self.* New York: International University Press

Kronfeld, A. 1922. Über schizophrene Veränderungen des Bewußtseins der Aktivität. *Z. ges. Neurol. Psychiat.,* **74,** 15–68

Kutter, P. 1967. Psychiatrische Krankheitsbilder. In *Die Krankheitslehre der Psychoanalyse,* ed. W. Loch. Stuttgart: Hirzel

Laplanche, J. and Pontalis, J.-B. 1973. *Das Vokabular der Psychoanalyse.* Frankfurt/M: Suhrkamp

Lebra, W. P. 1972. *Transcultural Research in Mental Health.* Honolulu: University Press of Hawaii

Lehmann, L. S. 1974. Depersonalisation. *Amer. J. Psychiat.,* **131,** 1221–4

Levita, J. E. de. 1971. *Der Begriff der Identität* (English: 1965). Frankfurt/M: Suhrkamp

Lidz, Th. 1970. *Das menschliche Leben.* (English: 1968). Frankfurt/M: Suhrkamp

Loch, W. 1967. *Die Krankheitslehre der Psychoanalyse.* Stuttgart: Hirzel
    1975. *Über Begriffe und Methoden der Psychoanalyse.* Berne: Huber

Mahler, M. S. 1951. On Child Psychosis and Schizophrenia: *Autistic and Symbiotic Infantile psychosis,* vol. VII, pp. 286–305. New York: International University Press
    1958. Autism and symbiosis, two extreme disturbances of identity. *Int. J. Psycho-Anal.,* **39,** 77–83
    1968. *On Human Symbiosis and the Vicissitudes of Individuation.* New York: International University Press
    1972. On the first three sub-phases of the separationindividuation process. *Int. J. Psycho-Anal.,* **53,** 333–8

Meyer, J.-E. 1959. *Die Entfremdungserlebnisse.* Stuttgart: Thieme
    1963. Depersonalisation und Derealisation. *Fortschr. Neurol. Psychiat.,* **31,** 438–50
    1968. *Depersonalisation.* Darmstadt: Wissenschaftliche Buchgesellschaft

Nunberg, H. 1971. *Allgemeine Neurosenlehre.* (1st edn. 1931) Berne: Huber
    1939. Ichstärke und Ichschwäche. *Int. Z. Psychoanal.,* **24,** 49–61

Parin, P. and Morgenthaler, F. 1964. Ego and orality in the analysis of West Africans. *Psychoanal. Stud. Soc.,* **3,** 197–202

Pohlen, M. 1969. *Schizophrene Psychosen: Ein Beitrag zur Strukturlehre des Ich.:* Berne: Huber

Rapaport, D. 1950 and 1967. On the psychoanalytic theory of thinking. In *The Collected Papers of David Rapaport*, ed. M. Gill, pp. 313–23. New York: Basic Books

Schafer, R. 1968. Mechanisms of defense. *Int. J. Psycho-Anal.*, **49**, 49–62

Scharfetter, Ch. 1973. Streifzüge in die Geschichte des Schizophrenenbegriffs. *Schweiz. Arch. Neurol. Neurochir. Psychiat.*, **112**, 75–85

Schilder. P. 1914. Selbstbewußtsein und Persönlichkeitsbewußtsein. In *Monographien aus dem Gesamtgebeit der Neurologie und Psychiatrie*, ed. M. Müller, H. Spatz, and P. Vogel, H. 9. Berlin: Springer

1925. *Entwurf zu einer Psychiatrie auf psychoanalytischer Grundlage*. (1st edn.) Frankfurt/M: Suhrkamp, 1973

Schneider, K. 1967. *Klinische Psychopathologie*. 8th edn. (10th edn. 1973). Stuttgart: Thieme

Sedman, G. 1970. Theories of depersonalisation. A reappraisal. *Brit. J. Psychiat.*, **117**, 1–14

1972. An investigation of certain factors concerned in the etiology of depersonalisation. *Acta psychiat. scand.*, **48**, 191–219

Semrad, E. V., Greenspoon, L. and Fienberg, St. E. 1973. Development of an ego profile scale. *Arch. gen. Psychiat.*, **28**, 70–7

Spitz, R. A. 1962. Autoerotism reexamined: The role of early sexual behaviour patterns in personality formation. In *The Psychoanalytic Study of the Child*, vol. XVII, pp. 283–315. New York: International University Press

1965. *The First Year of Life*. New York: International University Press

1972. *Eine genetische Feldtheorie der Ichbildung*. Frankfurt/M: Fischer (English: 1959. *A Genetic Field Theory of Ego Formation*. New York: International University Press)

Sullivan, H. St. 1962. Schizophrenia as a Human Process. New York: Norton

Vaillant, G. E. 1971. Theoretical hierarchy of adaptive ego mechanisms. *Arch. gen. Psychiat.*, **24**, 107–18

Winkler, W. Th. 1954. Zum Begriff der Ich-Anachorese beim schizophrenen Erleben. *Arch. Psychiat. Nervenkr.*, **192**, 234–40

1971. *Übertragung und Psychose*. Berne: Huber

Winkler, W. Th. and Wieser, St. 1959. Die Ichmythisierung als Abwehrmaßnahme des Ich, dargestellt am Beispiel des Wahneinfalles von der jungfräulichen Empfängnis und Geburt bei paraphrenen Episoden. *Nervenarzt*, **30**, 75–81

294 *Bibliography*

Wulff, E. 1972. Psychiatrischer Bericht aus Vietnam – Grundfra₍ der transkulturellen Psychiatrie. Sprachbarrieren als Hind nisse psychiatrischer Forschung. In *Psychiatrie und Klassen₍ sellschaft*. Frankfurt/M: (Athenäum) Fischer

Wylie, R. C. 1961. *The Self Concept*. Lincoln, Nebraska: Univers of Nebraska Press

4. CONSCIOUSNESS OF EXPERIENCE, REALITY TESTING

Blankenburg, W. 1971. *Der Verlust der natürlichen Selbstverstän lichkeit, ein Beitrag zur Psychopathologie symptomarm₍ Schizophrenien*. Stuttgart: Enke

Bleuler, E. 1969. *Lehrbuch der Psychiatrie*. 11th edn. rev. M. Bleule pp. 99–104. Berlin, Springer

Freud, S. 1911. Psychoanalytische Bemerkungen über einen autc biographisch beschriebenen Fall von Paranoia Dementia para noides). *Gesammelte Werke*, vol. VIII, Frankfurt/M: Fischeɪ 1968

Gadamer, H.-G. 1972. *Wahrheit und Methode*. 3rd edn. Tübingen Mohr

Holzhey, H. 1970. *Kants Erfahrungsbegriff*. Basle: Schwabe

Janet, P. 1903. *Obsession et la psychasthénie*. Paris: Alcan

Jaspers, K. 1912. Die Trugwahrnehmungen. *Z. ges. Neurol. Psychiat.*, **4**, 289–354

1925. *Psychologie der Weltanschauungen*. 3rd edn. Berlin: Springer

1959. *Allgemeine Psychopathologie*. 7th edn. Berlin: Springer

Kloos, G. 1938. *Das Realitätsbewußtein in der Wahrnehmung und Trugwahrnehmung*. Leipzig: Thieme

Laing, R. D. 1967. *Phänomenologie der Erfahrung*. Frankfurt/M: Suhrkamp

5. ORIENTATION

Pauleikhoff, B. 1955. Über Veränderungen des Situationsgefüges bei dementen Erscheinungsbildern. *Nervenarzt*, **26**, 510–15

Scheller, H. 1963. Über das Wesen der Orientierung. *Nervenarzt*, **34**, 1–4

6. EXPERIENCE OF TIME

7. MEMORY

8. ATTENTION AND CONCENTRATION

Adams, A. E. 1971. Informationstheorie und Psychopathologie des Gedächtnisses. In *Monographien-aus dem Gesamtgebiete der Psychiatrie*, ed. H. Hippius, W. Janzarik and M. Müller, vol. III. Berlin: Springer

Beringer, K. 1927. *Der Meskalinrausch*. (New edn. 1969) Berlin: Springer

Bilodeau, E. A. 1966. *Acquisition of Skill*. New York: Academic Press

Fischer, F. 1930. Raum-Zeit-Struktur und Denkstörung in der Schizophrenie. *Zbl. ges. Neurol. Psychiat.*, **124**, 241–56

Foppa, K. 1965. *Lernen, Gedächtnis, Verhalten. Ergebnisse und Probleme der Lernpsychologie*. Cologne: Kiepenheuer & Witsch

Fraisse, P. 1966. Zeitwahrnehmung und Zeitschätzung. In *Handbuch der Psychologie*, vol. I: *Allgemeine Psychologie*, 1. Der Aufbau des Erkennens, 1. Half-vol.: Wahrnehmung und Bewußtsein, ed. K. Gottschaldt, Ph. Lersch. F. Sander and H. Thomae, pp. 656–90. Göttingen: Hogrefe

Gebsattel, V. E. v. 1939. Die Störungen des Werdens und Zeiterlebens im Rahmen psychiatrischer Erkrankungen. In *Gegenwartsprobleme der psychiatrisch-neurologischen Forschung*, ed. Ch. Roggenbau. Stuttgart: Enke

Kloos, G. 1938. Störungen des Zieterlebens in der endogenen Depression. *Nervenarzt*, **11**, 225–44

Lhamon, W. T. and Goldstone, S. 1956. The time sense. *AMA (Chicago) Arch. Neurol. Psychiat.*, **76**, 625–9

McGhie, A. 1969. Pathology of Attention. *Sci. Behav.*, **10**, 12

Mierke, K. 1966. *Konzentrationsfähigkeit und Konzentrationsschwäche*. Berne: Huber, and Stuttgart: Klett

Minkowski, E. 1971 (orig. 1933). *Die gelebte Zeit*. Salzburg: Müller

Strauss, E. 1928. Das Zeiterlebnis in der endogenen Depression und in der psychopathischen Verstimmung. *Mschr. Psychiat. Neurol.*, **68**, 640–56

Swets, J. A. and Kristofferson, A. B. 1970. Attention. *Ann. Rev. Psychol.*, **21**, 339–66

Zeh, W. 1961. *Die Amnesien*. Stuttgart: Thieme

9. THOUGHT, LANGUAGE, SPEECH

10. INTELLIGENCE

Ambrose, A. 1969. *Stimulation in Early Infancy*. London: Academic Press

Arieti, S. 1955. *Interpretation of Schizophrenia*. New York: Brunner

Arnold, O. H. 1969. Inner Sprache und Begriffsbildung beim Schizophrenen. *Wien. Z. Nervenheilk.*, **26**, 213–22

Bleuler, E. 1927. *Das autistisch-undisziplinierte Denken in der Medizin und seine Uberwindung*. (5th edn. 1966) Berlin: Springer

Duncker, K. 1974. *Zur Psychologie des produktiven Denkens*. Berlin: Springer

Ellis, N. R. 1963. *Handbook of Mental Deficiency*. New York: McGraw-Hill

Eysenck, H. J. 1967. Intelligence assessment: a theoretical and experimental approach. *Brit. J. educ. Psychol.*, **37**, 81–98

1971. *Race, Intelligence, and Education*. London: Temple Smith

Flegel, H. 1965. *Schizophasie in linguistischer Deutung*. Berlin: Springer

Freund, H. 1953. Psychopathological aspect of stuttering. *Amer. J. Psychother.*, **7**, 689–705

Frosting, J. 1929. *Das schizophrene Denken*. Leipzig: Thieme

Furneaux, W. D. 1960. Intellectual abilities and problem-solving behavior. In *Handbook of Abnormal Psychology*, ed. H. J. Eysenck. London: Pitman

Goldstein, K. 1948. *Language and Language Disturbances*. New York: Grune & Stratton

Gottesmann, I. I. 1963. Genetic aspects of intelligent behavior. In *Handbook of Mental Deficiency*, ed. N. R. Ellis. New York: McGraw-Hill

Guilford, J. P. 1967. *The Nature of Human Intelligence*. New York: McGraw-Hill

HAWIE *1955. Wechsler, D. Die Messung der Intelligenz Erwachsener. Textband zum Hamburg-Wechsler-Intelligenztest für Ewachsene (HAWIE)*.(German: A. Hardesty and H. Lauber, ed. C. Bondy. 3rd edn. Berne and Stuttgart: Huber)

Heidegger, M. 1959. *Unterwegs zur Sprache*. Pfullingen: Neske

1971. *Was heißt denken?* Tübingen: Niemeyer

Hermann, T. 1972. Sprache. In *Einführung in die Psychologie*, ed. C. F. Graumann, vol. v. Berne: Huber

Hörmann, H. 1967. *Psychologie der Sprache*. (New impression, 1970) Berlin: Springer

Jäger, A. D. 1967. *Dimensionen der Intelligenz*. Göttingen: Hogrefe

Jahrreiss, W. 1928. Störungen des Denkens. In *Handbuch der Geisteskrankheiten*, ed. O. Bumke, vol. I. Berlin: Springer

Jaspers, K. 1964. *Die Sprache*. Munich: Piper

Kasanin, J. S. 1944. *Language and thought in Schizophrenia*. Berkeley/Calif.: University of California Press

Langen, D. 1957. Diagnostik, aus dem sprachlichen Ausdruck. *Dtsch. med. Wschr.*, **82**, 1006–9

Leischner, A. 1951. Über den Verfall der menschlichen Sprache. *Arch. Psychiat. Nervenkr.*, **187**, 250–67

Moses, P. J. 1956. *Die Stimme der Neurose*. Stuttgart: Thieme

Pawlik, K. 1968. *Dimensionen des Verhaltens*. Berne: Huber

Piaget, J. 1967. *Psychologie der Intelligenz*. 3rd edn. Zürich: Rascher
  1973. *Einführung in die genetische Erkenntnistheorie*. Frankfurt/M: Suhrkamp

Piro, S. 1960. La dissociation sémantique. *Ann. méd.-psychol.*, **118**, II, 407–36

Robinson, W. P. 1972. *Language and Social Behaviour*. Harmondsworth/Middlesex: Penguin

Schneider, C. 1930. *Die Psychologie der Schizophrenen*. Leipzig: Thieme

Slater, E. and Cowie, V. 1971. *The Genetics of Mental Disorders*. London: Oxford University Press

Spitz, R. 1967. *Vom Säugling zum Kleinkind*. Stuttgart: Klett

Spoerri, Th. 1964. *Sprachphänomene und Psychose*. Basle: Karger

Stockert, F. G. 1929. *Über Umbau und Abbau der Sprache bei Geistesstörung. Mschr. Psychiat. Neurol.*, Beih. **49**

Storch, A. 1922. *Das archaisch-primitive Erleben und Denken der Schizophrenen*. Berlin: Springer

Stransky, E. 1905. *Über Sprachverwirrtheit*. Halle: Marhold

Teulié, G. 1931. La schizophasie. *Ann. méd.-psychol.*, **89**, 113–23; 225–33

Thorndike, R. L. 1966. Intellectual status and intellectual growth. *J. educ. Psychol.*, **57**, 121–7

Thurstone, L. L. 1935. *Vectors of Mind*. Chicago. University of Chicago Press

Vetter, H. J. 1968. *Language Behavior in Schizophrenia*. Springfield/Ill: Thomas

Wechsler, D. 1961. *Die Messung der Intelligenz Erwachsener.* 2nd edn. Berne: Huber

Whorf, B. L. 1963. *Sprache, Denken, Wirklichkeit.* Hamburg: Rowohlt

Wiseman, S. 1967. *Intelligence and Ability.* Harmondsworth/ Middlesex: Penguin

11. PERCEPTION

12. APPERCEPTION

Allport, F. H. 1955. *Theories of Perception and the Concept of Structure.* New York: Wiley

Bartley, S. H. 1969. *Principles of Perception.* New York: Harper & Row

Bay, E. 1950. *Agnosie und Funktionswandel. Eine hirnpathologische Studie.* Berlin: Springer

Boring, E. G. 1942. *Sensation and Perception in the History of Experimental Psychology.* New York: Appleton-Century-Crofts

Conrad, K. 1951. Aphasie, Agnosie, Apraxie. *Fortsch. Neurol. Psychiat.*, **19**, 291–325

Frederiks, J. A. M. 1969. Agnosias. In *Handbook of Clinical Neurology*, ed. P. J. Vinken and G. W. Bruyn, vol. IV. Amsterdam: North-Holland Publishing Company

Freedman, B. J. 1974. The subjective experience of perceptual and cognitive disturbances in schizophrenia. *Arch. gen. Psychiat.*, **30**, 333–40

Goldstein, K. A. 1920. Psychologische Analysen hirnpathologischer Fälle auf Grund von Untersuchungen Hirnverletzter. *Z. Psychol. Physiol. Sinnesorg.*, **83**, 1–94

Hayos, A. 1972. *Wahrnehmungspsychologie. Psychophysik und Wahrnehmungsforschung.* Stuttgart: Kolhammer

Herrmann, Th. 1965. *Psychologie der kognitiven Ordnungen.* Berlin: de Gruyter

Jaspers, K. 1959. *Allgemeine Psychopathologie.* 7th edn. (9th edn. 1973) Berlin: Springer

Kandinski, V. 1885. *Kritische und klinische Betrachtungen im Gebiet der Sinnestäuchungen.* Berlin: Friedländer

Kloos, G. 1938. *Das Realitätsbewußtsein in der Wahrnehmung und Trugwahrnehmung.* Leipzig: 1938

Laing, R. D. 1967. *The Politics of Experience.* Harmondsworth/ Middlesex: Penguin (German: 1969. *Phänomenologie der Erfahrung.* Frankfurt/M: Suhrkamp)

Mayer-Gross, W. and Stein, J. 1928. Psychopathologie der Wahrnehmung. In *Handbuch der Geisteskrankheiten*, ed. O. Bumke. Berlin: Springer

Matussek, P. 1952. Untersuchungen über die Wahrnehmung. 1. Mitt. Veränderungen der Wahrnehmungswelt bei beginnendem, primärem Wahn. *Arch. Psychiat. Nervenkr.*, **189**, 279–319

1953. Untersuchungen über die Wahrnehmung. 2. Mitt. Die auf einem abnormen Vorrang von Wesenseigenschaften beruhenden Eigentümlichkeiten der Wahnwahrnehmung. *Schweiz. Arch. Neurol. Neurochir. Psychiat.*, **71**, 189–210

1963. Psychopathologie II: Wahrnehmung, Halluzination und Wahn. In *Psychiatrie der Gegenwart*, 1st edn., ed. H. W. Gruhle, R. Jung, and W. Mayer-Gross, vol. I/2, Grundlagen und Methoden der klinischen Psychiatrie, pp. 23–76. Berlin: Springer

Merleau-Ponty, M. 1966. *Phänomenologie der Wahrnehmung.* Berlin: de Gruyter

Metzger, W. 1966. Allgemeine Psychologie. 1. Der Aufbau des Erkennens. 1st Half-vol.: Wahrnehmung und Bewußtsein. In *Handbuch der Psychologie*, ed. K. Gottschaldt, Ph. Lersch, F. Sander and H. Thomae, vol. I. Göttingen: Hogrefe

Meyer, J.-E. 1959 *Die Entfremdungserlebnisse.* Stuttgart: Thieme

1968. *Depersonalisation.* Darmstadt: Wissenschaftliche Buchgesellschaft

Müller, C. 1956. Mikropsie und Makropsie. Basle: Karger

Murray, H. 1943. *Thematic Apperception Test.* Cambridge, Mass.: Harvard University Press

Piaget, J. 1973. *Einführung in die genetische Erkenntnistheorie.* Frankfurt/M: Suhrkamp

Piaget, J. and Inhelder, Bärbel. 1971. *Die Entwicklung des räumlichen Denkens beim Kinde.* Stuttgart: Klett

Powers,W. T. 1973. *Behaviour: The Control of Perception.* Chicago: Aldine

Reimer, F. 1970. *Das Syndrom der optischen Halluzinose.* Stuttgart: Thieme

Scheid, W. 1937. Über Personenverkennung. *Zbl. ges. Neurol. Psychiat.*, **157**, 1–16

Schneider, K. 1967. *Klinische Psychopathologie.* 8th edn. (10th edn. 1973) Stuttgart: Thieme

Schooler, C. and Feldman, S. E. 1967. *Experimental Studies of Schiziphrenia.* Goleta/California: Psychonomic Press

Schorsch, G. 1934. *Zur Theorie der Halluzinationen.* Leipzig: Barth
Sedman, G. 1966. A phenomenological study of pseudohallucinations
  and related experiences. *Acta psychiat. (Kbh),* **42,** 35–70
Séglas, M. J. 1892. De l'obsession hallucinatoire et de l'hallucination
  obsédante. *Ann. méd.-psychol.,* **50,** 119–29
Spitz, R. 1957. *Die Entstehung der ersten Objektbeziehungen.*
  Stuttgart: Klett
Straus, E. 1935. *Vom Sinn der Sinne.* Berlin: Springer
  1949. Die Ästhesiologie und ihre Bedeutung für das Verständnis
  der Halluzinationen. *Arch. Psychiat. Nervenkr.,* **182,** 301–32

13. DELUSION

Abraham, K. 1908. Die psychosexuellen Differenzen der Hysterie
  und der Dementia praecox. *Zbl. ges. Neurol. Psychiat.,* **31**
  (NF19), 521–33
Achté, K. A. 1971. Zum Einfluß der Kultur auf die schizophrenen
  Wahnvorstellungen. *Psychiat. fenn.* 45–50
Adler, A. 1920. *Praxis und Theorie der Individualpsychologie.*
  Munich: Bergmann
Baeyer, W. v. 1932. Über konformen Wahn. *Z. ges. Neurol. Psychiat.,*
  140, 398–438
Berner, P. 1965. Das paranoische Syndrom. In *Monographien aus
  dem Gesamtgebiet der Neurologie und Psychiatrie,* ed. M. Müller.
  H. Spatz and P. Vogel, H.110. Berlin: Springer
Bilz, R. 1967. Der Wahn in ethologischer Sicht. *Stud. gen.,* **20,**
  650–60
Binswanger, L. 1955. *Ausgewählte Vorträge und Aufsätze:* Berne:
  Francke
  1957. *Schizophrenie.* Pfullingen: Neske
  1965. *Wahn.* Pfullingen: Neske
Blankenburg, W. 1967. Die anthropologische und daseinsanalytische
  Sicht des Wahns. *Stud. gen.,* **20,** 639–50
  1971. *Der Verlust der natürlichen Selbstverständlichkeit; ein
  Beitrag zur Psychopathologie symptomarmer Schizophrenien.*
  Stuttgart: Enke
Blankenburg, W. and Zilly, A. 1973. Gestaltwandel im schizophrenen
  Wahnerleben? In *Gestaltwandel psychiatrischer Krankheits-
  bilder,* ed. J. Glatzel, pp. 129–43. Stuttgart: Schattauer
Bleuler, E. 1906. *Affektivität, Suggestibilität, Paranoia.* Halle:
  Marhold
  1911. Dementia praecox oder Gruppe der Schizophrenien. In

Handbuch der Psychiatrie, ed. G. Aschaffenburg, Spec. Pt. 4. Vienna: Deuticke

Boss, M. 1971. *Grundriß der Medizin*. Berne: Huber

1974. *Schizophrenes Kranksein im Lichte einer daseinsanalytischen Phänomenologie*. Vortrag, Japan, October.

Conrad, K. 1958. *Die beginnende Schizophrenie*. (3rd edn. 1971) Stuttgart: Thieme

Cotard, J. 1882. Du délire des négations. *Arch. Neurol. (Paris)*, **4**, 153; 282

Duden. 1963. *Etymologie*. Mannheim: Bibliographisches Institut

Ey, H. 1973. *Traité des hallucinations*. Paris: Masson

Feer, H. 1970. *Kybernetik in der Psychiatrie*. Basle: Karger

Fenichel, O. 1971. *The Psychoanalytic Theory of Neurosis*. (1st edn. 1946) London: Routledge & Kegan Paul

Freud, S. 1896. Weitere Bemerkungen über die Abwehr-Neuropsychosen. *Gesammelte Werke*, vol. I. Frankfurt/M: Fischer 1968

1906–1909. Der Wahn und die Träume in W. Jensens 'Gradiva'. *Gesammelte Werke*, vol. VII. Frankfurt/M: Fischer 1968

1911. Psychoanalytische Bemerkungen über einen autobiographisch beschriebenen Fall von Paranoia (Dementia paranoides). *Gesammelte Werke*, vol. VIII. Frankfurt/M: Fischer 1968

1913–1917. Zur Einführung des Narzißmus. *Gesammelte Werke*, vol. X. Frankfurt/M: Fischer 1968

1916–1917. Vorlesungen zur Einführung in die Psychoanalyse. *Gesammelte Werke*, vol. XI. Frankfurt/M: Fischer 1968

1920–1924. Über einige neurotische Mechanismen bei Eifersucht, Paranoia und Homosexualität. *Gesammelte Werke*, vol. XIII. Frankfurt/M: Fischer 1968

1932. Neue Folgen der Vorlesungen zur Einführung in die Psychoanalyse. *Gesammelte Werke*, vol. XV. Frankfurt/M: Fischer 1968

1932–1939. Konstruktion in der Analyse. *Gesammelte Werke*, vol. XVI. Frankfurt/M: Fischer 1968

Gaupp, R. 1920. Der Fall Wagner. Eine Katamnese, zugleich ein Beitrag zur Lehre von der Paranoia. *Z. ges. Neurol. Psychiat.*, **60**, 312–27

1938. Krankheit und Tod des paranoischen Massenmörders Hauptlehrer Wagner. Eine Epikrise. *Z. ges. Neurol. Psychiat.*, **163**, 48–82

1947. Die Lehre von der Paranoia. *Nervenarzt*, **18**, 167–9

Gittelson, N. L. and Dawson-Butterworth, K. 1967. Subjective experience of sexual change in female schizophrenics. *Brit. J. Psychiat.*, **113**, 491–4

Gittelson, N. L. and Levine, S. 1966. Subjective experience of sexual change in male schizophrenics. *Brit. J. Psychiat.*, **112**, 779–82

Gruhle, H. W. 1936. Über den Wahn bei Epilepsie. *Z. ges Neurol. Psychiat.*, **154**, 395

1951. Über den Wahn. *Nervenarzt*, **22**, 125

Haase, H. J. 1963. Zur Psychodynamik, und Pathoplastik paranoider und paranoidhalluzinatorischer Psychosen bei alleinstehenden Frauen. *Fortschr. Neurol. Psychiat.*, **6**, 308–22

Heidegger, M. 1927. *Sein und Zeit*. 1st edn. Tübingen: Niemeyer 1972

Heinrich, K. 1965. Zur Bedeutung der Stammesgeschichte des menschlichen Erlebens für Neurologie und Psychopathologie. *Homo*, **16**, 65–77

Helmchen, H. 1968. *Bedingungskonstellationen paranoid-halluzinatorischer Syndrome*. Berlin: Springer

Hofer, G. 1953. Zum Terminus Wahn. *Fortschr. Neurol. Psychiat.*, **21**, 93–100

1968. Der Mensch im Wahn. *Bibl. psychiat. neurol.* (*Basle*) **136**

Hole, G. 1971. Über das Gewißheitselement im Glauben und im Wahn. *Confin. psychiat.* (Basle), **14**, 65–90; 145–73

Huber, G. 1964. Wahn (1954–1963). *Fortschr. Neurol. Psychiat.*, **32**, 429–89

Janzarik, W. 1955. Der Wahn schizophrener Prägung in den psychotischen Episoden der Epileptiker und die schizophrene Wahnwahrnehmung. *Fortschr. Neurol. Psychiat.*, **23**, 533–46

1956. Der lebensgeschichtliche und persönlichkeitseigene Hintergrund des cycolothymen Verarmungswahns. *Arch. Psychiat. Nervenkr.*, **195**, 219–33

1959a. Zur Differentialtypologie der Wahnphänomene. *Nervenarzt*, **30**, 153–9

1959b. *Dynamische Grundkonstellationen in endogenen Psychosen. Ein Beitrag zur Differentialtypologie der Wahnphänomene.* Berlin: Springer

1967. Der Wahn in strukturdynamischer Sicht. *Stud. gen.*, **20**, 628–38

Jung C. G. 1968. Über die Psychologie der Dementia praecox. Der Inhalt der Psychose. Das Unbewußte in der Psychopathologie. Psychogenese bei Geisteskranken. Über die Psychogenese der Schizophrenie. Die Schizophrenie. In *Gesammelte Werke*, vol. III, Psychogenese der Geisteskrankheiten. Zürich: Rascher

Kahn, E. 1929. Über Wahnbildung. *Arch. Psychiat. Nervenkr.*, **88**, 435–54

Kant, O. 1927a. Beiträge zur Paranoiaforschung: I. Die objektive Realitätsbedeutung des Wahns. *Z. ges. Neurol. Psychiat.*, **108**, 625–44

1927b. Beiträge zur Paranoiaforschung: II. Paranoische Haltung in der Gesundheitsbreite. *Z. ges. Neurol. Psychiat.*, **110**, 558–79

1930. Beiträge zur Paranoiaforschung: III. Allgemeine Gedanken zum Wahnproblem. *Z. ges. Neurol. Psychiat.*, **127**, 615–59

Kehrer, F. 1922. Über Spiritismus, Hypnotismus und Seelenstörung, Aberglaube und Wahn. *Arch. Psychiat. Nervenkr.*, **66**, 381–438

1928. Paranoische Zustände. In *Handbuch der Geisteskrankheiten*, ed. O. Bumke, vol. VI, spec. pt. II, pp. 232–364. Berlin: Springer

Kempe, P., Schönberger, J. and Gross, J. 1974. Sensorische Deprivation als Methode in der Psychiatrie. *Nervenarzt*, **45**, 561–8

Kolle, K. 1931. *Die primäre Verrücktheit*. Leipzig: Thieme

Kranz, H. 1955. Das Thema des Wahns im Wandel der Zeit. *Fortschr. Neurol. Psychiat.*, **23**, 58–72

1967. Wahn und Zeitgeist. *Stud. Gen.*, **20**, 605–11

Kretschmer, E. 1963. *Medizinische Psychologie*. 12th edn. (13th edn. 1971) Stuttgart: Thieme

1966. *Der sensitive Beziehungswahn*. 4th edn. Berlin: Springer

Kuhn, R. 1963. Daseinsanalyse und Psychiatrie. In *Psychiatrie der Gegenwart*, ed. H. W. Gruhle, R. Jung, W. Mayer-Gross and M. Müller, vol. I/2: Grundlagen und Methoden der klinischen Psychiatrie, pp. 853–902. Berlin: Springer

Kulenkampff, C. 1955. Entbergung, Entgrenzung, Überwältigung als Weisen des Standverlustes. Zur Anthropologie der paranoiden Psychosen. *Nervenarzt*, **26**, 89–95

1956. Erblicken und Erblicktwerden. Das für-andere-Sein (J. P. Sartre) in seiner Bedeutung für die Anthropologie der paranoiden Psychosen. *Nervenarzt*, **27**, 2–12

Kunz, H. 1931. Die Grenze der psychopathologischen Wahninterpretationen. *Z. ges Neurol. Psychiat.*, **135**, 671–715

1962. Die eine Welt und die Weisen des In-der-Welt-seins. *Psyche (Stuttgart)*. **16**, 58–80, 142–49, 221–39

1972. Erfahrung, Wahngeschehen und Todesgewißheit. *Z. klin. Psychol. Psychother.*, **20**, 334–47

Laing, R. D. 1959. *The Divided Self*. London: Tavistock

Lange, E. and Poppe, G. 1964. Faktoren der sozialen Isolierung im

Vorfeld paranoider Beeinträchtigungssyndrome des höheren Lebensalters. *Nervenarzt*, **35**, 194–200

Langfeldt, G. 1961. The erotic jealousy syndrome. A clinical study. *Acta psychiat. scand.*, Suppl. **151**

Lenz, H. 1973. Glaube und Wahn. *Fortschr. Neurol. Psychiat.*, **41**, 341–59

Lewis, A. 1970. Paranoia and paranoid: a historical perspective. *Psychol. Med.*, **1**, 2–12

Lindemann, H. 1957. *Allein über den Ozean*. Frankfurt/M: Scheffler

Matussek, P. 1952. Untersuchungen über die Wahnwahrnehmung. 1. Mitt. Veränderungen der Wahrnehmungswelt bei beginnendem primären Wahn. *Arch. Psychiat. Nervenkr.* **188**, 279–319

1953. Untersuchungen über die Wahnwahrnehmung. 2. Mitt. Die auf abnormem Vorrang von Wesenseigenschaften beruhenden Eigentümlichkeiten der Wahnwahrnehmung. *Schweiz. Arch. Neurol. Neurochir. Psychiat.*, **71**, 189–210

1963. Psychopathologie II: Wahrnehmung, Halluzination und Wahn. In *Psychiatrie der Gegenwart*, 1st edn., ed. H. W. Gruhle, R. Jung, W. Mayer-Gross and M. Müller, vol. I/2: Grundlagen und Methoden der klinischen Psychiatrie, pp. 23–76. Berlin: Springer

Mayer-Gross, W. 1932. Die Klinik. In *Handbuch der Geisteskrankheiten*, vol. IX, spec. pt. 5: Die Schizophrenie, ed. O. Bumke, pp. 293–578. Berlin: Springer

Murphy, H. B. M. 1967. Cultural aspects of the delusion. *Stud. gen.*, **20**, 684–92

Neisser, C. 1897. Paranoia und Schwachsinn. *Allg. Z. Psychiat.*, **53**, 241–69

Nunberg, H. 1971. *Allgemeine Neurosenlehre*. (1st edn. 1931) Berne: Huber

Orelli, A. v. 1954. Der Wandel des Inhaltes der depressiven Ideen bei der reinen Melancholie. *Schweiz. Arch. Neurol. Neurochir. Psychiat.*, **73**, 217–87

Pauleikhoff, B. 1954. Statistische Untersuchung über Häufigkeit und Thema von Wahneinfällen bei der Schizophrenie. *Schweiz. Arch. Psychiat. Nervenkr.* **191**, 341–50

1967. Der Eifersuchtswahn. *Fortschr. Neurol. Psychiat.*, **35**, 516–39

1969. Der Liebeswahn. *Fortschr. Neurol. Psychiat.*, **37**, 251–79

Pfeiffer, W. M. 1970. *Transkulturelle Psychiatrie*. Stuttgart: Thieme

Ploog, D. 1964. Verhaltensforschung und Psychiatrie. In *Psychiatrie der Gegenwart,* 1st edn. vol. i/1b, ed. H. W. Gruhle, R. Jung, W. Mayer-Gross and M. Müller, p. 291. Berlin: Springer

Raskin, D. E. and Sullivan, K. E. 1974. Erotomania. *Amer. J. Psychiat.,* **131,** 1033–5

Scharfetter, Ch. 1970. *Symbiontische Psychosen.* Berne: Huber

Scheler, M. 1913. *Zur Phänomenologie und Theorie der Sympathiegefühle und von Liebe und Haß.* Halle: Niemeyer

Schilder, P. 1918. Wahn und Erkenntnis. In *Monographien aus dem Gesamtgebiete der Neurologie und Psychiatrie,* H. 15, ed. M. Müller, H. Spatz and P. Vogel. Berlin: Springer

Schmidt, G. 1940. Der Wahn im Deutschsprachigen Schrifttum der letzten 25 Jahre (1914–1939). *Zbl. ges. Neurol. Psychiat.,* **97,** 113–43

1951. Liebeswahn. *Fortschr. Neurol. Psychiat.,* **18,** 623–34

Schneider, K. 1949. Zum Begriff des Wahns. *Fortschr. Neurol. Psychiat.,* **17,** 26–31

1952. *Über den Wahn.* Stuttgart: Thieme

1967. *Klinische Psychopathologie.* Stuttgart: Thieme

Schulte, W. 1958. Die gesunde Umwelt und ihre Reaktion auf Psychosen und Psychopathien. In *Psychiatrie und Gesellschaft,* ed. H. Ehrhardt. D. Ploog and H. Stutte. Berne: Huber

1968. Die Auswirkungen der Schizophrenie auf ihre Umwelt. *Nervenarzt,* **39,** 98–104

Schulte, W. and Tölle, R. 1972. *Wahn.* Stuttgart: Thieme

Shepherd, M. 1961. Morbid jealousy: some clinical and social aspects of a psychiatric symptom. *Brit. J. Psychiat.,* **107,** 687–753

Stierlin, H. 1967. Die Gestaltung und Übermittlung des Wahns in der Familie. *Stud. Gen.,* **20,** 693–700

Storch, A. 1959. Beiträge zum Verständnis des schizophrenen Wahnkranken. *Nervenarzt,* **30,** 49–58

1965. Wege zur Welt und Existenz des Geisteskranken. In *Schriftenreihe zur Theorie und Praxis der Psychotherapie,* Vol. viii, ed. E. Wiesenhütter. Stuttgart: Hippokrates-Verlag

Wasserzieher, E. 1963. *Woher?* Bonn: Dümmler

Weber, A. 1938. *Über nihilistischen Wahn und Depersonalisation.* Basle: Karger

Willie, J. 1962. Die Schizophrenie in ihrer Auswirkung auf die Eltern. *Arch. Neurol. Neurochir. Psychiat.,* **89,** 426–63

Winkler, W. T. and Wieser, S. T. 1959. Die Ich-Mythisierung als Abwehrmaßnahme des Ich, dargestellt am Beispiel des Wahneinfalls von der jungfräulichen Empfängnis und der Geburt bei paraphrenen Episoden. *Nervenarzt*, 30, 75–81

Yarrow, M. R., Schwartz, Ch. G., Murphy, H. S. and Deasy, L. C. 1955. The psychological meaning of mental illness in the family. *J. soc. Issues*, 11, 12–24

Zutt, J. 1963. Versuch einer anthropologischen Grundlegung der psychiatrischen Erfahrung. In *Psychiatrie der Gegenwart*, 1st edn. ed. H. W. Gruhle, R. Jung, W. Mayer-Gross and M. Müller, vol. 1/2: Grundlagen und Methoden der klinischen Psychiatrie, pp. 763–852. Berlin: Springer

Zutt, J. and Kulenkampff, C. 1958. *Das paranoide Syndrom in anthropologischer Sicht*. Berlin: Springer

14. DRIVE, BASIC ACTIVITY

Baeyer, W. v. 1961. Erlebnisbedingte Verfolgungsschäden. *Nervenarzt*, 32, 534–8

Baeyer, W. v., Häfner, H. and Kisker, K. P. 1964. *Psychiatrie der Verfolgten*. Berlin: Springer

Bilz, R. 1960. Langeweile. *Nervenarzt*, 31, 433–43

Craig, W. 1918. Appetites and aversions as constituents of instincts. *Biol. Bull. Woods Hole*, 34, 91–107

Eibl-Eibesfeld, I. 1969. Grundriß der vergleichenden Verhaltensforschung. *Ethologie*, 2nd edn. Munich: Piper

1970. *Liebe und Haß; zur Naturgeschichte elementarer Verhaltensweisen*. Munich: Piper

Ernst, K. 1959. Die Prognose der Neurosen. In *Monographien aus dem Gesamtgebiete der Neurologie und Psychiatrie*, H. 85, ed. M. Müller, H. Spatz and P. Vogel. Berlin: Springer

Hartwig, P. and Steinmeyer, E. 1974. Experimentelle Untersuchungen und faktorenanalytische Interpretation zur Antriebsstruktur Hebephrener und Gesunder. *Zbl. ges. Neurol. Psychiat.*, 207, 328–9

Janzarik, W. 1959. Dynamische Grundkonstellationen in endogenen Psychosen. Ein Beitrag zur Differentialtypologie der Wahnphänomene. In *Monographien aus dem Gesamtgebiete der Neurologie und Psychiatrie*, H. 86, ed. M. Müller, H. Spatz and P. Vogel. Berlin: Springer

Jung, C. G. 1924. *Wandlungen und Symbole der Libido*. Vienna: Deuticke

Klages, W. 1967. *Der menschliche Antrieb*. Stuttgart: Thieme

Klages, W. and Behrends, K. 1961. Zur Structur der schizophrenen Antriebsstörung. *Arch. Psychiat. Nervenkr.*, **202**, 504–12

Kongreß in Kiel. 1961. *Zbl. ges. Neurol. Psychiat.*, **162**, 202–12

Kretschmer, E. 1940. Das apallische Syndrom. *Zbl. ges. Neurol. Psychiat.*, **169**, 576–9

1961. *Körperbau und Charakter*. 23rd edn. Berlin: Springer

Lorenz, K. 1963. *Das sogenannte Böse; zur Naturgeschichte der Aggression*. Vienna: Borotha-Schoeler

Matussek, P. 1971. Die Konzentrationslagerhaft und ihre Folgen. In *Monographien aus dem Gesamtgebiete der Psychiatrie*, vol. II, ed. H. Hippius, W. Janzarik and M. Müller. Berlin: Springer

Spitz, R. 1960. *Die Entstehung der ersten Objektbeziehungen*. Stuttgart: Klett

Tinbergen, N. 1952. *The Study Of Instinct*. Oxford: Clarendon Press (German: 1956: *Instinktlehre, vergleichende Erforschung angeborenen Verhaltens*. 3rd edn. Berlin: Parey)

15. AGGRESSION

Berkowitz, L. 1962. *Aggression. A Social Psychological Analysis*. New York: McGraw-Hill

Bilz, R. 1967. Menschliche Aggressivität. *Z. Psychother. med. Psychol.*, **17**, 157–78, 197–202

Böker, W. and Häfner, H. 1973. *Gewalttaten Geistesgestörter*. Berlin: Springer

Corning, P. A. and Corning, C. H. 1972. Toward a general theory of violent aggression. *Soc. Sci. Inform*, **11**, 7–36

Delgado, J. M. R. 1967. Aggression and defense under cerebral radio control. In *Aggression and Defense. Neural Mechanisms and Social Patterns, UCLA Forum in Medical Sciences*, ed. C. D. Clemente and D. B. Lindsley, pp. 171–93. Berkeley/Calif.: University of California Press

Eibl-Eibesfeld, I. 1969. *Grundriß der vergleichenden Verhaltensforschung. Ethologie*. 2nd edn. Munich: Piper

1970. *Liebe und Haß: Zur Naturgeschichte elementarer Verhaltensweisen*. Munich: Piper

Fromm, E. 1974. *Anatomie der menschlichen Destruktivität*. Stuttgart: Deutsche Verlagsanstalt

Ghysbrecht, P. 1961. *Doppelselbstmord*. Munich: Reinhardt

Heimann, P. and Valenstein, A. F. 1972. The psychoanalytical concept of aggression, an integrated summary. *Int J. Psycho-Anal.*, **53**, 31–5

Hess, W. R. 1962. *Psychologie in biologischer Sicht*. (2nd edn. 1968) Stuttgart: Thieme

Kummer, H. 1973. Aggression bei Affen. In *Der Mythos vom Aggressionstrieb*, ed. A. Plack, pp. 69–91. Munich: List

Lorenz, K. 1963. *Das sogenannte Böse; zur Naturgeschichte der Aggression*. Vienna: Borotha-Schoeler

1969. *Über tierisches und menschliches Verhalten*. Munich: Piper

Plack, A. 1973. *Der Mythos vom Aggressionstrieb*. Munich: List

Schmidbauer, W. 1972. *Die sogenannte Aggression*. Hamburg: Hoffman & Campe

Storr, A. 1969/70. *Human Aggression*. Harmondsworth/Middlesex: Penguin

Thomae, H. 1965a. Motivation. In *Handbuch der Psychologie*, vol. II, ed. K. Gottschaldt, Ph. Lersch, E. Sander and H. Thomae. Göttingen: Hogrefe

1965b. *Die Motivation menschlichen Handelns*. Cologne: Kiepenheuer & Witsch

Tinbergen, N. 1952. *The Study of Instinct*. Oxford: Clarendon Press (German: *Instinktlehre, vergleichende Erforschung angeborenen Verhaltens*. Berlin: Parey 1956)

16. THE MOTOR SYSTEM

Binswanger, L. 1955. Vom anthropologischen Sinn der Verstiegenheit. In *Ausgewählte Vorträge und Aufsätze*, vol. II, ed. L. Binswanger. Berne: Francke

Glatzel, J. 1970. Die akute Katatonie. *Acta psychiat. scand.*, **46**, 151–79

Kahlbaum, K. L. 1874. *Die Katatonie oder das Spannungsirresein*. Berlin: Hirschwald

Kläsi, J. 1922. *Über die Bedeutung der Stereotypien*. Berlin: Karger

Kraepelin, E. 1909–1915. *Psychiatrie. Ein Lehrbuch für Studierende und Ärzte*. 4 vols. Leipzig: Barth

Kretschmer, E. 1953. Der Begriff der motorischen Schablonen und ihre Rolle in normalen und pathologischen. Lebensvorgängen. *Arch. Psychiat. Nervenkr.*, **190**, 1–3

1958. *Hysterie, Reflex und Instinkt*. 6th edn. Stuttgart: Thieme

Mucha, H. 1972. Der Katalepsie-Begriff von Kahlbaum bis zur Gegenwart. *Psychiat. chir.*, **5**, 330–49

Pauleikhoff, P. 1969. Die Katatonie (1868–1968). *Fortschr. Neurol. Psychiat.*, **37**, 461–96
Payk, Th. R. 1973. Mimik und Physiognomie in der Psychopathologie. *Psychiat. clin.*, **6**, 271–87
Straus, E. 1930. Die Formen des Räumlichen. Ihre Bedeutung für die Motorik und die Wahrnehmung. *Nervenarzt*, **3**, 633–56
1960. Gesammelte Schriften: Die aufrechte Haltung. Eine anthropologische Studie. In *Psychologie der menschlichen Welt*, ed. E. Straus. Berlin: Springer
Wieser, St. and Itil, T. 1954. Die Aufbaustufen der primitiven Motorik. *Arch. Psychiat. Nervenkr.* **191**, 450–62

17. OBSESSIONS AND PHOBIAS

Boss, M. 1971. *Grundriß der Medizin*. Berne: Huber
Frankl, V. E. 1956. *Theorie und Therapie der Neurosen*. Vienna: Urban & Schwarzenberg
Freud, S. 1906–1909. Bemerkungen über einen Fall von Zwangsneurose. *Gesammelte Werke*, vol. VII. Frankfurt/M: Fischer 1968
Gebsattel, V. E. v. 1928. Zeitbezogenes Zwangsdenken in der Melancholie. *Nervenarzt*, **1**, 275–87
Marks, I. M. 1969. Fears and Phobias. In *Personality and Psychopathology Series*, vol. v. New York: Academic Press
1970. The origins of phobic states. *Amer. J. Psychother.*, **24**, 652–76
Quint, H. 1971. *Über die Zwangsneurose; Studie zur Psychodynamik des Charakters und der Symptomatik*. Göttingen: Vandenhoeck & Ruprecht
Rümke, H. C. 1967. Über die Klinik und Psychopathologie der Zwangserscheinungen. In *Eine blühende Psychiatrie in Gefahr*, ed. H. C. Rümke. Berlin: Springer
Schneider, K. 1918. Die Lehre vom Zwangsdenken in den letzten 12 Jahren. *Z. ges. Neurol. Psychiat.*, **16**, 113–46
Straus, E. 1960. Ein Beitrag zurt Pathologie der Zwangserscheinungen. In *Psychologie der menschlichen Welt*, ed. E. Straus. Berlin: Springer
Weitbrecht, H. J. 1963. *Psychiatrie im Grundriß*. 1st edn. (3rd edn. 1973) Berlin: Springer
Zerbin-Rüdin, E. 1953. Ein Beitrag zur Frage der Zwangskrankheit, insbesondere ihrer hereditären Beziehungen. *Arch. Psychiat. Nervenkr.* **191**, 14–54

18. IMPULSIVE ACTS

Boor, W. de 1955. Zur Psychologie und Psychopathologie der Brandstiftung. *Fortschr. Neurol. Psychiat.*, **23**, 367–78

Bräutigam, W. 1973. Stichwort Kleptomanie. In *Lexikon der Psychiatrie*, ed. C. Müller. Berlin: Springer

Göppinger, H. and Witter, H. 1972. *Handbuch der forensischen Psychiatrie.* Berlin: Springer

Kraepelin, E. 1896. *Psychiatrie. Ein Lehrbuch für Studierende und Ärtzte.* 5th edn. Leipzig: Barth

Thiele, R. 1953. Zum Begriff und zur Pathologie der Drangserscheinungen. *Psychiat. Neurol. med. Psychol. (Lpz.)*, **5**, 51–9

Többen, H. 1971. *Beiträge zur Psychologie und Psychopathologie der Brandstifter.* Berlin: Springer

19. AFFECTIVITY

Baeyer, W. v., Häfner, H. and Kisker, K. P. 1964. *Psychiatrie der Verfolgten.* Berlin: Springer

Battegay, R. 1970. *Angst und Sein.* Stuttgart: Hippokrates-Verlag

Binswanger, L. 1945. Über die manische Lebensform. In *Ausgewählte Vorträge und Aufsätze*, vol. II, ed. L. Binswanger. Berne: Francke 1955

1960. *Melancholie und Manie.* Pfullingen: Neske

Bleuler, E. 1911. Dementia praecox oder Gruppe der Schizophrenien. In *Handbuch der Psychiatrie*, spec. pt. 4, ed. G. Aschaffenburg. Vienna: Deuticke

Bräutigam, W. 1956. Analyse der hypochondrischen Selbstbeobachtung. Beitrag zur Psychopathologie und zur Pathogenese mit Beschreibung einer Gruppe von jugendlichen Herzhypochondern. *Nervenarzt*, **27**, 409–18

Eitinger, L. 1964. *Concentration Camp Survivors in Norway and Israel.* London: Allen & Unwin

Eysenck, H. J. 1957. *The Dynamics of Anxiety and Hysteria.* London: Routledge & Kegan Paul

Feldmann, H. 1972. Hypochondrie. In *Monographien aus dem Gesamtgebiete der Psychiatrie*, vol. VI, ed. H. Hippius, W. Janzarik and M. Müller. Berlin: Springer

Fischer-Homberger, E. 1970. *Hypochondrie, Melancholie bis Neurosen.* Berne: Huber

Freud, S. 1894. Über die Berechtigung, von der Neurasthenie einen bestimmten Symptomenkomplex als Angstneurose abzutrennen. *Gesammelte Werke*, vol. I, Frankfurt/M: Fischer 1968

1926. Hemmung, Symptom, Angst. *Gesammelte Werke*, vol. XIV. Frankfurt/M: Fischer 1968

Gebsattel, V. E. v. 1959. Die phobische Fehlhaltung. In *Handbuch der Neurosenlehre und Psychotherapie*, vol. II, ed. V. E. Frankl, V. E. v. Gebsattel and J. H. Schultz. Munich: Urban & Schwarzenberg

Häfner, H. 1959. Hypochondrische Entwicklungen. *Nervenarzt*, **30**, 529–39

Janzarik, W. 1957. Die hypochondrischen Inhalte der cyclothymen Depression in ihren Beziehungen zum Krankheitstyp und zur Persönlichkeit. *Arch. Psychiat. Nervenkr.*, **195**, 351–71

1959. Zur Klinik und Psychopathologie des hypochondrischen Syndroms. *Nervenarzt*, **30**, 539–45

Kielholz, P. 1967. *Angst*. Berne: Huber

1971. *Diagnose und Therapie der Depressionen für den Praktiker*. Munich: Lehmanns

Kisker, K. P. 1964. Kernschizophrenie und Egopathien. Bemerkungen zum heutigen Stand der Forschungen und zur Methodologie. *Nervenartz*, **35**, 286–94

Kohn, R. 1958/59. Wohlbefinden und Mißbefinden. *Psyche (Heidelberg)*, **12**, 33–49

Kretschmer, E. 1958. *Hysterie, Reflex und Instinkt*. Stuttgart: Thieme

1971. *Medizinische Psychologie*. 13th edn. Stuttgart: Thieme

Kulenkampff, C. and Bauer, A. 1960. Über das Syndrom der Herzphobie. *Nervenarzt*, **31**, 443–54, 496–507

Ladee, G. A. 1966. *Hypochondriacal Syndromes*. Amsterdam: Elsevier

Lader, M. H. 1969. Studies of anxiety. *Brit. J. Psychiat.*, Spec. Publ. No. 3

Lersch, Ph. 1966. *Aufbau der Person*. 10th edn. Munich: Barth

Lewis, A. 1967. Problems presented by the ambiguous word 'anxiety' as used in psychopathology. *Israel Ann. Psychiat.*, **5**, 105–21

Matussek, P. 1971. Die Konzentrationslagerhaft und ihre Folgen. In *Monographien aus dem Gesamtgebiete der Psychiatrie*, vol. II, ed. H. Hippius, W. Janzarik and M. Müller. Berlin: Springer

Petrilowitsch, N. and Baer, R. 1970. Zyklothymie 1964–1969. *Fortschr. Neurol. Psychiat.*, **38**, 601–92

Plügge, H. 1958. Zur Phänomenologie des Leiberlebens besonders bei inneren Krankheiten. *Jb. Psychol. Psychotherap.*, **5**, 155–68
1960. Hypochondrische Patienten in der inneren Medizin. *Nervenarzt*, **31**, 13–19
Riemann, F. 1961. *Grundformen der Angst*. Munich: Reinhardt
Rümke, H. C. 1924. *Zur Phänomenologie und Klinik des Glücksgefühls*. Berlin: Springer
Ruffin, H. 1959. Leiblichkeit und Hypochondrie. *Nervenarzt*, **30**, 195–203
Scheler, M. 1913. Zur Phänomenologie und Theorie der Sympathiegefühle und von Liebe und Haß. Halle: Niemeyer
Schneider, K. 1935. *Psychopathologie der Gefühle und Triebe*. Leipzig: Thieme
Weitbrecht, H.-J. 1951. Über die Hypochondrie. *Dtsch. med. Wschr.* **76**, 313–15
1968. *Psychiatrie im Grundriß*. 2nd edn. (1st edn. 1963). Berlin: Springer
Wolpe, J. 1952. Experimental neuroses as learned behaviour. *Brit. J. Psychol.*, **43**, 243–68
Wulff, E. 1958. Der Hypochonder und sein Leib. *Nervenarzt*. **29**, 60–71

20. CONATIVE FUNCTIONS, DRIVES

Berning, D., Meyer, J. E. and Pudel, V. 1972. Psychogene Polydipsie. *Arch. Psychiat. Nervenkr.*, **215**, 396–406
Hess, W. R. 1962. *Psychologie in biologischer Sicht*. 2nd edn. 1968 Stuttgart: Thieme
Jores, A. 1954. Die Anorexia nervosa als endokrinologisches Problem. *Acta endocr. (Kbh.)*, **17**, 206–10
Kuhn, R. 1951. Zur Daseinsanalyse der Anorexia mentalis. *Nervenarzt*, **22**, 11–13
1953. *Nervenarzt*, **24**, 191–8
Meyer, J.-E. 1965, *Anorexia nervosa*. Stuttgart: Thieme
Peters, G., Fitzsimons, J. T. and Peters-Haefeli, I. 1974. *Control Mechanisms of Drinking*. Berlin: Springer
Thomä, H., 1961. *Anorexia nervosa*. Stuttgart: Klett
Zutt, J. 1948. Das psychiatrische Bild der Pubertätsmagersucht. *Arch. Psychiat. Nervenkr.*, **180**, 776

21. SEXUALITY

Abraham, K. 1971. Psychoanalytische Studien. In *Gesammelte Werke*, ed. J. Cremerius. Frankfurt/M: Fischer

Allen, C. 1969. *A Textbook of Psychosexual Disorders*. London: Oxford University Press

Boss, M. 1966. *Sinn und Gehalt der sexuellen Perversionen*. Berne: Huber

Bräutigam, W. 1972. Die sexuellen Verirrungen. In *Psychiatrie der Gegenwart*, 2nd edn., vol. II/1, ed. K. P. Kisker, J. E. Meyer, M. Müller and E. Strömgren, pp. 523–86 Berlin: Springer

Dörner, G. 1972. *Sexualhormonabhängige Gehirndifferenzierung und Sexualität*. Vienna: Springer

Feldman, M. P. and McCulloch, M. J. 1971. *Homosexual Behaviour: Therapy and Assessment*. Oxford: Pergamon Press

Fenichel, O, 1931. *Perversionen, Psychose, Charakterstörungen*. Vienna: Internationaler Psychoanalytischer Verlag

Ford, C. S. and Beach, F. A. 1968. *Formen der Sexualität*. Hamburg: Rowohlt

Frankl, V. E. 1959. Psychogene Potenzstörungen. In *Handbuch der Neurosenlehre und Psychotherapie*, vol. II, ed. V. E. Frankl, V. E. v. Gebsattel and J. H. Schultz, pp. 610–32. Munich: Urban & Schwarzenberg

Freud, S. 1904–1905. Drei Abhandlungen zur Sexualtheorie. *Gesammelte Werke*, vol. v. Frankfurt/M: Fischer 1968

1920. Über die Psychogenese eines Falles von weiblicher Homosexualität. *Gesammelte Werke*, vol. XII. Frankfurt/M: Fischer 1968

1924. Das ökonomische Probleme des Masochismus. *Gesammelte Werke*, vol. XIII. Frankfurt/M: Fischer 1968

1924. Über einige neurotische Mechanismen bei Eifersucht, Paranoia und Homosexualität. *Gesammelte Werke*, vol. XIII. Frankfurt/M: Fischer 1968

1925–1932. Fetischismus, *Gesammelte Werke*, vol. XIV. Frankfurt/M: Fischer 1968

1920–1924. Jenseits des Lustprinzips. *Gesammelte Werke*, vol. XIII. Frankfurt/M: Fischer 1968

Freund, K. 1969. *Homosexualität*. Hamburg: Rowohlt

Gebsattel, V. E. v. 1929. Über Fetischismus. *Nervenarzt*, **2**, 8–20

Giese, H. 1958. *Der homosexuelle Mann in der Welt*. Stuttgart: Enke

1962. *Psychopathologie der Sexualität*. Stuttgart: Enke

1971. *Die Sexualität des Menschen. Handbuch der medizinischen Sexualforschung.* Stuttgart: Enke

Green, R. and Money, J. 1969. *Transsexualism and Sex Reassignment.* Baltimore: John Hopkins Press

Hentig, H. v. 1962. *Soziologie der zoophilen Neigung. Beiträge zur Sexualforschung.* Hamburg: Rowohlt

Hirschfeld, M. 1926. *Geschlechtskunde.* Stuttgart: Püttmann

Johnson, J. 1973. Psychopathia sexualis. *Brit. J. Psychiat.*, **122**, 211–18

Kinsey, A. C., Pomeroy, W. B. and Martin, C. E. 1948. *Sexual Behaviour in the Human Male.* Philadelphia: Saunders. (German: *Das sexuelle Verhalten des Mannes.* 1954. Frankfurt/M: Fischer)

Kinsey, A. C., Pomeroy, W. B., Martin, C. E. and Gebhard, P. H. 1953. *Sexual Behaviour in the Human Female.* Philadelphia: Saunders. (German: *Das sexuelle Verhalten der Frau.* 1954. Frankfurt/M: Fischer)

Klein, Melanie 1932. *Die Psychoanalyse des Kindes.* Vienna: Internationaler Psychoanalytischer Verlag

Kockott, G. and Dittmar, F. 1973. Verhaltenstherapie sexueller Störungen: Diagnostik und Behandlungsmethoden. *Nervenarzt*, **44**, 173–83

Krafft-Ebing, R. v. 1918. *Psychopathia Sexualis.* 15th edn. Stuttgart: Enke

Kunz, H. 1942. Zur Theorie der Perversion. *Mschr. Psychiat. Neurol.*, **105**, 1–103

Malinowski, B. 1962. *Geschlecht und Verdrängung in primitiven Gesellschaften.* Hamburg: Rowohlt

Marshall, D. S. and Suggs, R. C. 1971. *Human Sexual Behaviour.* New York: Basic Books

Masters, W. H. and Johnson, V. E. 1966. *Human Sexual Response.* Boston: Little, Brown & Co.

Maters, W. H.: and Johnson, V. E. 1970. *Human Sexual Inadequacy.* Boston: Little, Brown & Co. (German: *Funktionelle Sexualstörungen.* 1972. Frankfurt/M: Akademische Verlagsgesellschaft)

Matussek, P. 1959. Störungen des Sexuallebens. In *Handbuch der Neurosenlehre und Psychotherapie*, vol. II, ed. V. E. Frankl, V. E. v. Gebsattel and J. H. Schulz, pp. 580–98. Munich: Urban & Schwarzenberg

Mead, Margaret 1949. *Male and Female. A Study of the Sexes in a*

Changing World. New York: Morrow (German: 1958. *Mann und Weib. Das Verhältnis der Geschlechter in einer sich wandelnden Welt.* Hamburg: Rowohlt)

1959. Geschlecht und Temperament in primitiven Gesellschaften. Hamburg: Rowohlt

Orthner, H. 1971a. *Zentralnervöse Sexualsteuerung (Symposium 1969).* Vienna: Springer

1971b. Anatomie und Physiologie der Steuerungsorgane der Sexualität. In *Die Sexualität des Menschen, Handbuch der medizinischen Sexualforschung,* ed. H. Giese, pp. 446–545. Stuttgart: Enke

Overzier, C. 1961. *Die Intersexualität.* Stuttgart: Thieme

Reich, W. 1971. *Die sexualle Revolution.* Frankfurt/M: Fischer

1972. *Die Entdeckung des Orgons. Die Funktion des Orgasmus.* Frankfurt/M: Fischer

Rutter, M. 1971. Normal psychosexual development. *J. Child Psychol.,* **11,** 259–63

Schätzing, E. 1959. Die weibliche Impotenz. Das Frigidätsproblem. In *Handbuch der Neurosenlehre und Psychotherapie,* vol. II, ed. V. E. Frankl, V. E. v. Gebsattel and J. H. Schultz, pp. 599–609. Munich: Urban & Schwarzenberg

Schelsky, H. 1955. *Soziologie der Sexualität.* Hamburg: Rowohlt

Schorsch, G. 1971. *Sexualstraftäter.* Stuttgart: Enke

Sigusch, V. 1972. *Ergebnisse zur Sexualmedizin.* Basle: Karger

Spoerri, T. 1959. *Nekrophilie.* Basle: Karger

Stoller, R. J. 1973. Overview: The impact of new advances in sex research on psychoanalytic theory. *Amer. J. Psychiat.,* **130,** 241–51

Straus, E. 1930. *Geschehnis und Erlebnis, zugleich eine historiologische Deutung des psychischen Traumas und der Rentenneurose.* Berlin: Springer

Wolff, Charlotte. 1973. *Psychologie der lesbischen Liebe.* Hamburg: Rowohlt

APPENDICES TO BIBLIOGRAPHY

Handbooks

Arieti, S. 1974. *American Handbook of Psychiatry.* 2nd edn. New York: Basic Books

Aschaffenburg, G. 1911. *Handbuch der Psychiatrie.* Vienna: Deuticke

Bumke, O. 1928. *Handbuch der Geisteskrankheiten.* Berlin: Springer
Frankl, V. E., Gebsattel, V. E. v. and Schultz, J. H. 1959. *Handbuch der Neurosenlehre und Psychotherapie.* Munich: Urban & Schwarzenberg
Freedman, A. M. and Kaplan, H. I. 1967. *Comprehensive Textbook of Psychiatry.* Baltimore: Williams & Wilkins
Gottschaldt, K., Lersch, Ph., Sander, F. and Thomae, H. 1966. *Handbuch der Psychologie*, vol. I: Allgemeine Psychologie, I. Der Aufbau des Erkennens, 1 Half-vol.: Wahrnehmung und Bewußtsein, ed. W. Metzger. Göttingen: Hogrefe
Gruhle, H. W., Jung, R., Mayer-Gross, W. and Müller, C. 1960–1967. *Psychiatrie der Gegenwart.* 1st edn. Berlin: Springer
Kisker, K. P., Meyer, J. E., Müller, M. and Strömgren, E. 1972. *Psychiatrie der Gegenwart.* 2nd edn. Berlin: Springer

Dictionaries

Birnbaum, K. 1930. *Handwörterbuch der medizinischen Psychologie.* Leipzig: Thieme
Hinsie, L. E. and Campbell, R. J. 1970. *Psychiatric Dictionary.* 4th edn. London: Oxford University Press
Moore, Lise. 1969. *Lexique français-anglais-allemand des termes usuels en psychiatrie, neuro-psychiatrie infantile et psychologie pathologique.* 2nd edn. Paris: L'expansion Scientifique Française
Müller, C. 1973. *Lexikon der Psychiatrie.* Berlin: Springer
Neugebauer, J. and Weil, C. 1971. *Common psychiatric terms in 4 languages (World Psychiatric Association).* Basle: Sandoz
Peters, U. H. 1974. *Wörterbuch der Psychiatrie und medizinischen Psychologie.* Munich: Urban & Schwarzenberg

NOTES

PREFACE

1 Denoted in the text by the word Protocol plus a number. Most of the examples have been taken from my dealings with schizophrenics. Some are used more than once, to illustrate different points under discussion. For other detailed examples see Bash (1955), Conrad (1958). Autobiographical accounts are given in Kaplan (1964), Sommer and Osmond (1960, 1961).

2 See in particular Gottschaldt *et al.* (1966).

3 For the literature see Benedetti (1973), Chalmers *et al.* (1971), Delay and Pichot (1966), Eccles (1970), Hassler (1967), Hess (1962), R. Jung (1967), Perret (1973), Peters (1967).

4 For the literature see, for example, Argelander (1970), Kind (1973), Meerwein (1974); further indications on p. 25.

5 For a review of the literature see Eysenck (1973), Schraml and Baumann (1975), Brickenkamp (1975).

6 For the literature see Schooler and Feldman (1967), Cohen and Meyer-Osterkamp (1974), Meyer-Osterkamp and Cohen (1973).

CHAPTER 1

1 I.e. devoted entirely to the individual man.

2 I.e. looking for laws of general validity.

3 Cf. Freud (1931) in the Foreword to Nunberg (1959): 'when speculation never abandons the guiding-line of experience'. Fenichel (1971, p. 416): 'The "microscopic" studies of psycho-analysis presuppose the "macroscopic" studies of psychiatry, in the same way that histology presupposes anatomy.'

4 For the literature see Rosenthal *et al.* (1968), Rosenthal (1970).

5 Boss (1971).

6 Kiev (1972), Lebra (1972), Pfeiffer (1970), Wulff (1972), Zubin and Hunt (1967). The two most important transcultural journals are: *Journal of Cross-cultural Psychology*, London/Washington, and *Transcultural Psychiatric Research Review*, Quebec, Canada.

7 In war killing is normal, in peace it is not – in our culture. In a headhunting society certain killings are normal, in others it is normal to kill old people and unwanted children.

8 To disburb means to confuse, break up, stir up, destroy established order.

9 For the theme of 'Genius and Insanity', see Lange-Eichbaum (1967); Kretschmer (1948); Benedetti (1975).

317

10 The concept of normality is again implicit here.

11 Symptom comes from the Greek συμπί πτειν, i.e. to happen, to come to pass, to arise simultaneously, hence σύμπτωμα = sign of illness.

12 In the transitional state between waking and sleeping, in fatigue, in sensory deprivation (Zubek, 1969), in tense expectation, in emotionally charged situations (Hocking, 1970), in loneliness (e.g. after loss of a spouse), in hypnosis, in autogenic training, in meditation, in dreams, under the influence of hallucinations (see Tart, 1969).

13 This may be done either by clinical empiricism (expertise) or according to scientific method (see p. 25).

14 We would draw attention to the issue of causality as a concept in the natural sciences. As a rule one must satisfy oneself with regularly demonstrable connections (correlations), working therefore with the logical sequence of 'if so and so...then so and so'.

15 Any activity that involves classifying human beings may be abused, including the diagnostic process.

16 For the literature see Argelander, 1970; Jacob, 1962; McKinnon and Michels, 1971; Meerwein, 1974; Stevenson, 1971; Sullivan, 1955.

17 For the literature see Bochenski, 1954; Boss, 1971; Gadamer, 1972, Habermas, 1973; Kuhn, 1973; Lorenzer, 1973, 1974; Meerwein, 1965; Perrez, 1972; Popper, 1959; Rapaport, 1970; Savigny, 1974; Scharfetter, 1973, 1974; Seiffert, 1971; Slater, 1972, 1973, 1975; and the further literature contained in the collective volumes put out by Zimmerli, 1974; and Holzhey, 1974.

18 For pre-Freudian history see Ellenberger, 1970. For the existential significance of psycho-analysis see Kunz, 1930, 1956, 1975a, b.

19 It is the danger of leaping to conclusions.
Cf. also Goethe (Maxim No. 428): 'Theories are usually the overhasty conclusions of an impatient mind which would like to be free of the phenomena and therefore puts in their place images, concepts and often even only words.'
Nietzsche (1955): 'What is unknown brings in its train danger, unrest, worry – our first instinct is to get rid of these painful conditions... Evidence of desire ('power') as a criterion of truth.'

CHAPTER 2

1 This corresponds also to the etymological sense of *Bewußtsein* as *bi-bei-wizan*: *bei* = at something – the directedness, intentionality of consciousness. Thus one says of a fully conscious man: 'he is "himself"' (*bei sich*) and of someone who is recovering from a disturbance of consciousness: 'he is coming to himself again'.

2 A foundation is a necessary condition of the effect in question but is not by itself sufficient to produce that effect.

3 According to this view, conscious and unconscious are not contradictory terms but extremes in a continuum.

4 The term 'rational' twilight state is self-contradictory; rationality is the outcome of clear, conscious reflection and implies a complete review of inner and outer events and their orderly arrangement.

5 The borderline between this and a twilight state is blurred.

6 The distinction still commonly drawn between confusional state (*Verwirrtheit*) in psychoses associated with physical illness and confusion (*Verworrenheit*), a schizophrenic or, more rarely, a manic incoherence, is not terminologically justified.

CHAPTER 3

1 Jaspers touches on this concept in his 'awareness of one's own existence' (*Daseinsbewußtsein*) (1959, p. 101).

2 The concept is covered partially by Jaspers' 'awareness of one's own performance' (*Vollzugsbewußtsein*) (1959, p. 102), by Gruhle's impulse quality (Impulsqualität) (1956) and by K. Schneider's 'myness' (*Meinhaftigkeit*) (1967); see also Kronfeld, 1922.

3 From the Latin *idem*, the same, one and the same. For this concept see in particular Erikson (1966). For review and history of the concept see Levita (1965). Be careful not to confuse identity with role, or identity with individuality.

4 Self-image can in part be measured by scales of self-estimation (Collett, 1972; Wylie, 1961).

5 Hartmann (1964a) also pointed out the frequent confusion caused by using the explanatory terms of psycho-analysis for purposes of description.

6 E.g. Fenichel (1971, p. 440): 'In psychoses loss of reality *causes* the pathological result.' (my italics).

7 Personal communication (quoted by Bellak, 1973, p. 59).

8 According to Federn this was his own idea, according to Bellak it was jointly conceived by Federn and Tausk.

9 See Ackner, 1954; Brauer, 1970; Burger, 1910; v. Gebsattel, 1937; Glatzel, 1971; Göppert, 1960; Lehmann, 1974; Meyer, 1959, 1963, 1968; Sedman, 1970, 1972.

10 Such symptoms may also occur to a rudimentary degree in the healthy, e.g. repetition of words or gestures, when bored, puzzled or embarrassed.

11 Do not confuse with heautoscopy (experience of having a *doppelgänger*), which is the rare optical phenomenon of seeing oneself outside oneself yet at the same time retaining one's ego-experience intact.

12 This theme may come to the patient in a dream.

13 Do not confuse with alternating personality: hysterical patients may (very rarely) experience another personality for a time and claim to have no memory for their former life. In this succession of personalities there is always ego-consciousness, but there is no ego-continuity throughout life (for a review of the literature see Cutler and Reed, 1975).

14 Cf. Bleuler's concept of schizophrenia (1908, 1911) and its history (Scharfetter, 1973).
15 The dynamic interpretation of schizophrenia in terms of latent homosexuality (Freud, 1911, later taken up by Pohlen, 1969, and others) need not concern us here.
16 My italics.
17 The difference between Freud and Federn is a purely theoretical one. The key issue for both is the helpless weakness of the schizophrenic individual.
18 For a discussion of regression, narcissism and the therapeutic problems involved, see Balint (1973).

CHAPTER 4

1 Jaspers (1912, 1959) in connection with Janet's (1903) *fonction du réel*.
2 The philosophical question of the nature of our knowing is not dealt with here.
3 For the philosophy and history of the concept of experience see, for example, Gadamer (1972), Holzhey (1970).
4 N.B. Not to be confused with Freud's reality principle (1911). Freud's reality principle, the distinction between internal and external, is, on the contrary, a part of consciousness of experience and reality testing as described here (see *Ego-demarcation*).
5 In the same way a dreamer often knows that he is dreaming and even struggles to understand the dream experience.
6 Cf. Jaspers (1925), *Psychologie der Weltanschauungen*, p. 300: 'When what is self-evident is cut away from under our feet'. Cf. also Blankenburg (1971).

CHAPTER 7

1 The definition of an immediate memory (direct retention for about ten seconds) is of little practical clinical significance and it is difficult to distinguish between this and attention and concentration.

CHAPTER 10

1 As opposed to instinctive action.
2 In severe cases we may find the clinical picture that used to be called *dementeia ex separatione* (cf. wolf children).

CHAPTER 11

1 See Philosophy: the theory of knowledge.
2 Greek: χοινός = common, i.e. general, bodily feelings.

CHAPTER 13

1 For the difference between delusion and faith see Hole (1971), between this and superstition, see Kehrer (1922) and O. Kant (1927b).

2 'Determined' has been put in inverted commas because it is not certain that the life history and situation alone – without predisposing factors – can lead to delusion.

3 Freud in his earlier works on defence neuropsychosis had already pointed out that the sense of a delusion clearly corresponded to a need. From the recognition of a delusion as biographically meaningful to its formulation as a 'necessity of life' (O. Kant, 1927a, p. 643) one can draw a straight line.

4 See Kehrer (1928) and O. Kant (1930) on 'The need for social communion and the inability to surrender.' These authors have contributed much to the final understanding of delusion. See also Kahn (1929).

5 Many such cases are difficult to explain without the additional assumption of other predisposing (genetic) factors.

CHAPTER 14

1 Cf. the concepts of libido in C. G. Jung's sense (1924), vital energy, *élan vital* (H. Bergson).

2 The neurological procedure of leucotomy (lesions in the *gyrus cinguli*, in the fronto-thalamic pathways, etc.) aims at producing this numbing effect when the patient is tormented by depressive moods, or when he suffers from compulsive activities or very severe, persistent pain for which there is no other remedy.

CHAPTER 15

1 For violence in the mentally ill, see Böker and Häfner (1973). Three per cent of all the perpetrators of violence examined were mentally ill in the broad sense of this term. This corresponds to the incidence of mental illness in the adult population. The mentally ill and the mentally retarded are no more liable than the mentally normal to commit acts of violence. Among those mentally ill who did commit violent acts, schizophrenics headed the list.

CHAPTER 17

1 Not to be confused with hydrophobia, which is an older name for rabies (lyssa).

CHAPTER 19

1 The isolation of affect as 'reactive' feeling is artificial and unnecessary.
2 In common speech intuition is also classed as a feeling: 'I have a feeling that...'
3 The use of the term dysthymia in this sense is misleading. Dysthymia implies a variety of mood upsets, mostly depressive.

INDEX